Skin Diseases of the Dog and Cat

THIRD EDITION

Skin Diseases of the Dog and Cat

THIRD EDITION

NICOLE A. HEINRICH, DVM, DACVD
McKeever Dermatology Clinics
Eden Prairie and Inver Grove Heights
Minnesota, USA

MELISSA EISENSCHENK, MS, DVM, DACVD
Pet Dermatology Clinic
Maple Grove
Minnesota, USA

RICHARD G. HARVEY, BVSc, DVDF, Dip. ECVD, FRSB, PhD, MRCVS
The Veterinary Centre
Coventry, UK

TIM NUTTALL, BSc, BVSc, PhD, CertVD, CBiol, MRSB, MRCVS
Head of Dermatology
The Royal (Dick) School of Veterinary Studies
The University of Edinburgh
Roslin, UK

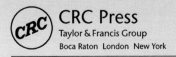

CRC Press
Taylor & Francis Group
Boca Raton London New York

CRC Press is an imprint of the
Taylor & Francis Group, an **informa** business

CRC Press
Taylor & Francis Group
6000 Broken Sound Parkway NW, Suite 300
Boca Raton, FL 33487-2742

© 2019 by Taylor & Francis Group, LLC
CRC Press is an imprint of Taylor & Francis Group, an Informa business

International Standard Book Number-13: 978-1-4822-2596-9 (Hardback)
International Standard Book Number-13: 978-1-138-30870-1 (Paperback)

Library of Congress Cataloging-in-Publication Data

Names: Nuttall, Tim, 1967- author. | Eisenschenk, Melissa, author. |
Heinrich, Nicole A., author. | Harvey, Richard G., author.
Title: Skin diseases of the dog and cat / Tim Nuttall, Melissa Eisenschenk,
Nicole A. Heinrich, Richard G. Harvey.
Other titles: A colour handbook of skin diseases of the dog and cat
Description: Third edition. | Boca Raton : CRC Press, [2018] | Preceded by A
colour handbook of skin diseases of the dog and cat / Tim Nuttall, Richard
G. Harvey, Patrick J. McKeever. 2nd ed. c2009. | Includes bibliographical
references and index.
Identifiers: LCCN 2017033713 (print) | LCCN 2017035548 (ebook) | ISBN
9781315118147 (Master eBook) | ISBN 9781138308701 (pbk. : alk. paper) |
ISBN 9781482225969 (hardback : alk. paper)
Subjects: LCSH: Dogs--Diseases. | Cats--Diseases. | Veterinary dermatology. |
MESH: Skin Diseases--veterinary | Dog Diseases | Cat Diseases
Classification: LCC SF992.S55 (ebook) | LCC SF992.S55 M37 2018 (print) | NLM
SF 992.S55 | DDC 636.7/08965--dc23
LC record available at https://lccn.loc.gov/2017033713

Visit the Taylor & Francis Web site at
http://www.taylorandfrancis.com

and the CRC Press Web site at
http://www.crcpress.com

CONTENTS

PREFACE

A *Colour Handbook of Skin Diseases of the Dog and Cat* was first published in 1998. It was one of the first books to bring key information about skin diseases to first-opinion clinicians in an easy to use problem-orientated format. By 2009 the huge growth in knowledge about skin conditions necessitated an updated and almost completely rewritten second edition. Subsequent exponential growth in veterinary dermatology has led to the discovery of new conditions, development of new approaches to management and effective new treatment options. In this third edition, we have completely revised and updated the chapters while retaining the problem-based approach. We hope that this new edition will continue to provide key information about the diagnosis and management of skin conditions in a format that is easily accessible to busy clinicians.

ACKNOWLEDGEMENTS

The authors thank all the referring veterinarians and owners that have entrusted the care of their animals to us so that we could accumulate the knowledge and experience necessary to write this book.

A special thanks to Patrick McKeever DVM, DACVD for invaluable mentorship.

TREATMENT RECOMMENDATIONS AND PROFESSIONAL RESPONSIBILITIES

Wherever possible, the treatment recommendations in this book are evidence based, following published data and therapeutic guidelines. Where such data are lacking, we have based the recommendations on consensus opinion and personal experience. The treatment options may include off-label or off-cascade suggestions. The prescribing veterinarian has complete responsibility for any decision on treatment protocols for a particular case, taking into account the diagnosis, potential for adverse effects, underlying conditions and any concurrent therapy. Veterinarians must also be aware of relevant medicines legislation and whether it is legal to administer certain treatments in their country or province of work.

CHAPTER 1

BASICS

TERMINOLOGY USED IN THE DESCRIPTION OF DERMATOLOGICAL LESIONS[1]

Primary lesions

Primary lesions are directly associated with the disease process. They are not necessarily pathognomonic, but give a valuable clue as to the type of disease process occurring.

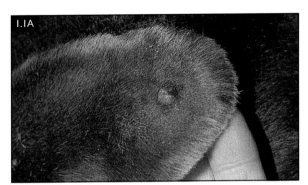

Papules are solid, elevated lesions up to 1 cm in diameter associated with cell infiltration and/or proliferation, in this case a mast cell tumour (**Fig. 1.1**).

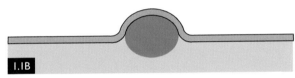

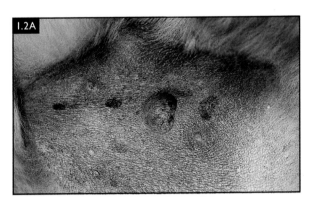

A **nodule** is a solid elevation of the skin >1 cm in diameter, located primarily in the dermis or subcutis. The nodule illustrated in **Fig. 1.2** is a mast cell tumour on the abdomen of a dog.

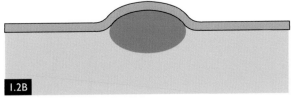

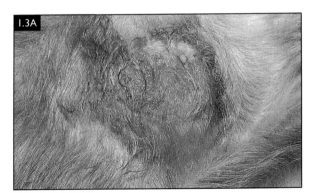

A **plaque** is a flat, solid, circumscribed, elevated lesion of >1 cm in diameter, again associated with cell infiltration and/or proliferation (**Fig. 1.3**). A plaque may result from a coalescence of papules. The lesions illustrated are eosinophilic plaques on a cat.

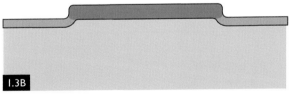

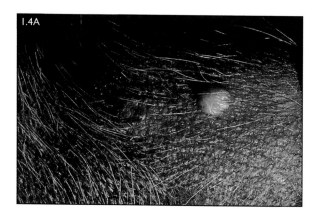

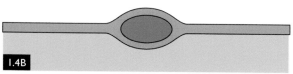

A **pustule** is a circumscribed skin lesion containing purulent material (**Fig. 1.4**). This consists of degenerate inflammatory cells (most commonly neutrophils) with or without microorganisms or other cells (e.g. acanthocytes in pemphigus foliaceus). Pustules and vesicles rapidly rupture in dogs and cats to form crusts.

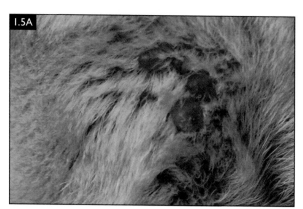

A **vesicle** is a circumscribed elevation of the skin up to 1 cm in diameter filled with liquid (clear, serous or haemorrhagic). A bulla describes the same lesion >1 cm in diameter. These lesions usually quickly rupture to leave ulcers and/or crusts. **Fig. 1.5** shows vesicles due to cutaneous mucinosis in a Shar Pei.

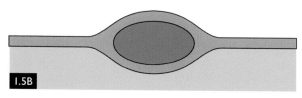

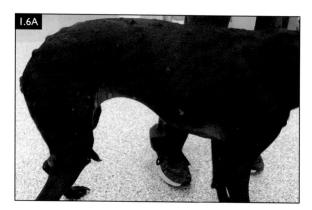

A **cyst** is an enclosed cavity with an epithelial lining that contains liquid or semi-solid matter. **Fig. 1.6** is of multiple follicular infundibular cysts in a dog.

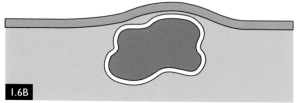

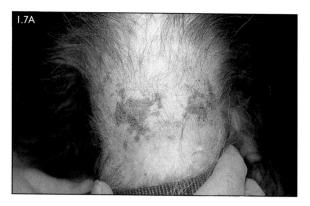

Macules are flat, non-palpable areas of circumscribed discoloration up to 1 cm in diameter (**Fig. 1.7**). Patches are >1 cm in diameter. Changes can involve increased blood flow (erythema), extravasated blood (haemorrhagic petechiae and ecchymoses) or pigment changes. Erythema can be distinguished from haemorrhage by blanching on digital pressure or using a glass slide (Diascopy, see page 11).

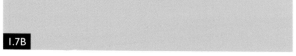

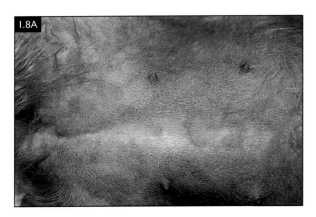

A **weal** is a transient elevation of the skin due to dermal oedema (**Fig. 1.8**). The weals in this case were acute, transient and of unknown aetiology.

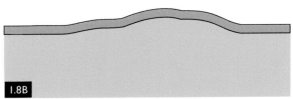

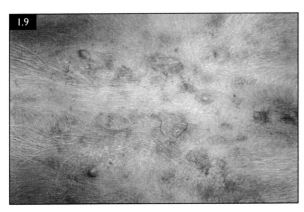

Epidermal collarettes are circular rings of scale with an erythematous, often slightly raised, margin and a clear, often slightly pigmented, centre. They may expand and coalesce to form large, interlinked and irregular lesions. They are most commonly associated with exfoliative staphylococcal pyoderma. **Fig. 1.9** shows papules, pustules and epidermal collarettes on the ventral abdomen of a dog with a staphylococcal pyoderma.

Secondary lesions

Secondary lesions are a result of trauma, time and degree of insult to the skin. Often, primary lesions evolve into secondary lesions. Thus papules become pustules, which become focal encrustations, often hyperpigmented. Secondary lesions are much less specific than primary lesions.

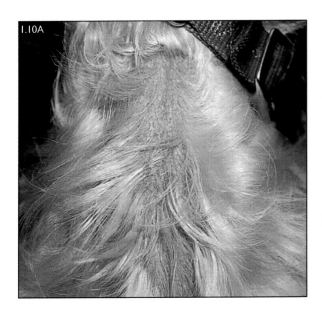

Erythema is reddening of the skin due to increased blood flow, usually secondary to inflammation. The pattern of erythema may be diffuse to generalised (e.g. atopic dermatitis) or maculopapular (e.g. pyoderma or ectoparasites). In this Springer Spaniel the erythema is due to a *Malassezia pachydermatis* infection (**Fig. 1.10**).

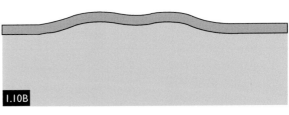

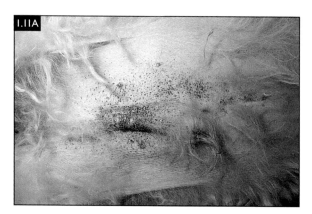

Comedones are the result of sebaceous and epidermal debris blocking a follicle. They may be seen in many diseases that affect hair follicles, but are often very prominent in cases of hyperadrenocorticism (**Fig. 1.11**).

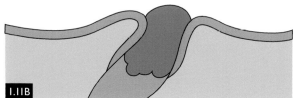

Scale results from altered keratinisation and accumulations of keratin forming a flat plate or flake. This is usually caused by an underlying condition (secondary scaling) but may be associated with inherent changes in skin turnover (primary scaling). In this case there is an epidermal collarettes (see above) surrounding a postinflammatory patch of hyperpigmentation. This presentation is frequently seen in cases of superficial pyoderma and other pustular diseases (**Fig. 1.12**).

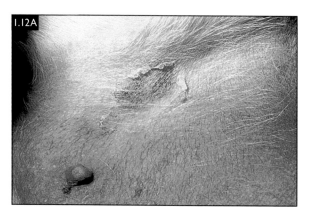

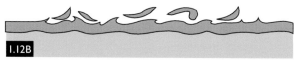

Crust is composed of cells and dried exudates. It may be serous, sanguineous, purulent or mixed. The dog in **Fig. 1.13** has a staphylococcal dermatitis secondary to allergies.

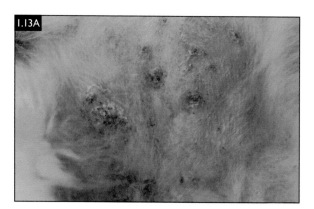

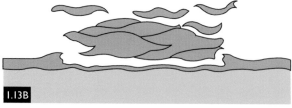

An **excoriation** is loss of epidermis and potentially part of the dermis that results from trauma, either self-trauma or an injury. They are often linear and parallel. The dog in **Fig. 1.14** has allergies causing pruritus and scratching of the axilla.

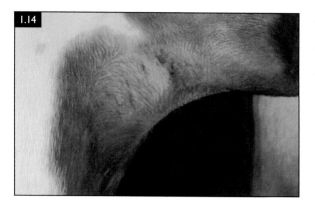

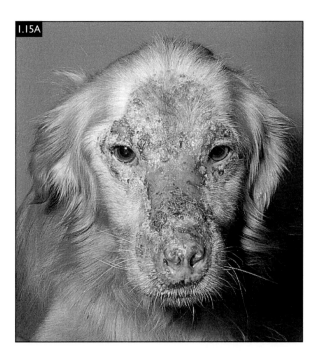

An **erosion** is a loss of a portion or of the entire epidermis as on the face of the dog in **Fig. 1.15** with discoid lupus erythematosus. Erosions usually heal by re-epithelisation.

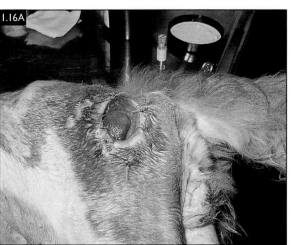

An **ulcer** is a full-thickness loss of the epidermis and part of the dermis. This is a decubital ulcer overlying the bony prominence of the hip (**Fig. 1.16**). Ulcers often result in a scar.

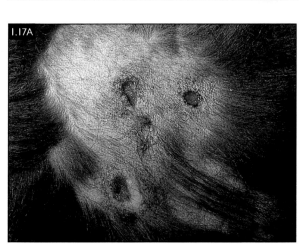

A **fistula** is an abnormal congenital or acquired passage from an abscess or hollow organ to the skin surface. A **sinus** is a tract leading from a deeper focus to the skin surface. The dog in **Fig. 1.17** has panniculitis and there are draining fistulae on the flank.

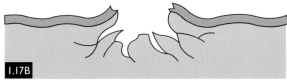

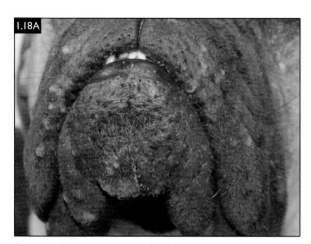

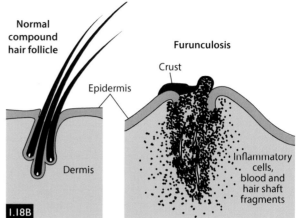

Furunculosis results from the inflammatory reaction to hair follicles rupturing under the skin, causing draining sinuses, crusting and bullae. **Fig. 1.18A** shows furunculosis due to chin acne in a Mastiff. **Fig. 1.18B** shows a normal hair follicle (left) and a hair follicle that has undergone furunculosis characterised by swelling and infiltration of neutrophils (right).

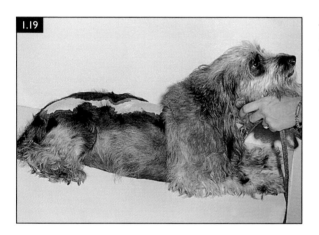

A **scar** results from the abnormal fibrous tissue that replaces normal tissue after an injury, such as a burn as in the case in **Fig. 1.19**.

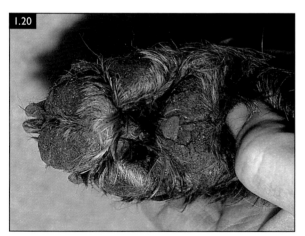

A **fissure** is a linear vertical disruption of the stratum corneum that may extend into the deeper epidermis or into the dermis. **Fig. 1.20** shows fissures on the foot of a dog with necrolytic migratory erythema.

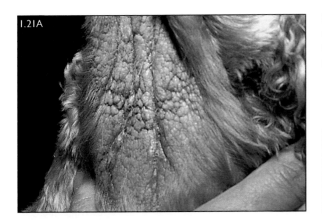

Lichenification is a thickening of the epidermis causing accentuation of normal skin markings that occurs after chronic inflammation. **Fig. 1.21** is a case of *Malassezia pachydermatis* infection.

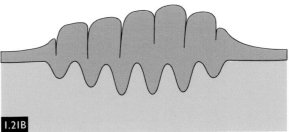

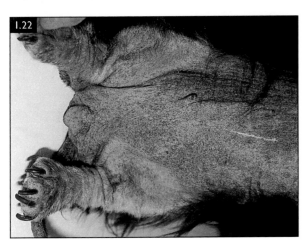

Hyperpigmentation, an increase in cutaneous pigmentation, usually occurs after chronic inflammation, as with the dog in **Fig. 1.22** with chronic atopic dermatitis. This form of hyperpigmentation has a characteristic lace-like pattern, with areas of normal skin between the pigmented patches. More solid hyperpigmentation may be associated with an endocrinopathy.

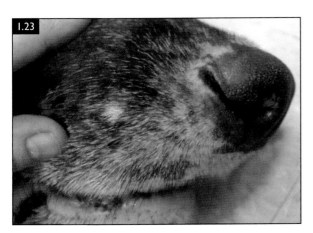

Hypopigmentation is a decrease in cutaneous pigmentation and **depigmentation** is a loss of pigmentation. These changes may be postinflammatory, infiltrative or genetic. The German Shepherd dog in **Fig. 1.23** shows **leukoderma** (white skin) due to vitiligo.

Reference

1 Nast A, Griffiths CEM, Hay R, Sterry W, Bolognia JL. The 2016 International League of Dermatological Societies' revised glossary for the description of cutaneous lesions. *Br J Dermatol* 2016; **174**: 1351–1358.

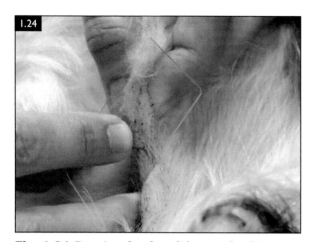

Fig. 1.24 Pressing the glass slide onto the skin.

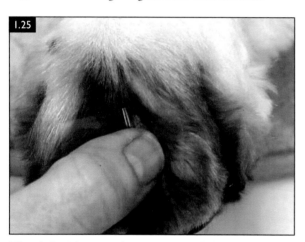

Fig. 1.25 Tape cytologies are very helpful to collect a sample from between the toes or other body folds.

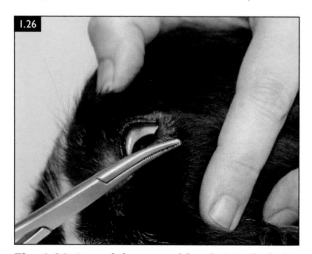

Fig. 1.26 Around the eyes and feet, hair is plucked for a trichogram because a skin scraping would be difficult in these areas.

DERMATOLOGICAL SAMPLING TECHNIQUES

Impression cytology is performed to look for organisms such as yeast or bacteria on the surface of the skin. A glass slide is pressed to the skin several times (**Fig. 1.24**). This works best when the sampled area is moist, so lifting crusts or scraping off the surface of pustules first is helpful. Impressions can also be made from the underside of fresh crusts. If the surface is greasy, heat fixing is useful to help adhere material to the slide before staining with a DiffQuik®-type stain.

Tape cytology is useful to sample dry or scaly areas, or areas where a slide cannot be pressed (such as interdigital spaces) (**Fig. 1.25**). It is highly effective unless the skin is moist, when the tape will not stick. Clear acetate tape is pressed sticky side down on to the sample area, then dipped into eosinophilic (pot 2) and basophilic dyes (pot 3) of a DiffQuik®-type stain (skip the fixative [pot 1] because this will remove the tape adhesive). The tape is then pressed to a slide where hydrostatic pressure holds the tape in place. Excess moisture is pressed out against tissue paper. The tape is viewed under 100× objective with oil immersion. There is often excessive keratin debris to look through, so bacteria may take some skill to reliably find. Non-stained tape-strips are also useful to look for surface parasites such as *Cheyletiella* spp. and fragments of flea faeces in pruritic animals. *Demodex* spp. can be found by very firmly squeezing the skin and then applying adhesive tape.

One-stain techniques are very quick and intensely stain microorganisms, although there is a more monochromatic blue stain compared with the two-stain methods described above. For impression smears, simply place one drop of the basophilic stain (pot 3) on the sample and apply a cover slip. For adhesive tape samples, place one drop of the stain on a microscope slide, stick the tape down over the drop and blot the excess stain away with tissue paper.

Trichograms are performed to look at the roots of hair shafts or other abnormalities in the structure of hair (**Fig. 1.26**). It can be useful to observe hairs infected with dermatophytes, hair growth abnormalities, hair shaft defects or *Demodex* spp. present at the root of the hairs. Usually telogen hairs are

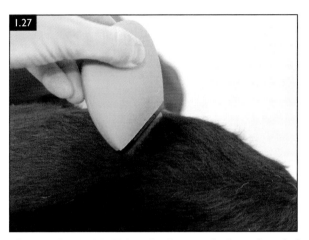

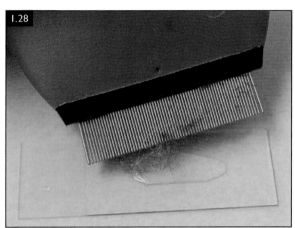

Figs. 1.27, 1.28 Using the fine-toothed comb and placing the sample on the slide.

seen only with hair plucks because they most easily fall out. Hairs are usually viewed unstained at low power in mineral oil with a cover slip over the top. Lactophenol cotton blue stain can highlight dermatophytes, and spores are best seen at 40× or greater.

Flea combing is a great way to look for fleas, flea dirt, *Cheyletiella* mites or lice (**Figs. 1.27, 1.28**). A fine-toothed comb is used to collect quantities of scale, debris and hair that can be viewed at low power (4× to 10×) with mineral oil and a coverslip.

Skin scrapings with oil are used to look for microscopic ectoparasites and are performed by placing mineral oil onto a glass slide, scooping some of the mineral oil onto a dulled no. 10 scalpel blade, and placing the oil onto the area of the skin to be sampled. Squeezing the skin may help to retrieve contents of a hair follicle (**Figs. 1.29, 1.30**). The entire blade

should be used to firmly scrape the skin in several locations, scooping up contents of the scrape onto the scalpel and placing on the slide at each location. The material should be homogenised in the oil on the slide and a coverslip applied. Skin scrapings are usually visualised on the 4× or 10× objective of the microscope, with the condenser closed to enhance contrast and bring into focus a wider field of view, which makes unstained parasites stand out more.

Dry skin scrapings are most commonly used to identify yeast organisms from a lichenified or greasy area of the skin. No oil is used because it will interfere with staining and visualising, and the material smeared from the scalpel to the slide is often heat fixed before staining. Yeast should be stained with DiffQuik®-type stains and are best visualised using the 100× oil objective.

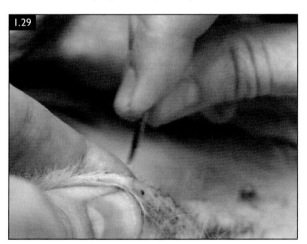

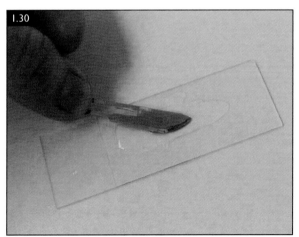

Figs. 1.29, 1.30 Using the scalpel blade to take a skin scraping and placing the sample on the slide.

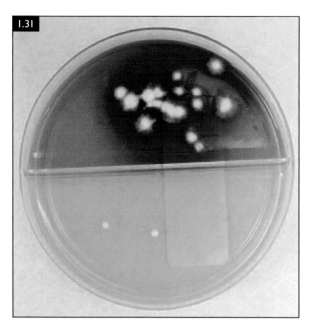

Fig. 1.31 Culture of *Microsporum canis*.

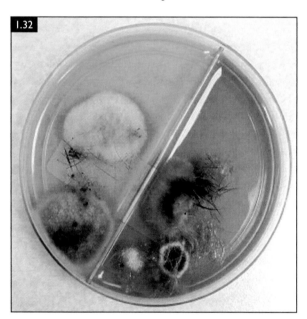

Fig. 1.32 Fungal contaminants.

Bacterial culture for antibiotic resistant staphylococci should be performed as soon as possible where there is any suspicion of antibiotic resistance (e.g. postoperative infections, clinic-acquired infections, after multiple antibiotic course and/or treatment failure). There is no need to withdraw use of oral antibiotics before sampling. Swabs are best taken from a primary lesion such as a ruptured

pustule, but samples can also be taken from under crusts, the margin of epidermal collarettes or draining sinus tracts. All deep infections should be cultured. Samples from deep locations can be obtained by inserting swabs into draining tracts or squeezing the skin to exude pus for sampling. Aspirates or pieces of tissue should be obtained and isolated from oxygen if anaerobic organisms (such as *Actinomyces* spp.) are suspected.

Fungal culture samples to look for dermatophytosis are collected by sampling hair and scales from the affected inner rims of lesions. Sometimes dry scrapings are used to collect scale or crusts because not all dermatophytes infect hair shafts. Dermatophyte culture plates are incubated for 1–3 weeks in the dark at room temperature or slightly warmer to determine which species is present (**Figs. 1.31, 1.32**). Growth may be prolonged if a pet is on antifungal therapy. Dermatophytes always form white or slightly off-white fluffy or powdery colonies and cause rapid red colour change in the dermatophyte test medium (DTM) agar. White growth without colour change is not typical of a dermatophyte, but can be seen with *Trichophyton* spp. Any grey, green or blackish colonies are not dermatophytes. To determine the species of the fungus, clear acetate tape can be gently pressed to the growth and then pressed down on a small drop of lactophenol cotton blue on a slide. The hyphae can be observed at 40× to look for macroconidia, which help with identification. If no macroconidia are found, other features may indicate the species, but it is best to wait several more days and resample the culture because macroconidia may take a week to form after colony growth has been observed. Subculture onto Sabouraud's agar may be necessary for definitive speciation.

McKenzie toothbrush technique is used to obtain material or a fungal culture if the pet is being treated for dermatophytosis and no obvious lesions are present. It can also be used to detect carriers of dermatophytosis, although a positive culture indicates only environmental contamination of the hair and not necessarily infection. A new, clean toothbrush is combed through the hair in the locations of previous lesions (**Fig. 1.33**). Hair and scale obtained are pressed into the dermatophyte culture.

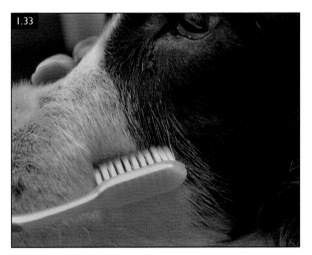

Fig. 1.33 Combing the hair using a new, clean toothbrush.

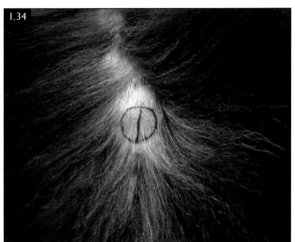

Fig. 1.34 This dog has cutaneous histiocytosis. The circle marks where lidocaine was infused; the line with the direction of hair growth helps the pathologist orientate the sample for processing.

For culture at an external laboratory, the toothbrush and sample can be placed in a small plastic bag and double bagged with a larger one for transport.

Skin biopsy is a useful technique to diagnose or rule out many diseases. It is best performed when infection is controlled. Corticosteroids can alter the appearance of biopsy samples and, for the most accurate diagnosis, biopsy should be obtained before starting on steroids, or steroids withdrawn to allow new lesions to form before biopsy. Do not withdraw steroids before biopsy for severe conditions. Most pets do not need sedation for obtaining biopsies, only local anaesthesia with 0.5–1 ml lidocaine injected subcutaneously (**Fig. 1.34**). Exceptions would be nose, face, ear, tail or foot lesions, which often require sedation or general anaesthesia to obtain good samples. A minimum of two 6-mm punches should be obtained for most skin conditions unless the lesion is solitary and tiny; a 4-mm punch can be used for areas that bleed a lot like the nose or feet. Multiple samples should be taken from the newest stages of primary lesions (e.g. pustules) if possible and slightly older lesions (e.g. crusts). The hair should not be clipped too short and the skin should not be scrubbed in any way. If the crust falls off during the biopsy process, it can be added to the formalin jar with a note to the pathologist. Ideally, samples should be obtained from non-eroded or ulcerated areas because an intact epidermis is critical for the diagnosis of many conditions. It is very rare that an area of normal skin would be helpful in the diagnosis of a condition, so normal skin should not be included in a biopsy. The biopsy punch should be rotated in one direction only while pressing to the skin. A new punch should be used for each animal, because dull punches give poor results. Incisional wedge biopsies can be used for deeper lesions affecting the subcutaneous tissues. Do not squeeze the sample in a forceps; the tissue should be gently lifted and immediately placed into formalin – any drying of the biopsy at all is harmful. The biopsy site should be sutured after the sample is in formalin. A monofilament non-absorbable suture is preferred for most biopsy situations because it is less irritating than absorbable suture. Samples should be fixed in formalin for 24 hours before shipping if there is a risk of freezing during shipping. A history and all information about the pet should be included for the pathologist, and photos can be very helpful as well.

Diascopy is a technique used to distinguish erythema from haemorrhage. A glass slide is pressed against the lesion. The skin will blanche under the slide if the redness is due to erythema. The redness will persist under the slide if the redness is due to haemorrhage or vascular congestion.

DERMATOLOGICAL HISTORY AND PHYSICAL EXAM

Preparation for visit

It is best if the pet is not bathed and that no ear flushing or ear medications are used the day of the appointment. It is also best that the pet has not eaten for at least 6 hours in case blood work or sedation is needed.

In dermatology, as in most diseases in medicine, the history is a key part of the patient evaluation. Some important dermatological history questions are given below. Not all can be answered by the client and may necessitate reading through the previous medical records. Instead of asking 'Is your pet itchy?', it is better to ask specifics, for example: 'Does your pet lick its feet or legs, or any other areas?' or 'Does he scoot his hind end on the ground?'. Specific questions must be asked because many owners do not recognise other behaviours as being itchy other than scratching, and will erroneously answer 'no' to the question about itching if the dog is licking the feet. You may also get more accurate answers if you ask open-type questions, e.g. 'how itchy is your dog?' rather than 'is he very itchy?', and 'how often did you give the tablets?' rather than 'did you give them twice daily?'. Always remember to check the pet's general health – there may be systemic complications, concurrent conditions and other treatment that you will need to be aware of.

Reason for visit

- What areas of the body are affected?
- When did the problem start? Describe the progression.
- What were the first lesions? How have these changed?
- Itching: is your pet scratching, rubbing, licking, biting at any part of the body? Any scooting of the hind end?
- How severe are the above symptoms: not licking or scratching, mild, moderate, severe?
- Is the problem year-round, seasonal only, unknown; worst time of year: spring, summer, autumn, winter.
- Ears: is your pet scratching its ears, shaking its head, has a foul ear smell, or discharge from the ears?

- Other current symptoms: coughing, sneezing, vomiting, diarrhoea, not eating well, weight loss, weight gain, excessive drinking, excessive urination, low energy, eye discharge, lameness, neurological problems or behavioural change (list).
- List past illnesses or conditions.
- When was the last blood work performed?
- Environment: indoors only, indoor/outdoor, on leash only, outdoors, farm/woods, swims, hunting dog.
- List other animals in contact. Are they also affected? Are they on flea control? Any contact with wild animals?
- Is your pet currently on flea/tick preventive? List name and frequency, when last used.
- Do any humans in the household have a skin problem?
- What is your pet's current diet? Has a food trial been done? Which foods? Length of trial? Strict?
- List treats and supplements.
- How frequently do you bathe and with what? Is bathing helpful?
- List any known food or drug sensitivity.
- List current and past drugs and dosages. What treatments seem to help? Any adverse effects?

All areas of the body should be examined. Move from the front of the patient to the back. Examine the oral cavity, chin and lip folds, ears (check the pinnal–pedal reflex and otoscopic exam), under the neck (lift the collar), axillae, interdigital skin (noting footpads), abdomen, perineal and vulva area. Part the hair down the dorsum, and examine closely the caudal dorsum for fleas or flea dirt. It is often very helpful to lift up or roll the patient on its side or back so the entire ventrum can be properly evaluated. Discuss the physical exam findings as you go to give value to your examination to the client and so these findings can be noted by an assistant. Take samples of representative areas for diagnostics. Taking photos can help track progress at rechecks, especially if there are multiple veterinarians in a practice. Finally, remember that skin disease does not occur in isolation – always do a thorough general examination to detect any systemic complications or concurrent conditions.

ACRAL LICK DERMATITIS
(Acral lick granulomas)

Definition
Acral lick dermatitis is an ulcerated lesion, usually on the lower legs, caused by self-trauma due to licking or gnawing. It is not a disease, but a symptom of an underlying condition.

Aetiology and pathogenesis
Acral lick lesions are caused by self-trauma. There are many reasons for a dog to lick obsessively at the legs, the most common reason being pruritus. Pruritus of the legs is most often caused by atopic dermatitis, but ectoparasites should be ruled out as well. In addition, abnormal sensory perception is a possible reason for licking. Acral lick lesions have been reported over surgical implants,[1] at arthritic joints and following nerve pathways, indicating that pain plays a role in some cases. Excessive licking can be a sign of gastrointestinal or dental disease.[2] Anxiety or compulsive disorders may play a role in some dogs, by either causing this condition or exacerbating it[3] (see Behavioural dermatoses, page 15). It is important to recognise that these are not mutually exclusive and many dogs have multiple triggers. In some cases, a small initial injury to the skin may be a focus of licking, causing a secondary bacterial folliculitis and furunculosis, which leads to more pain or pruritus, causing more licking and enlarging the lesion.

Clinical features
Middle-aged to older and large breed dogs are predisposed. Lesions are plaque like, firm and often ulcerated on the surface. A rim of hyperpigmented, lichenified skin and saliva-stained hair usually surrounds the lesion. Dogs start these lesions on the dorsal lower legs and feet and, where the dog has a

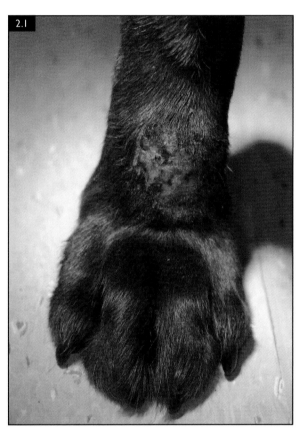

Fig. 2.1 A well-developed acral lick granuloma with well-demarcated swelling, erythema, alopecia, erosions and hyperpigmentation.

favourite limb that is focused on, the front limbs are often preferred (**Fig. 2.1**). Atopic dermatitis and/or a food allergy is the most common underlying reason for this condition, and so other symptoms such as pododermatitis, otitis and skin infections may be concurrent. Other causes typically have no skin lesions other than those created by the animal. Very precise and focal lesions (e.g. single digits) often have a neuropathic cause, especially if bilateral.

Differential diagnoses

- Neoplasia.
- Ulcerated sebaceous hyperplasia.
- Foreign body.
- Deep bacterial or fungal infection.

Diagnosis

These lesions are usually easy to diagnose visually; it is the underlying cause of the condition that can be more difficult to establish, especially if the dog has no other signs or history of atopic dermatitis. A careful history and thorough physical examination is required to rule out systemic illness, musculoskeletal problems, neuropathies and behavioural factors. These lesions almost always involve a deep staphylococcal bacterial infection,[4] so cytology and deep bacterial culture/sensitivity is ideal. Multiple biopsies or surgical removal with histopathology may be needed to confirm diagnosis and rule out infectious or neoplastic causes of this condition.

Treatment

This condition can be very frustrating to manage if an underlying condition is not found and if owners are not compliant. Owners should be warned of the low likelihood of curing the condition once it has become chronic, especially if an underlying condition is not found and, no matter what, it is likely that the dog will need some form of long-term management:

- In mild cases, start by treating the secondary staphylococcal infections (usually for 6–8 weeks), and investigate and treat the underlying condition (see Aetiology and pathogenesis section). It is best to be very diligent to make sure that the lesions are resolving well with your choice of treatment, to stop them becoming chronic and severe.
- For pruritus and atopic dermatitis work-up and treatments, see pages 18 and 41.
- For suspected neurogenic pruritus, see page 63.
- When all other medical conditions are ruled out, and a true behavioural component is suspected, see page 15.
- In severe cases, no matter the underlying reason, the following protocol can be attempted using

all medications and barriers constantly until resolution (smooth, non-lichenified skin and hair regrowth), which usually takes 1–2 months. Bear in mind that glucocorticoids frequently mask underlying diseases, so diagnostics should be performed before starting therapy. Also remember that glucocorticoid therapy has many adverse side effects:

- Prednisone/prednisolone 0.5–1 mg/kg per day.
- Oral antibiotics based on culture; topical antibiotics may be sufficient for less severe lesions.
- Twice-daily topical DMSO/fluocinolone 1 drop per cm of ulceration, followed by a thin layer of antibiotic/antifungal/steroid ointment.
- An Elizabethan (e-)collar and/or other barrier method (wrapping, basket muzzle, sock, etc.) is essential to break the self-trauma cycle.
- Naltrexone (2 mg/kg po q12–24 h) or hydrocodone (0.25 mg/kg po q8–12 h) can be used to help break a compulsive cycle, if suspected.

- Topical 0.25% capsaicin, peppermint and tea tree ointments may provide short-term relief.
- Ciclosporin and topical 0.1% tacrolimus may help in cases that fail to respond or those that do not tolerate topical or oral glucocorticoids.
- Recalcitrant lesions can be removed surgically or with a laser or cautery. Caution should be used as without strict barriers and controlling the underlying cause, the surgical site will usually become a new target of self-trauma.
- There should be a plan in place for long-term management of the underlying condition, which may include: more exercise, enrichment with chew toys, anxiety treatments, food trials, or long-term treatment of allergies, neuropathies or arthritis. If not, the condition will commonly rapidly recur when steroid and antibiotic treatments are stopped.

Key point

- Underlying causes of acral lick dermatitis must be diagnosed and treated long term.

References
1 Denerolle P, White SD, Taylor TS, Vandenabeele SI. Organic diseases mimicking acral lick dermatitis in six dogs. *J Am Anim Hosp Assoc* 2007; **43**: 215–220.
2 Bécuwe-Bonne, V, Bélanger, M-C, Frank D, Parent J, Hélie P. Gastrointestinal disorders in dogs with excessive licking of surfaces. *J Vet Behav Clin Appl Res* 2012; **7**: 194–204.
3 Virga V. Behavioral dermatology. *Vet Clin North Am Small Anim Pract* 2003; **33**: 231–251.
4 Shumaker AK, Angus JC, Coyner KS, Loeffler DG, Rankin SC, Lewis TP. Microbiological and histopathological features of canine acral lick dermatitis. *Vet Dermatol* 2008; **19**: 288–298.

BEHAVIOURAL DERMATOSES

Definition

Behavioural dermatoses involve skin or hair damage caused by compulsive actions of the animal. These include acral lick dermatitis, flank sucking, nail biting, tail biting, tail sucking, anal/genital licking and feline psychogenic overgrooming.

Aetiology and pathogenesis

Most dermatological conditions that appear to be behavioural have an underlying painful, pruritic, endocrine or neurogenic disease associated with them. Pure behavioural dermatoses with no underlying or contributing condition are very rare. Some exceptions to this that are almost always purely behavioural appear to be flank and tail sucking.

Compulsive disorders arise from frustration as a result of lack of or changes in environmental stimulation or social interaction. Strictly indoor cats appear to be predisposed to psychogenic alopecia.[1] There are breed and genetic predispositions for many compulsive disorders, e.g. Doberman Pinschers[2] and Siamese cats appear to be predisposed to compulsive disorders, and large breed dogs appear to be predisposed to acral lick dermatitis.[1] Many behaviours are attention seeking.[1]

Clinical features

Acral lick dermatitis (see page 13) is a firm ulcerated plaque on the lower limbs or feet, caused by excessive licking. **Flank sucking** is seen most frequently in Doberman Pinschers. **Tail sucking** is most common in Siamese cats, and usually involves the tip of the tail. **Tail biting** is seen most commonly in young, long-tailed, long-haired dogs where they chase the tail and bite the tip. **Anal/genital licking** is seen most commonly in Poodles and is often very upsetting for the owner. Attention-seeking behaviours should cease when the owner or other people are absent. Constantly traumatised skin may become alopecic, lichenified and hyperpigmented with secondary infections, which may be pruritic and worsen the problem. However, a lack of inflammation does not rule out compulsive behaviour.

Psychogenic overgrooming in cats is very rare (**Figs. 2.2, 2.3**), and other causes of overgrooming are much more common.[3] The barbering is often bilaterally symmetrical and can be patchy or well demarcated, most commonly on the abdomen, inner fore- and hindlimbs and flanks. Occasionally, cats persistently damage the skin, resulting in erosions and ulceration. The clinical signs are very similar to those caused by allergic dermatitis or *Demodex gatoi*.

Feline hyperaesthesia syndrome is considered a compulsive disorder, although it can be associated with generalised neuropathies and systemic disease. It is most commonly seen in young cats (age 1–5 years), and Siamese, Burmese, Persian and Abyssinian cats are more predisposed.[4] Common symptoms include mydriasis, aggression, staring at and attacking the tail and flanks and biting the tail base, forelegs and paws. Cats may run wildly around the house during these bouts. Petting may trigger this behaviour. Ruling out pruritus from other diseases such as from fleas, mites or allergy is very important. If treatment trials with ectoparasiticides are not helpful, a glucocorticoid trial can be helpful because these symptoms are most commonly related to pruritic diseases. In contrast, compulsive disorders are less likely to respond to glucocorticoids.

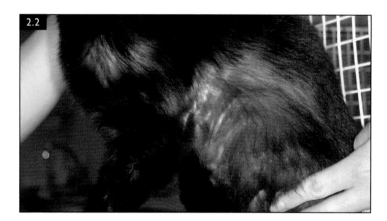

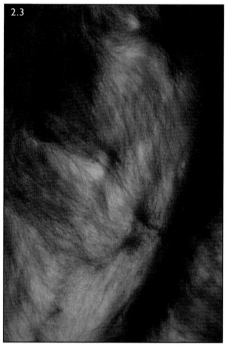

Figs. 2.2, 2.3 Self-induced alopecia of the flanks, lateral limbs (**Fig. 2.2**) and ventral body (**Fig. 2.3**) of an anxious cat in a multi-cat household.

Differential diagnoses

- Flank and tail sucking are characteristic and do not have differentials.
- For acral lick dermatitis (see page 13), differentials include any painful (arthritis), pruritic (atopic, food or parasitic), endocrine (hypothyroidism) or neurogenic (sensory neuropathy) condition.
- For feline psychogenic overgrooming and feline hyperaesthesia syndrome, differentials include pruritic (allergic, parasitic, dermatophytic), painful (arthritis, urinary tract disease), neuropathic or endocrine (hyperthyroidism) condition. Allergic dermatitis will sometimes manifest with scratching or otitis as well as overgrooming, indicating that the issue is unlikely to be psychogenic. In an older cat with sudden dramatic abdominal alopecia, consider paraneoplastic alopecia (see page 110).
- For nail biting, differentials include allergic dermatitis, yeast pododermatitis, lupoid onychodystrophy, nailbed neoplasia and peripheral neuropathies. In puppies, this behaviour can indicate acral mutilation syndrome (see page 242).

- For tail biting, differentials include atopic dermatitis, parasites, sensory neuropathy, tail dock neuroma and anal sacculitis.
- For anal/genital licking, differentials include atopic dermatitis, pain (anal sacculitis or perineal fistulae), incontinence, external or internal parasites and bacterial or yeast infections. Anal/genital licking along with scratching or scooting indicates that the behaviour has an atopic or anal sac component.

Diagnosis

Diagnosis of a compulsive condition is made by ruling out all other possible explanations for a behaviour. For licking/biting/overgrooming behaviours this includes the following:

- Full blood work including thyroid profiles and urinalysis.
- Radiographs to determine underlying arthritic diseases.
- Musculoskeletal and neurological examinations.
- Cytology, and/or fungal and bacterial cultures, and treatment of any infections.

- Treatment trials for ectoparasites, even if none are found.
- Investigation of atopic dermatitis and/or food allergies, including several different, appropriately dosed, treatment trials (for cats see page 41; for dogs see page 18).

Treatment

- It is rare that drugs alone can successfully treat behavioural dermatoses, and the owner must be willing to put in time for environmental enrichment and positive attention that does not inadvertently reward the behaviour. Desensitisation to or alleviation of anxiety-inducing stimuli should be performed if possible. Vigorous exercise, social interactions and mental stimulation can be very helpful for dogs.
- For cats, creating a stable consistent environment is helpful. This may include regular feeding times, play sessions and redirecting behaviour with positive reinforcement.[4] Stressful social interactions with other cats must be investigated and improved. Homes should be zoned into territories for each social unit in multi-cat households, each with feeding stations, litter trays and elevated resting sites.
- Punishing behaviours is almost never helpful, and often makes them worse.
- Secondary bacterial or yeast infections must be effectively managed.
- Muzzles and e-collars may be useful to prevent self-trauma in severe cases.
- For management of acral lick dermatitis, see page 14. Where there is a strong suspicion of a behavioural component, behavioural drugs (see below) can be considered.
- Drugs may be helpful for anxiety or behaviour modification in combination with increased enrichment, allowing 3–4 weeks for assessment of effectiveness. All of these drugs should be used with care, because they may lower thyroid hormone concentrations, worsen cardiac arrhythmias, lower seizure threshold and cause hepatotoxicity. There are many possible side effects and interactions that are not covered in this book and clinicians should research these carefully.

- Dogs:[1,5]
  - Clomipramine (1 mg/kg po q12 h increasing to 1.0–3.5 mg/kg q12 h over 3–4 weeks); amitriptyline (1–2 mg/kg po q12 h increasing to 1–4 mg/kg q12 h over 3–4 weeks); doxepin (1 mg/kg po q12 h increasing to 1–5 mg/kg q12 h over 3–4 weeks).
  - Fluoxetine (1 mg/kg po q12–24 h); sertraline (1 mg/kg po q24 h).
  - Diazepam (0.55–2.2 mg/kg po q12–24 h); alprazolam (0.05–0.25 mg/kg po q12–24 h); lorazepam 0.025–0.25 mg/kg po q12–24 h); oxazepam (0.2–1.0 mg/kg po q12–24 h); clonazepam (0.05–0.25 mg/kg po q12–24 h).
  - Naltrexone (2 mg/kg po q12–24 h); hydrocodone (0.25 mg/kg po q8–12 h); dextromethorphan (2 mg/kg po q12 h).
- Cats:[1,4]
  - Clomipramine (0.5–1.0 mg/kg po q24 h); amitriptyline (0.5–1.0 mg/kg po q12–24 h); doxepin (0.5–1.0 mg/kg po q12–24 h, up to 25 mg/cat).
  - Fluoxetine (0.5–2.0 mg/kg po q24 h); sertraline (0.5–1.0 mg/kg po q24 h).
- Collars, sprays, diffusers and/or foods with pheromones, herbs and amino acids can also be helpful, especially for cats.

Key point

- Always strive to find an underlying disease when presented with an abnormal behaviour.

References

1 Virga V. Behavioral dermatology. *Vet Clin North Am Small Anim Pract* 2003; **33**: 231–251.
2 Ogata N, Gillis TE, Liu X *et al.* Brain structural abnormalities in Doberman pinschers with canine compulsive disorder. *Prog Neuropsychopharmacol Biol Psychiatry* 2013; **45**: 1–6.
3 Waisglass SE, Landsberg GM, Yager JA, Hall JA. Underlying medical conditions in cats with presumptive psychogenic alopecia. *J Am Vet Med Assoc* 2006; **228**: 1705–1709.
4 Ciribassi JJ. Understanding behavior – feline hyperesthesia syndrome. *Compend Contin Educ Vet* 2009; **31**: E10.
5 White SD. Naltrexone for treatment of acral lick dermatitis in dogs. *J Am Vet Med Assoc* 1990; **196**: 1073–1076.

ATOPIC DERMATITIS IN DOGS

Definition

Atopic dermatitis is a common hypersensitivity reaction pattern that is associated with a typical history and characteristic clinical signs:

- Classic atopic dermatitis (AD) is associated with sensitisation to environmental allergens (pollens, dusts and/or moulds). The patient may or may not produce immunoglobulin E (IgE) antibodies to allergens.
- Food-induced atopic dermatitis (FIAD) is used to describe cases where food is one of the triggers for the skin condition. Dogs with FIAD may or may not have concurrent sensitisation to environmental allergens.

Aetiology and pathogenesis

The development of atopic dermatitis is a complex interaction between genetics and the environment involving poor skin barrier function, abnormal skin inflammation and sensitisation to environmental and/or food allergens. Subsequent self-trauma, altered cutaneous microflora populations and secondary staphylococcal and *Malassezia* skin and ear infections drive chronic inflammatory changes. Some dogs become sensitised to staphylococcal and *Malassezia* proteins and glycoproteins, which then act as endogenous allergens.

Most known allergens are proteins, but carbohydrates are likely also to play a role. There is evidence that constant exposure to certain allergens (such as flea saliva) at a young age may impart tolerance, whereas intermittent exposure or exposure later in life often triggers an allergic response.

T lymphocytes are the main cells involved in atopic dermatitis. Exposure to allergens is by inhalation, ingestion or cutaneous penetration. These allergens are presented by Langerhans' cells causing sensitisation of memory T cells. Subsequent allergen exposure and T-cell activation release inflammatory mediators that cause skin barrier dysfunction, skin inflammation and pruritus. Secondary yeast and bacterial infections greatly intensify the symptoms. The cascade of inflammatory mediators recruits and activates other cells (e.g. mast cells, eosinophils, neutrophils, macrophages and keratinocytes) that contribute further to the skin inflammation and skin barrier dysfunction.

Clinical features

The clinical features of canine atopic dermatitis are extremely variable, with no single physical or historical finding that definitively diagnoses the disease. The true incidence of canine atopic dermatitis is unknown and probably varies by geographical region, but it is thought to affect nearly 10% of all dogs (and more in predisposed breeds). There are well-recognised breed predispositions, although these vary regionally and any breed or cross can be affected.

Generally, clinical signs are first seen when dogs are between 1 and 3 years of age, and at least some signs should be present before age 6 years. However, the disease has been noted in very young (3 months old) and older (7 years old) animals.

Seasonal disease or seasonal flares are commonly associated with pollen allergies, and the clinical signs should match local pollen production (although seasonal parasites such as *Neotrombicula autumnalis* should be eliminated). Year-round clinical signs are associated with sensitivity to indoor allergens and/or foods.

About 7–25% of allergic dogs have a food allergy,[1] alone or in combination with an environmental allergy. Clinical signs before 1 year of age, non-seasonal symptoms and concurrent gastrointestinal symptoms are often associated with allergy to foods. Dogs with food allergy tend to react to more than one food. Beef, lamb, chicken, dairy products, maize, wheat, soy and eggs all seem to be common allergens in canine food allergy,[2] although the data are poor and this may reflect feeding patterns.[3] Food allergic dogs may have a higher incidence of gastrointestinal signs, although more subtle abnormalities (e.g. more than three bowel movements/day, borborygmi, flatulence, variable faecal consistency, straining, blood and mucus) are more common than vomiting or diarrhoea.[4]

Pruritus and erythema are the primary lesions in atopic dermatitis (**Figs. 2.4–2.7**). The degree of pruritus and erythema varies from very mild to intense and may be generalised or localised. Some animals, particularly with acute disease, have no primary lesions and show only pruritus. Erythema may be localised to ears, periocular skin, muzzle, ventral neck, axilla, groin, flank, feet (especially the interdigital webs) and flexor surfaces (under the tail, elbow, carpus and tarsus).

Secondary staphylococcal (see Superficial pyoderma, page 65) **and** *Malassezia* (see Malassezia dermatitis, page 30) **skin and ear infections** are very common, and greatly intensify the pruritus and inflammation (**Figs. 2.8–2.10**). Chronic or recurrent yeast and/or bacterial otitis (see page 267) is seen in 80% of atopic dogs and may be the only or most prominent clinical sign in up to 20% of cases. Protracted inflammation leads to hyperplasia of the

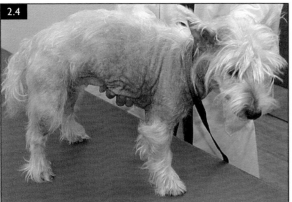

Fig. 2.4 Extensive erythema and alopecia on the ventral trunk, flanks and proximal limbs of a West Highland White Terrier.

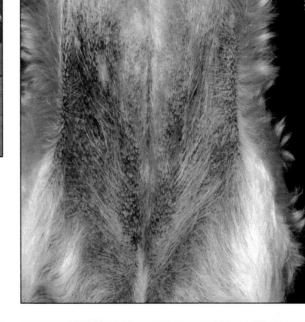

Fig. 2.5 Erythema and hyperpigmentation of the ventral abdomen in an atopic West Highland White Terrier.

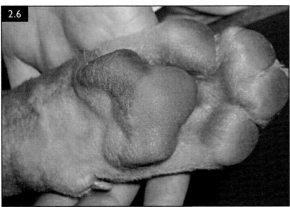

Fig. 2.6 Diffuse metacarpal and interdigital erythema in an atopic Bull Terrier.

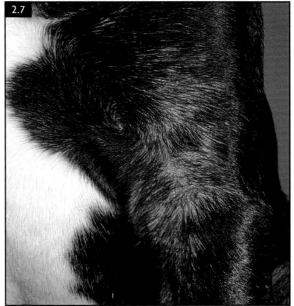

Fig. 2.7 Inflammation of the flexor surface of the elbow in an atopic Staffordshire bull terrier.

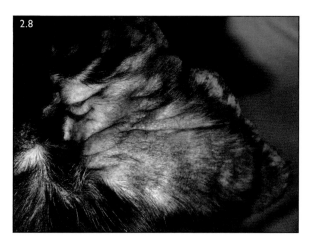

Fig. 2.8 Severe chronic erythroceruminous otitis externa in an atopic Labrador.

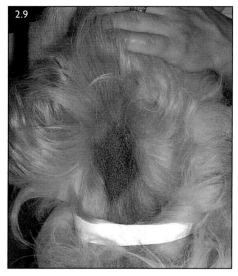

Fig. 2.9 Focal hyperpigmentation, alopecia, lichenification and erythema on the ventral neck of a Golden Retriever due to secondary *Malassezia pachydermatis*.

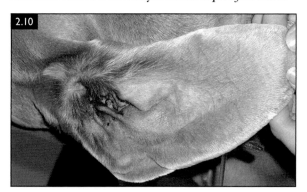

Fig. 2.10 Malassezia otitis externa in a Weimeraner with a cutaneous adverse food reaction.

tissues on the inside of the pinnae and the ear canals. It also predisposes to sebaceous and ceruminous hyperplasia, resulting in excess wax accumulation and stenosis, which predisposes to further infection.

Periocular dermatitis results in varying degrees of erythema, alopecia, excoriation and lichenification about the eyes. Conjunctivitis is seen in about 80% of atopic dogs, and they may scratch at their eyes or rub them along furniture or the floor (**Figs. 2.11–2.14**). It may occur as the only sign or together with other features of allergic dermatitis. Some dogs develop meibomian adenitis with granulomatous thickening of the eyelid margins, crusting and draining tracts.

Acral lick dermatitis (see page 13). Atopic dermatitis more commonly triggers acral lick dermatitis than anxiety, although concurrent psychogenic issues may make some atopic dogs more likely to develop acral lick lesions. These lesions almost always involve a secondary staphylococcal infection and sometimes become obsessive. These lesions are very difficult to resolve without treatment of the underlying cause.

Interdigital furunculosis or cysts (see page 216) are a common and complex problem, and atopic dermatitis is the most common primary trigger. Inflammation in the interdigital skin results in the walls of the hair follicles becoming hyperplastic and hyperkeratotic. A follicle may become plugged and expand as sebaceous and apocrine gland secretions continue to be secreted into it. Finally, it ruptures into the dermis, resulting in a foreign body reaction to sebum, keratin and hair. Bacteria in the hair follicles may lead to secondary infection. The papules or nodules may break open and drain a serosanguineous fluid. In many cases these lesions will develop spontaneously and then disappear. Single or multiple feet may be affected.

Perianal dermatitis is often misdiagnosed as either intestinal parasitism or anal sacculitis (see page 34). Lesions occur in the skin under the tail as well as in the skin of the perianal area. Erythema may be the only finding in some cases, but in others the affected skin can become chronically inflamed and hyperplastic. Animals will lick excessively, drag their perineal areas across the floor or spin in circles while sitting to relieve the pruritus. Chronic changes

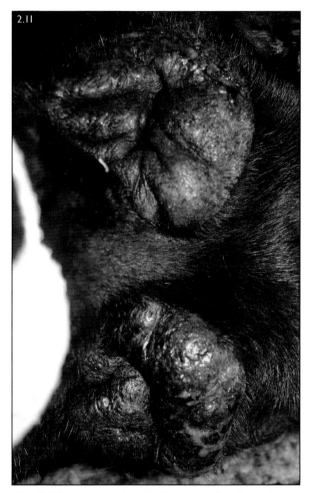

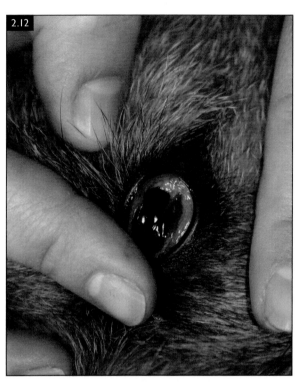

Fig. 2.12 Atopic conjunctivitis in a Border Terrier.

Fig. 2.11 Severe conjunctivitis causing facial excoriation and periocular pyoderma in an atopic Labrador.

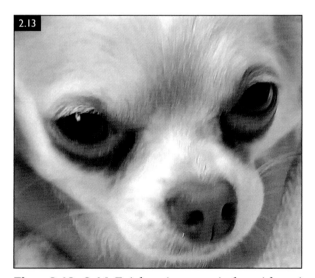

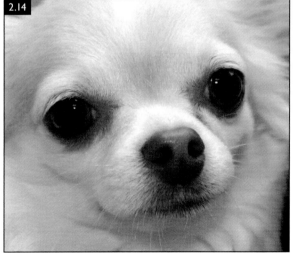

Figs. 2.13, 2.14 Epiphora in an atopic dog with conjunctivitis (Fig. 2.13), and the same dog after treatment (Fig. 2.14).

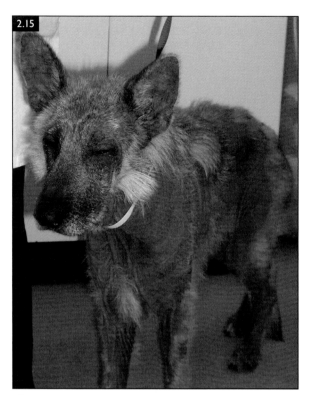

Fig. 2.15 Severe generalised atopic dermatitis with excoriation, alopecia, hyperpigmentation and seborrhoea in a German Shepherd dog.

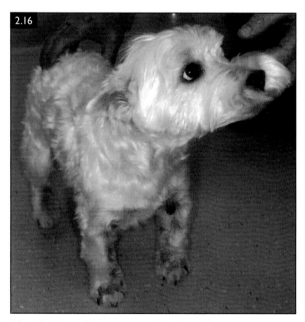

Fig. 2.16 Inflammation of the feet, flexor surfaces, medial limbs and ventral body in a West Highland White Terrier with food-induced atopic dermatitis.

and bacterial colonisation may predispose to anal sac impaction and infection.

Excoriations, hyperpigmentation, lichenification, seborrhoea, scaling, thinning hair and alopecia result from chronic skin inflammation, infections and self-trauma (licking, biting, chewing, rubbing and/or rolling) (**Figs. 2.15, 2.16**). However, these are non-specific and can be associated with any chronic dermatitis.

Differential diagnoses

- Parasites (fleas, mites and lice).
- Yeast or bacterial infection caused by other disease.
- Dermatophytosis (see page 115).
- Epitheliotrophic lymphoma (seen in older animals, see page 38).
- Pemphigus foliaceus (see page 81).
- When affecting the ears only: ear mites, foreign body or middle-ear disease (see page 267).
- When affecting periocular skin only: demodicosis, dermatophytosis, staphylococcal pyoderma, meibomian gland adenitis and other causes of conjunctivitis.
- For acral lick dermatitis lesions only, see page 13.
- When symptoms affect the interdigital areas of feet only (see Diseases of paws and nails, page 215): hookworm dermatitis, interdigital cysts, demodicosis, contact dermatitis, necrolytic migratory erythema.

Diagnosis[5]

Figure 2.17 outlines the basic principles of the diagnostic work-up. Atopic dermatitis is diagnosed by history, clinical findings, ruling out other diseases and response to therapy. Hair plucks, tapestrips and skin scrapings should be taken from multiple affected locations to rule out demodicosis, *Cheyletiella* and *Neotrombicula* spp. and lice, and possibly find sarcoptic mange. A fungal culture should be obtained if this is suspected, although it is rarely pruritic in dogs. Cytology for yeast and bacterial infections should be taken from several affected locations, especially the ears and feet (if affected). Infections should be treated and cleared, and an 8-week broad-spectrum treatment trial for fleas,

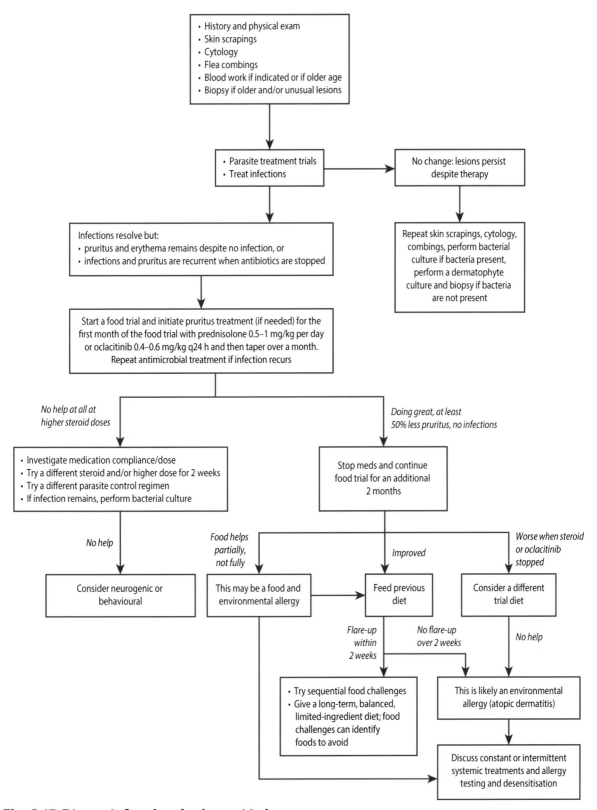

Fig. 2.17 Diagnostic flow chart for the pruritic dog.

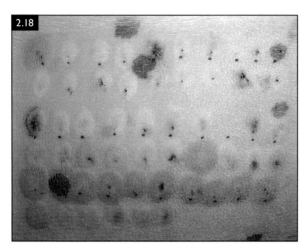

Fig. 2.18 Positive intradermal allergen test in a dog with atopic dermatitis. The positive test sites show erythema and swelling.

lice and mites should be performed. If the pruritus is year-round, an 8-week food trial should be started. If the pruritus persists then intradermal or serological allergen tests to identify allergens for allergen-specific immunotherapy can be considered (**Fig. 2.18**). Positive intradermal or serological tests for staphylococcal and/or *Malassezia* allergens should prompt rigorous topical antimicrobial therapy to reduce microbial burdens on the skin and in the ears.

Diagnosis of food allergy

The diagnosis of a food allergy is based on feeding a restricted diet composed of unique ingredients to which the animal has never, or only very rarely, been exposed. It is therefore critically important to obtain a full dietary history including data on commercial diets, scraps or leftovers, biscuits or chews, flavoured medicines and any vitamin or mineral supplements. However, this may be difficult where the owner cannot recall which foods have been fed or is unaware of the ingredients in commercial foods because over-the-counter and even prescription diets may contain ingredients not on the label.[6,7]

Serological food allergen tests are of limited value.[8] Very few have been validated, and the positive predictive values are low (30–70%). However, the negative predictive values tend to be higher (approximately 80%), so they could be used to identify foods

suitable for inclusion in a diet trial. Closed-cup patch tests with fresh foods are more accurate but are difficult to perform outside specialist centres.

Diet trials are ideally performed using home-cooked diets or commercially prepared hydrolysed or limited-ingredient prescription diets. Home-cooked diets are in theory better because the foods can be very restricted, but they are not nutritionally balanced for very young animals, dogs with specific nutritional needs and long-term use and are labour intensive, and may (depending on the ingredients) be more expensive. Commercial single protein diets are easier to feed and should be nutritionally balanced, but it may be difficult to find a diet with suitable ingredients. It is important not to confuse 'novel' with 'exotic', e.g. dogs sensitised to beef are likely to react to closely related species such as water buffalo, bison, antelope and sheep, but are unlikely to react to less closely related species such as horse and rabbit. Hydrolysed foods avoid some of these problems, but these diets must be completely hydrolysed to avoid reactions, and a few dogs may still react to the high-molecular-weight maize-starch allergens present in these foods. These diets may also be more expensive and less palatable. In short, there is no single ideal approach to a food trial. The trial and the diet should be selected carefully, considering the owners' wishes and abilities. Treat options (e.g. limited ingredient treats, shaped and cooked kibble or tinned food, and/or crisps, liver cake or jerky from novel sources) must be given where necessary to encourage compliance. Other problems can include scavenging, flavoured medications, dropped food, licking other animals' 'empty' food bowls and coprophagia.

The length of a diet trial necessary to confirm an adverse reaction to food is controversial, but, for dogs, most authorities now recommend at least 8 weeks (and sometimes 10 weeks) for a good response.[9] However, it is useful to follow cases carefully because gastrointestinal signs will improve more rapidly than acute dermatitis, which improves quicker than chronic dermatitis. For example, if there are still gastrointestinal problems after two weeks, check compliance and/or consider changing the diet. In contrast, rapid resolution of the gastrointestinal signs should encourage persisting with the food trial.

As allergy symptoms commonly fluctuate, an animal that improves with a restricted diet should be challenged with its original diet, which should include all treats, scraps, biscuits, chews and dietary supplements. If a food allergy is involved, there will be an increase in pruritus within 7 days of the dietary challenge (again gastrointestinal signs often relapse sooner). If there is no increase in pruritus after the dietary challenge, then a food allergy can be ruled out and the apparent improvement was probably the result of some other effect. If there is recrudescence of pruritus with the dietary challenge, then the restricted diet should be reinstituted and there should once again be resolution of the pruritus. It is helpful to identify the specific foods to which the animal is reacting using a series of sequential food challenges, with 2 weeks between each new food item.

Failure to recognise and treat secondary infections and ectoparasites during a dietary trial is a common cause of problems. Another major reason for poor compliance during a dietary trial is continued pruritus. One solution is to allow the use of short courses of glucocorticoids or oclacitinib for the first 3–4 weeks of the trial and then taper to see if the improvement can be maintained. Alternatively, the owners can give 3- to 7-day courses of glucocorticoids or oclacitinib at their discretion to manage unacceptable pruritus during the food trial.

Treatment[10]

Management of allergic dermatitis can be very complex and frustrating. It is very important to emphasise to the client that this condition cannot be cured, but will need to be managed when the symptoms are present and treatment will probably be lifelong. Treatment of allergic dermatitis must be tailored to the specific signs and secondary changes or complications present in an individual animal. Owners need to be aware that it is not possible to predict initially which animal will respond to a particular therapy. They also need to understand that clinical manifestations frequently change, resulting in the need to adjust the therapy. Also, it is necessary for the owner to appreciate the time and financial commitment needed for the management of atopic dermatitis.

Parasite prevention
Long-term flea and parasite prevention should be instituted.

Avoidance of allergens
If a food allergy is deemed to be all or part of the dog's problem, the offending foods must be eliminated from the diet. It may be possible to avoid some environmental allergens, but this is usually difficult and of limited benefit.

Topical therapy
Topical steroids are very useful for short- or long-term intermittent management of localised lesions. Combinations of steroids with antibiotics and antifungals are very helpful for infected areas, such as the ears, feet or under the neck. Using topical steroids for over 2 months can cause significant skin thinning and hair loss, which may take years to resolve. Ideally animals should be maintained on less potent products (e.g. hydrocortisone or hydrocortisone aceponate) that are less likely to cause side effects and the frequency should be tapered to the lowest frequency needed. Nevertheless, some pets will still have systemic absorption and side effects, and animals on long-term treatment should have regular rechecks. Owners should wear gloves to apply these products.

Topical 0.1% tacrolimus is expensive, but can be very useful to avoid cutaneous atrophy or systemic absorption. Owners should wear gloves and use twice daily until improvement, before tapering to the lowest frequency that maintains remission (ideally twice weekly).

Topical antibiotics and antifungals work well to spot treat small areas but are very difficult for larger areas. Sprays, ointments, creams or lotions would need to be used twice daily to resolve an infection. Topical sensitivities can occasionally develop.

Shampooing is a very useful and important therapy in pruritic, greasy and/or infected skin. Bathing with lukewarm water with or without a shampoo is also helpful to rinse off allergens before they are absorbed percutaneously. Whirlpool baths are more effective than showers. The shampoo formulation and frequency should be based on cytology and coat greasiness. Bathing should typically be performed one to three times weekly until the clinical signs are controlled. Chlorhexidine products are the most effective antimicrobials, but may be drying and topical sensitisation can occur, including sensitisation in owners. Dogs with pruritic dry skin should be treated with an emollient product with proven antipruritic efficacy. Antiseborrhoeic shampoos can be used in dogs with greasy skin, although care should be taken to avoid over-drying the coat. Emollient leave-on lotions, foams and conditioners can be used where necessary to prevent dryness after or between baths. Owners should be discouraged from scrubbing or picking at the skin, and should not rub against the grain of the hair because this may cause folliculitis in a sensitive dog.

Spot-on therapies can help restore the skin barrier in localised areas of chronic cases. This may be more helpful for some dogs than others. There is only a mild-to-moderate improvement, and frequent use and several doses per pet are needed.

Ears (see page 267 for management of ear infections). Ear infections respond best to topical medications in the short term. Topical steroids can be used two to three times weekly to prevent recurrent inflammation. These can be used alone or combined with cleaning where necessary.

Conjunctivitis can be effectively managed with glucocorticoid-containing ophthalmic preparations (e.g. 1% prednisolone or 0.1% dexamethasone) used three to four times daily to remission, and then tapered for maintenance. Ciclosporin 0.2% ointment applied twice daily to remission and then tapering the frequency is also effective.

Systemic control of infections

Recurrent yeast and bacterial infections indicate that the atopic dermatitis is not controlled. Efforts should be made to better control the underlying problem and use topical antimicrobials to minimise the repeated use of systemic antimicrobials.

Antibacterial agents (see Superficial pyoderma, page 65) for secondary staphylococcal infections include cefalexin (25 mg/kg po q12 h), cefpodoxime proxetil (5–10 mg/kg po q24 h), oxacillin or dicloxacillin (20 mg/kg po q12 h), clindamycin (5.5–11 mg/kg po q12 h), lincomycin (22 mg/kg po q12 h) and clavulanic acid–potentiated amoxicillin (25 mg/kg po q12 h).

Antifungal agents to control secondary *Malassezia* infection include ketoconazole, itraconazole and fluconazole (5–10 mg/kg po q24 h).

Systemic anti-inflammatory therapy

There are a variety of treatment options, but those with good evidence of high efficacy thus far are broad-spectrum agents that target lymphocytes and inflammatory pathways (steroids, oclacitinib and ciclosporin) or precise pruritus pathways (interleukin [IL]-31 monoclonal antibody). Other agents are rarely effective by themselves and are most useful as adjunctive therapy.

Essential fatty acid (EFA)-rich diets or supplements may help coat texture and skin barrier function, but most have unproven efficacy in controlling symptoms of atopic dermatitis.

Antihistamines may be effective in some dogs with mild pruritus but are mostly used to reduce the dose and/or frequency of other treatments. They are most effective given before and not after a flare. The sedative effect may help reduce sleep deprivation in pruritic dogs (and their owners). Adverse effects are uncommon but include sedation, excitation and gastrointestinal upsets. The second-generation drugs can induce potentially fatal cardiac arrhythmias. Antihistamines may lower the seizure threshold. Two-week trials with different antihistamines may help determine which is most useful:

- Chlorpheniramine (0.4 mg/kg po q8 h).
- Diphenhydramine (2–4 mg/kg po q8 h).
- Hydroxyzine (2 mg/kg po q8 h).
- Clemastine fumarate (0.05 mg/kg po q8 h).
- Ketotifen (2–4 mg/kg po q8 h).

Glucocorticoids rapidly and reliably control acute or severe symptoms of allergic dermatitis. Methylprednisolone (0.4–0.8 mg/kg) is the drug of choice. Prednisolone and prednisone may also be used (0.5–1.0 mg/kg), but they are more likely to cause polyuria/polydipsia and polyphagia in some dogs. Induction doses should be given twice daily for 7 days or until remission, then once daily in the morning for 7 days, and then on alternate mornings. The dose can then be reduced to the lowest required to control the clinical signs. Injectable steroids may be warranted if only one to three injections are needed per year to control a seasonal allergy, and if the client finds it impossible to administer oral medications. As a result of potential adverse effects of glucocorticoids, long-term use is not recommended unless other treatments cannot be used. Adverse effects of systemic glucocorticoids are numerous, including (but not limited to) polyuria, polydipsia, polyphagia, weight gain, panting and mood changes (including aggression). The onset of iatrogenic hyperadrenocorticism is dose and duration dependent, but varies between individual dogs. Regular monitoring is necessary to ensure that appropriate doses are being given and that the dog is not developing iatrogenic Cushing's syndrome. Regular urinalysis and blood pressure monitoring are advisable.

Ciclosporin is a calcineurin inhibitor and immunomodulating agent that is useful for lymphocytic and granulomatous inflammation, including atopic dermatitis. The recommended dose for dogs is 4–7 mg/kg po q24 h. Ciclosporin is best suited to chronic use because it can take 2–6 weeks to see clinical improvement.[11] Oral steroids or oclacitinib can be coadministered for 2–3 weeks to give initial relief. Once disease has been controlled on ciclosporin alone, the frequency of dosing can be changed to every other day for 1 month and then, if still controlled, to twice weekly. A rough guideline would be that approximately 30% of cases can be maintained on alternate-day dosing and another 15–20% can be maintained with every third day dosing.[11] The dose can be tapered in dogs that require ongoing daily therapy. Satisfactory control of lesions will occur in approximately 60–80% of the cases treated with ciclosporin.[11] Urine samples should be checked every 6–12 months but routine blood work is not needed. Emesis is a major side effect of this treatment and is reported to occur in 14–40% of cases.[11] In most cases, an animal will tolerate the drug after a few days and giving the drug after a meal will help. The problem may also be reduced by giving a partial dose after a meal for 3 days, then increasing the dose every 3 days until the recommended dose is reached. Metoclopramide (0.2–0.4 mg/kg po), sucralfate (0.5–1.0 g/dog po), ranitidine (1 mg/kg po) or cimetidine (5–10 mg/kg po) given 30 minutes before dosing may also decrease the frequency of emesis. Some animals will not tolerate the drug and it has to be discontinued. Other less common side effects are diarrhoea, gingival hyperplasia, papilloma-type lesions of the epidermis, hirsutism and a psoriasiform–lichenoid-like dermatitis with coccoid bacteria. In rare instances, diabetes mellitus, pinnal erythema, lameness and muscle pain may be observed.[11] Ciclosporin is contraindicated in the presence of neoplasia, although there is no evidence that it induces neoplasia. Ciclosporin is metabolised by the liver, so caution should be used if the animal to be treated has liver disease, because very high blood levels will develop. In these cases, blood level assays should be performed and the dose adjusted accordingly. In animals without liver disease, blood levels are fairly consistent, so monitoring is not necessary. Drugs that inhibit cytochrome P450 microsomal enzyme activity (e.g. ketoconazole, itraconazole, fluconazole, erythromycin and allopurinol) can result in very high blood levels of ciclosporin and potentiate possible toxicity or other side effects. Ketoconazole (2.5–5 mg/kg with ciclosporin) or fluconazole (5 mg/kg with ciclosporin) have been used commonly to divide the dose of ciclosporin in half to save on cost, and have the same effectiveness. Conversely, drugs that increase cytochrome P450 metabolism (e.g. phenobarbital and trimethoprim–sulphonamides) may reduce plasma levels of ciclosporin.

Oclacitinib (Apoquel®, Zoetis) should be given at a dose of 0.4–0.6 mg/kg twice daily for 14 days and then once daily thereafter. If symptoms are completely controlled, this drug should be further tapered to the lowest dose needed, although most dogs will still require once-daily therapy. The pruritus often worsens when the dose is reduced to once daily, and some dogs require long-term treatment every 12 hours. It is recommended to check complete blood count, serum biochemistry and urinalysis before therapy, at the 2-month point and then at least yearly. Bone marrow suppression is a rare but possible side effect. This drug is not approved for dogs aged less than 12 months. Skin and ear infections, demodicosis, weight gain, aggression or anxiety and pneumonia have been seen while dogs are on this drug (especially if long-term, twice daily medication is required). Oclacitinib is contraindicated in the presence of neoplasia, although there is no evidence that it induces neoplasia.

IL-31 monoclonal antibody (Cytopoint™, Zoetis) effectively reduces pruritus in about 80% of dogs with atopic dermatitis. The antibody blocks IL-31, which is an important cytokine involved in early inflammation and pruritus in canine atopic dermatitis. The effectiveness peaks at day 7 and then declines, with repeated treatment required every 25–35 days in most cases. Long-term studies of safety had not been performed by the time of this publication, but it seems to have very few side effects and is well tolerated.

Recombinant canine interferon-γ or feline interferon-ω, given orally or subcutaneously, appears to be somewhat effective in the management of some long-term cases,[12,13] but availability is limited for many countries. The benefits may take several months to become apparent. No large studies have been performed.

Allergen testing and allergen-specific immunotherapy

Current allergen tests detect the presence of allergen-specific IgE antibodies. Not all atopic dogs produce IgE in response to allergens. If properly performed, intradermal allergen testing will result in positive results that concur with the history in approximately 85% of cases. To prevent inaccurate test results, antihistamines (including behavioural medications) should be discontinued 7 days before testing, oral and topical steroids 2 weeks before testing[14] and repository injectable steroids 6–8 weeks before testing. There are no withdrawals needed for ciclosporin, oclacitinib, IL-31 monoclonal antibody or EFAs. If this procedure is not performed routinely, or if the clinician has not had appropriate training, referral is recommended.

Serum tests (radioallergosorbent test [RAST], enzyme-linked immunosorbent assay [ELISA] and liquid-phase immunoenzymatic assay) are simpler to perform in practice and can be used to detect increased concentrations of allergen-specific IgE. The major problem with these tests is lack of specificity. Almost all non-allergic dogs react to at least one and sometimes many allergens.[15] There is moderate intra- and interlaboratory variability in results.[16] However, in some situations, serological testing may be helpful in the selection of allergens for immunotherapy. Serological testing for food allergens is neither accurate nor recommended, and food trials must be performed for diagnosis of food allergy.

Allergen-specific immunotherapy (ASIT) by subcutaneous injection (SCIT), intralymphatic injection (ILIT) or sublingual immunotherapy (SLIT) drops has been reported to result in at least a 50% improvement in 65–70% of atopic dogs,[10] although most dogs will not completely respond to ASIT alone. It may take animals as long as 6–12 months (and sometimes longer) to respond to immunotherapy and, therefore, critical clinical evaluation should not take place until a year of therapy has been completed.[10] Other concurrent therapy is therefore appropriate. Adverse effects are uncommon. Injection site reactions and anaphylactic shock are rare, and most dogs tolerate the injections with little discomfort. Mild reactions can generally be prevented by pretreating with antihistamines 1–2 hours before the injection if necessary. The intervals between injections can be individualised to the needs of each animal. Using SLIT avoids injections and is very safe, but it needs to be given every 12 hours. Little research on the effectiveness of SLIT has been performed in dogs. Discussing the pros and cons of each form of ASIT will help owners choose the format that best suits them and their dog. Dogs that fail to respond to one form of ASIT may still respond to another.

ASIT works by inducing tolerance to the allergens. It therefore prevents flares associated with future exposure to the allergens, rather than acting as an anti-inflammatory. Regular treatment is often necessary to maintain tolerance, but it is possible to make permanent changes and taper therapy off after 2–4 years of treatment in some dogs. Some dogs, however, will relapse on weaning of ASIT. Retesting may reveal new sensitivities in dogs that relapse while on ASIT, and reformulating their ASIT can be beneficial.

Key points

- The diagnosis of atopic dermatitis is based on a characteristic history, the typical clinical signs, ruling out other pruritic diseases and the response to therapy.
- Allergy tests are not diagnostic for the disease – food trials and allergy tests are used to determine the food and/or environmental allergens to which each dog is sensitised.
- Therapy is typically multi-modal and needs to be constantly modified to best suit each dog's symptoms. Typically, treatment is based around skin barrier care, allergen avoidance and ASIT, and anti-inflammatory therapy.
- Proactive therapy that maintains remission is more effective than simply reacting to recurrent flares.
- Most dogs with recurrent staphylococcal or *Malassezia* skin and ear infections have unmanaged atopic dermatitis.

References

1 Picco F, Zini E, Nett C et al. A prospective study on canine atopic dermatitis and food-induced allergic dermatitis in Switzerland. *Vet Dermatol* 2008; **19**: 150–155.
2 Gaschen FP, Merchant SR. Adverse food reactions in dogs and cats. *Vet Clin North Am Small Anim Pract* 2011; **41**: 361–379.
3 Mueller RS, Olivry T, Prélaud P. Critically appraised topic on adverse food reactions of companion animals (2): common food allergen sources in dogs and cats. *BMC Vet Res* 2016; **12**: 9.
4 Stetina KM, Marks SL, Griffin CE. Owner assessment of pruritus and gastrointestinal signs in apparently healthy dogs with no history of cutaneous or noncutaneous disease. *Vet Dermatol* 2015; **26**: 246–e54.
5 Hensel P, Santoro D, Favrot C, Hill P, Griffin C. Canine atopic dermatitis: detailed guidelines for diagnosis and allergen identification. *BMC Vet Res* 2015; **11**: 196.
6 Ricci R, Granato A, Vascellari M et al. Identification of undeclared sources of animal origin in canine dry foods used in dietary elimination trials. *J Anim Physiol Anim Nutr* 2013; **97**, 32–38.
7 Willis-Mahn C, Remillard R, Tater K. ELISA testing for soy antigens in dry dog foods used in dietary elimination trials. *J Am Anim Hosp Assoc* 2014; **50**: 383–389.
8 Bethlehem S, Bexley J, Mueller RS. Patch testing and allergen-specific serum IgE and IgG antibodies in the diagnosis of canine adverse food reactions. *Vet Immunol Immunopathol* 2012; **145**: 582–589.
9 Olivry T, Mueller RS, Prélaud P. Critically appraised topic on adverse food reactions of companion animals (1): duration of elimination diets. *BMC Vet Res* 2015; **11**: 225.
10 Olivry T, DeBoer DJ, Favrot C et al. Treatment of canine atopic dermatitis: 2015 updated guidelines from the International Committee on Allergic Diseases of Animals (ICADA). *BMC Vet Res* 2015; **11**: 1.
11 Palmeiro BS. Cyclosporine in veterinary dermatology. *Vet Clin North Am Small Anim Pract* 2013; **43**: 153–171.
12 Carlotti DN, Boulet M, Decret J et al. The use of recombinant omega interferon therapy in canine atopic dermatitis: a double-blind controlled study: Recombinant omega interferon therapy in canine atopic dermatitis. *Vet Dermatol* 2009; **20**: 405–411.
13 Litzlbauer P, Weber K, Mueller RS. Oral and subcutaneous therapy of canine atopic dermatitis with recombinant feline interferon omega. *Cytokine* 2014; **66**: 54–59.
14 Olivry T, Saridomichelakis M, for the International Committee on Atopic Diseases of Animals (ICADA). Evidence-based guidelines for anti-allergic drug withdrawal times before allergen-specific intradermal and IgE serological tests in dogs. *Vet Dermatol* 2013; **24**: 225–e49.
15 Plant JD. The reproducibility of three in vitro canine allergy tests: a pilot study. In: *Proceedings of the Members' Meeting of the American Academy of Veterinary Dermatology and American College of Veterinary Dermatology, Charleston, USA*, 1994: pp. 16–18.
16 Thom N, Favrot C, Failing K et al. Intra- and interlaboratory variability of allergen-specific IgE levels in atopic dogs in three different laboratories using the Fc-ε receptor testing. *Vet Immunol Immunopathol* 2010; **133**: 183–189.

MALASSEZIA DERMATITIS
(Cutaneous yeast infection)

Aetiology and pathogenesis

Similar to staphylococci, the yeasts *Malassezia* spp. are normal commensals in most dogs and cats. Cutaneous defence mechanisms normally limit colonisation and infection. Malassezia dermatitis is therefore usually secondary to an underlying condition such as atopic dermatitis. The vast majority of canine infections are associated with *M. pachydermatis*, although *M. furfur* has also been isolated.[1] A wider variety of species including *M. pachydermatis*, *M. sympodialis* and *M. furfur* have been isolated from cats.[2,3]

Clinical features

Clinical signs in dogs include otitis externa, pruritus (often unresponsive to corticosteroids), erythema, a rancid, musty or yeasty odour, seborrhoea, scaling, alopecia, lichenification and hyperpigmentation (**Figs. 2.19, 2.20**). Clinical signs can be focal or generalised, diffuse or well demarcated. Commonly affected sites include the ears, lips, muzzle, feet, ventral neck, axilla, medial limbs and perineum. *Malassezia* spp. can also cause paronychia, with a waxy exudate and discoloration of the nails.[4,5]

Pruritus is less common in feline malassezia dermatitis. Clinical signs include otitis externa, feline acne, seborrhoeic and scaling facial dermatitis, generalised scaling and erythema, and paronychia with discoloration of the nails (**Fig. 2.21**). Generalised erythema and scaling have been associated with malassezia dermatitis in cats with thymoma, lymphocytic mural folliculitis and paraneoplastic alopecia.[6]

Carriage of *M. pachydermatis* in dog owners has been demonstrated.[7] This should not be a concern in healthy individuals, but there are reports of zoonotic infections in immunocompromised neonates and adults.[8,9]

Differential diagnoses

A variety of other skin conditions can mimic malassezia dermatitis, but this is complicated by the fact that many of these can also be a trigger for a secondary *Malassezia* infection.[10] Primary malassezia dermatitis has been suspected in basset hounds and Devon Rex cats (particularly paronychia).

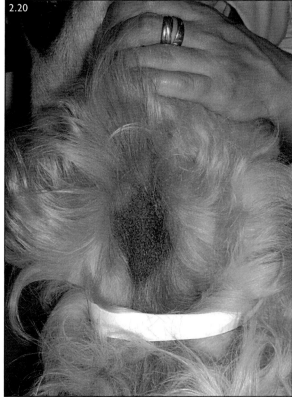

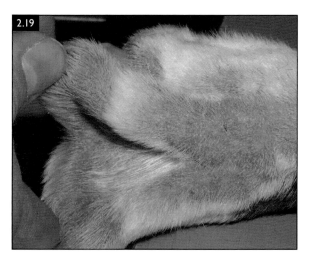

Fig. 2.19 Malassezia dermatitis affecting the foot of an atopic Boxer with erythema, alopecia and scaling.

Fig. 2.20 Alopecia, lichenification and hyperpigmentation of the ventral neck caused by malassezia dermatitis in an atopic Golden Retriever.

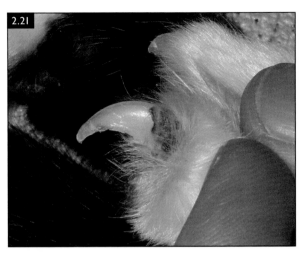

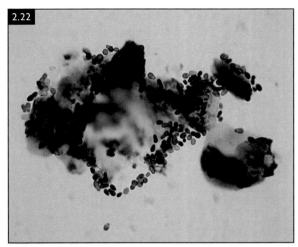

Fig. 2.21 Paronychia with tightly adherent, brown, waxy discharge associated with *Malassezia* in a cat with superficial necrolytic dermatitis.

Fig. 2.22 Numerous oval to peanut-shaped budding *Malassezia* surrounding corneocytes in an impression smear from otitis externa in a dog. Note the variable pink to purple staining (Diff-Quik®, ×400).

Diagnosis

No agreed criteria for diagnosis have been established, but demonstration of elevated numbers of *Malassezia* spp. with a good clinical and mycological response to antifungal treatment is diagnostic.[4] *Malassezia* spp. are easily visible as small oval to peanut or snowman shapes, often forming rafts on the surface of squames, cytology of tape-strips and direct or indirect impression smears. They most frequently stain blue–purple, but can appear red–pink or pale blue (**Fig. 2.22**). Some *Malassezia* spp. fail to stain, but their refractile cell wall can be picked out with a closed condenser. There is no standard accepted cut-off value to diagnose malassezia dermatitis, especially as they may not be uniformly distributed across a slide. In practice, only occasional *Malassezia* yeasts are found on healthy skin.

M. pachydermatis will grow on Sabouraud's medium, although the lipid-dependent species require supplemented media such as modified Dixon's agar.[11] However, as *Malassezia* spp. are commensal organisms, isolation, particularly of small numbers, is not necessarily significant.[4] *Malassezia* spp. can also be found in skin biopsies, but they may be removed by processing and a lack of *Malassezia* spp. on a biopsy report does not rule them out.

Research has shown that a proportion of atopic dogs develop specific IgE titres and intradermal tests to *Malassezia* extracts, suggesting that they may act as allergens.[12–14] *Malassezia*-specific serology and intradermal tests are available, and, although the clinical significance of *Malassezia* hypersensitivity in canine atopic dermatitis is unclear, some dogs appear to benefit from *Malassezia*-specific immunotherapy.[15]

Treatment

- The underlying condition for a yeast infection needs to be identified and addressed or the infection will recur.
- Localised areas may be treated with twice-daily application of an antifungal cream or lotion (miconazole, clotrimazole, nystatin or others).
- Antifungal shampoos are effective in local or generalised cases used once or twice weekly to remission. Regular use may also help prevent recurrent overgrowth in susceptible dogs. Chlorhexidine and/or antifungal-containing products are the most effective.
- Generalised, interdigital, multi-focal and/or non-responsive infections may need systemic antifungals. There may be several drug interactions with antifungal medications, so caution is needed if concurrent medications are used. Improvement is seen in 7–14 days, but treatment should be continued until recheck in 30 days. Treatment should be stopped if

gastrointestinal upset or inappetence occurs, because this may be a sign of liver damage.

- Ketoconazole (5–10 mg/kg po q 24 h):[16] give with food, do not use in cats.
- Fluconazole (5–10 mg/kg po q24 h).
- Itraconazole (5 mg/kg po q24 h).
- Terbinafine (30 mg/kg po q24 h)[17] has given variable results with *Malassezia* spp.

Key point

- The underlying condition for a yeast infection needs to be identified and addressed or the infection will recur.

References

1   Nardoni S, Mancianti F, Corazza M *et al*. Occurrence of *Malassezia* species in healthy and dermatologically diseased dogs. *Mycopathologia* 2004; **157**: 383–388.

2   Bensignor E, Weill FX, Couprie B. Population sizes and frequency of isolation of *Malassezia* yeasts from healthy pet cats. *Journal de Mycologie Medicale* 1999; **9**: 158–161.

3   Raabe P, Mayser P, Weiss R. Demonstration of *Malassezia furfur* and *M. sympodialis* together with *M. pachydermatis* in veterinary specimens. *Mycoses* 1998; **41**: 493–500.

4   Akerstedt J, Vollset I. *Malassezia pachydermatis* with special reference to canine skin disease. *Br Vet J* 1996; **152**: 269–281.

5   Mason KV, Evans AG. Dermatitis associated with *Malassezia pachydermatis* in 11 dogs. *J Am Anim Hosp Assoc* 1991; **27**: 13–20.

6   Mauldin EA, Morris DO, Goldschmidt MH. Retrospective study: the presence of *Malassezia* in feline skin biopsies. A clinicopathological study. *Vet Dermatol* 2002; **13**: 7–13.

7   Morris DO, O'Shea K, Shofer FS *et al*. *Malassezia pachydermatis* carriage in dog owners. *Emerg Infect Dis* 2005; **11**: 83–88.

8   Fan YM, Huang WM, Li SF *et al*. Granulomatous skin infection caused by *Malassezia pachydermatis* in a dog owner. *Arch Dermatol* 2006; **142**: 1181–1184.

9   Chang HJ, Miller HL, Watkins N *et al*. An epidemic of *Malassezia pachydermatis* in an intensive care nursery associated with colonization of health care workers pet dogs. *N Engl J Med* 1998; **338**: 706–711.

10 Bond R, Ferguson EA, Curtis CF *et al*. Factors associated with elevated cutaneous *Malassezia pachydermatis* populations in dogs with pruritic skin disease. *J Small Anim Pract* 1996; **37**: 103–107.

11 Bond R, Collin NS, Lloyd DH. Use of contact plates for the quantitative culture of *Malassezia pachydermatis* from canine skin. *J Small Anim Pract* 1994; **35**: 68–72.

12 Chen TA, Halliwell REW, Pemberton AD *et al*. Identification of major allergens of *Malassezia pachydermatis* in dogs with atopic dermatitis and *Malassezia* overgrowth. *Vet Dermatol* 2002; **13**: 141–150.

13 Nuttall TJ, Halliwell REW. Serum antibodies to *Malassezia* yeasts in canine atopic dermatitis. *Vet Dermatol* 2001; **12**: 327–332.

14 Morris DO, DeBoer DJ. Evaluation of serum obtained from atopic dogs with dermatitis attributable to *Malassezia pachydermatis* for passive transfer of immediate hypersensitivity to that organism. *Am J Vet Res* 2003; **64**: 262–266.

15 Farver K, Morris DO, Shofer F *et al*. Humoral measurement of type-1 hypersensitivity reactions to a commercial *Malassezia* allergen. *Vet Dermatol* 2005; **16**: 261–268.

16 Bensignor E. An open trial to compare two dosages of ketoconazole in the treatment of *Malassezia* dermatitis in dogs. *Annales de Medecine Veterinaire* 2001; **145**: 311–315.

17 Guillot J, Bensignor E, Jankowski F *et al*. Comparative efficacies of oral ketoconazole and terbinafine for reducing *Malassezia* population sizes on the skin of Basset Hounds. *Vet Dermatol* 2003; **14**: 153–157.

URTICARIA
(Hives)

Definition
Urticaria is associated with raised dermal welts caused by histamine release.

Aetiology and pathogenesis
Allergens, infectious agents or other triggers cause mast cells and basophils to release histamine and other inflammatory mediators. These mediators cause vasodilatation, plasma extravasation and nerve activation, which result in weals, erythema and sometimes pruritus. Common triggers of urticaria are vaccines,[1] insects, foods and drugs.[2]

Clinical features
Short-haired dogs appear to be predisposed to urticaria. Females may also be predisposed. Raised domes or plaques sometimes coalesce into serpiginous patterns on the skin. The oedematous skin causes the hair to stand erect in short-haired dogs. Urticarial lesions are commonly erythematous and sometimes pruritic (**Fig. 2.23**). This reaction can occur with other signs of anaphylaxis such as angio-oedema of the legs, face or ears (**Fig. 2.24**), vomiting, diarrhoea, collapse, hypotension, respiratory distress, heart failure and death. Urticaria can be acute or chronic. Lesions blanch when pressed (diascopy).

Differential diagnoses
- Bacterial folliculitis.
- Vasculitis.
- Erythema multiforme.
- Cutaneous histiocytosis.
- Staphylococcal folliculitis.

Diagnosis
Lesions are usually easily recognisable. Biopsy with histopathology should be performed for chronic or unresponsive lesions to rule out other causes.

Treatment
- If known, causative agents should be avoided.
- Most cases of urticaria resolve spontaneously in 12–48 hours.[3]

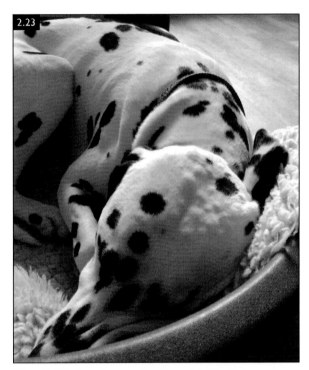

Fig. 2.23 Pruritus, urticaria and folliculitis on the head and trunk of a food-allergic Dalmatian.

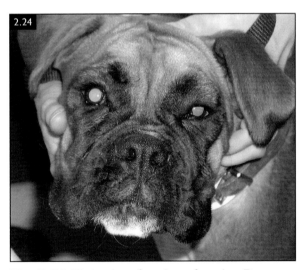

Fig. 2.24 Urticaria and angio-oedema in a Boxer following methadone administration.

- Acute and severe patients should be monitored in the clinic until weals begin to resolve and the patient is showing no signs of developing anaphylaxis.
- Owners should be instructed on how to monitor for signs of anaphylaxis.

- Adrenaline (1:1000 0.1–0.5 ml sc or im) will help reverse symptoms if the dog is showing any other signs of anaphylaxis.
- Dexamethasone (0.05–0.1 mg/kg iv) works rapidly to resolve urticaria, pruritus and erythema. Usually, only one dose is needed.
- Prednisone (1 mg/kg po q24 h and taper) for 3–5 days is typically curative within a day or two.
- Oral or injectable steroids can be combined with antihistamines such as diphenhydramine (2.2 mg/kg po q8–12 h), chlorpheniramine (0.4 mg/kg po q8–12 h) or hydroxyzine (2.2 mg/kg po q8–12 h). Antihistamines are most helpful to prevent new lesions rather than resolve existing lesions, but are safer than prednisone for long-term use if needed.
- The treatment for chronic urticaria depends on the underlying cause; these cases should be biopsied and may need work-ups and treatments similar to vasculitis (see pages 85 and 221) and atopic dermatitis (see page 18).

Key point

- Urticaria in dogs is common and typically rapidly responsive to treatment.

References

1   Moore GE, Guptill LF, Ward MP et al. Adverse events diagnosed within three days of vaccine administration in dogs. J Am Vet Med Assoc 2005; 227: 1102–1108.
2   Rostaher A, Hofer-Inteeworn N, Kümmerle-Fraune C, Fische NM, Favrot C. Triggers, risk factors and clinico-pathological features of urticaria in dogs – a prospective observational study of 24 cases. Vet Dermatol 2017; 28: 38–e9.
3   Hill P. Canine urticaria and angioedema. Vet Allergy 2013: pp. 195–200.

ANAL SAC DISEASE
(Anal sac impaction, sacculitis or abscessation)

Definition

Anal sac impaction is caused by blockage of the ductal outflow of anal sac secretion. Anal sacculitis is an inflammation of the anal sacs. Abscessation occurs when the anal sacs rupture under the skin and cause an abscess that usually forms a draining tract.

Aetiology and pathogenesis

Anal sac disease can be caused by many inflammatory factors that may cause closure of the ductal opening, including atopic dermatitis, food allergy, colitis, obesity, conformation, perianal fistulae, masses, anal hyperplasia and trauma.

Clinical features

Dogs and cats scoot, lick or show pain in the area of the affected anal sac. Pain can be intense during defecation or when the tail is raised. Enlargement of the glands may be palpated externally or by rectal exam. Draining tracts with purulent or haemorrhagic discharge, inflammation and cellulitis may be present over the inflamed abscessed gland.

Differential diagnoses

- Atopic dermatitis and food allergies commonly cause perineal pruritus, licking and scooting.
- Colitis or inflammatory bowel disease causing chronic diarrhoea may cause anal licking and scooting.
- Perineal fistulae cause draining tracts around the anus and into the anal sac.
- Faecal parasites.

Diagnosis

All pets with anal sac issues should have a rectal exam to make sure that there are no masses or other causes of the symptoms. Palpation of an enlarged anal sac and the resolution of symptoms by emptying the sac, are diagnostic for impaction. If painful, sedation or anaesthesia will be needed for thorough evaluation. Blood in the anal sacs is not a normal finding and indicates anal sacculitis.[1,2] An inflamed, painful anal sac that has abscessed under the skin with or without a draining tract is fairly characteristic, but if several draining tracts are present consider perineal fistulae, especially in German Shepherd dogs. Cytology of anal sac contents of normal dogs shows neutrophils, intracellular bacteria and yeasts, and so cytology may be of limited benefit.[3,4] Bacterial culture may be necessary if the infection fails to respond to treatment.

Treatment

- Underlying causes of anal sac inflammation should be looked for and treated, which may include diet trials for colitis and atopic dermatitis.
- Increased fibre diets to increase the bulk and firmness of the faeces can be tried.
- Impacted anal sacs should be carefully expressed and the underlying cause addressed. Follow-up cases to ensure that symptoms resolved after the anal sacs were expressed.
- Bloody discharge from the anal sac duct needs to be treated with anal sac lavage and instillation of medications. All cats and some dogs need sedation for this procedure. This involves cannulating the anal sac duct with a tom-cat catheter, a 22-gauge intravenous catheter (without needle) or a 5-Fr red rubber catheter, and lavaging repeatedly with saline. If lavage fluid cannot be sucked into the syringe the catheter should be withdrawn and the anal sac manually but gently expressed to remove debris. When the lavage fluid is mostly clear, the sac should be emptied completely and filled with a topical steroid/antibiotic/antifungal ear product. This process should be repeated every 10–14 days until the anal sac is no longer bloody; usually two treatments are needed. The case should be re-evaluated if more than four treatments are needed. Oral antibiotics are probably not helpful in these cases.
- If the anal sac is abscessed, has formed a draining tract to the outside and is draining well, only pain medication and oral antibiotics

may be needed, depending on the severity of the condition. If the abscess has not penetrated to the outside, or if a pocket of fluid has formed below the draining tract, the animal can be anaesthetised and the abscess opened at the point area most dependent and furthest from the anal opening, to obtain a sample for bacterial culture, and for flushing. The opening should be left open to drain and heal by second intention. These openings typically heal well with oral antibiotics and pain medications. Cases should be rechecked when less painful to ensure that there are not underlying causes for anal sac inflammation.

- Chronic anal sac disease that is painful and recurrent may warrant surgical removal of the anal sacs.[2] Bear in mind that removal of the anal sacs will not help with scooting or licking of the anus if these symptoms are due to other diseases – owners should be warned about this beforehand or they may be disappointed in the results. Faecal incontinence, anal stricture and fistulation are possible complications.[1]

Key point

- The underlying causes of anal sac inflammation must be addressed to prevent recurrence.

References

1 Hill, LN, Smeak DD. Open versus closed bilateral anal sacculectomy for treatment of non-neoplastic anal sac disease in dogs: 95 cases (1969–1994). *J Am Vet Med Assoc* 2002; **221**: 662–665.

2 Culp WT. Anal sac disease. *Small Anim Soft Tissue Surg* 2013: pp. 399–405.

3 Lake AM, Scott DW, Miller WH, Erb HN. Gross and cytological characteristics of normal canine anal-sac secretions. *J Vet Med Ser A* 2004; **51**: 249–253.

4 James DJ, Griffin CE, Polissar NL, Neradilek MB. Comparison of anal sac cytological findings and behaviour in clinically normal dogs and those affected with anal sac disease: canine anal sac cytology. *Vet Dermatol* 2011; **22**: 80–87.

CONTACT DERMATITIS
(Irritant contact dermatitis, allergic contact dermatitis)

Definition

Allergic contact dermatitis (ACD) and irritant contact dermatitis (ICD) are two very similar conditions mediated by direct contact with environmental substances.[1]

Aetiology and pathogenesis

ACD requires previous sensitisation. It is a type 4 (cell-mediated) hypersensitivity reaction to small, low-molecular-weight chemicals (haptens) that bind to host proteins. Haptenated proteins are phagocytosed, processed and presented by antigen-presenting cells, especially epidermal Langerhans' cells, to T cells bearing the appropriate T-cell receptors. These recirculate to the skin and, on subsequent exposure to the hapten, trigger a cell-mediated immune response.[2] ICD, in contrast, is not antigen specific and is directly triggered by noxious compounds[2] that damage keratinocytes. The effector stages and inflammation in ACD and ICD share similar immunological pathways, resulting in almost identical clinical signs and histopathology.[1,2]

Clinical features

The refractory period for ACD is reported to rarely be less than 2 years, so one would not expect it to appear in very young animals.[1] However, the inquisitive nature of puppies and, perhaps, their juvenile pelage, might predispose them to exposure to irritants and, therefore, ICD. German Shepherd dogs comprised 50% of the dogs in one series of confirmed ACD cases.[3] ACD requires multiple exposures, whereas ICD will occur on first exposure.[2] ACD usually affects individual animals, but ICD can affect all in-contact animals.[2] Most cases of ACD and ICD are perennial, although it does depend on the timing of exposure, and seasonal examples will be met, typically to vegetative allergens/irritants.[1,2,4,5]

Acute and severe ACD/ICD may result in erythema, oedema, vesicles, and even erosion or ulceration (**Figs. 2.25, 2.26**).[1–3,5,6] Primary lesions include erythematous macules, papules and occasionally vesicles. Secondary lesions (e.g. excoriation, alopecia, lichenification and hyperpigmentation) tend to mask these primary lesions. There is usually a well-defined margin between affected and normal skin (**Fig. 2.27**). Pruritus is variable, but may be intense.[1–3,6]

The distribution of the lesions reflects the exposed contact areas and, therefore, hairless dogs and cats

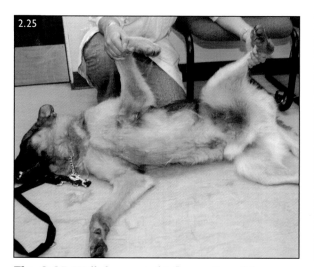

Fig. 2.25 Well-demarcated inflammation of the hairless skin of the axillae and groin in a German Shepherd dog with a contact reaction to a cleaning fluid.

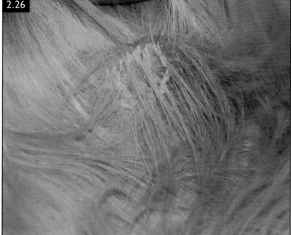

Fig. 2.26 Marked erythema and exfoliation in the axilla of a cross-bred dog after a reaction to a shampoo.

are at more risk.[7] Clinical signs are usually confined to sparsely haired skin, but prolonged contact will result in extension to adjacent areas and, with time, the chin, ventral pinna, ventral neck and medial limbs, and the entire ventrum will be affected.[1,5] Generalised reactions may be seen in cases of reactions to shampoos.[1,5] Chronic otitis externa may result from sensitivity to topical neomycin or other potential irritants and sensitisers.[5,8,9] Other potential substances include metals, plastics, fibres, leather, dyes, oils and cleaning fluids.[1–3,5–7]

Differential diagnoses
- Atopic dermatitis and/or food allergies.
- Sarcoptic mange.
- Demodicosis.
- *Neotrombicula* (harvest mite or berry bug) or chigger infestation.
- Bacterial or yeast dermatitis.
- Hookworm dermatitis.

Diagnosis
A tentative diagnosis can be based on history and clinical signs, and elimination of the differential diagnoses.[2] Histopathology from primary lesions or acute cases may reveal intraepidermal spongiosis or vesiculation and keratinocyte necrosis, but most biopsies are non-specific.[1,2,10]

If the environment is suitable, exclusion trials are useful tests. These can include: avoiding carpets, grass or concrete (wet concrete is a common irritant); plain cotton bedding; cleaning with water only; glass or ceramic food and water bowls; avoiding rubber or plastic toys; and avoiding topical medications. If the dermatitis goes into remission, provocative exposure may allow identification of the allergen/irritant.

Closed-patch testing for specific allergens may be indicated if exclusion trials are unrewarding, but this is a specialist procedure and referral is advised (**Fig. 2.28**).[1,2,7,9,11]

Treatment
If the allergen or irritant can be identified, and if exposure can be restricted, then the prognosis is good. Failure to identify the cause or prevent access results in reliance on symptomatic therapy, usually with systemic glucocorticoids. Topical therapy

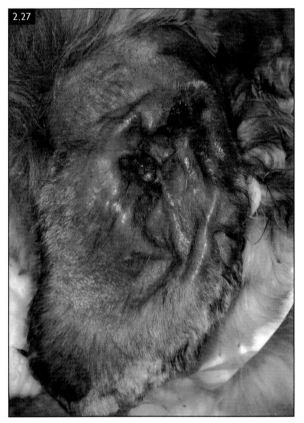

Fig. 2.27 Severe suppurative otitis in a dog that developed a reaction to commercial ear products.

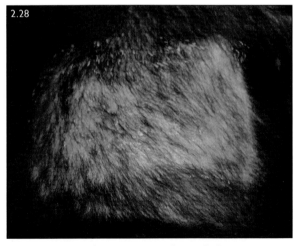

Fig. 2.28 Erythematous papules and plaques at a positive patch test site.

can be appropriate with localised lesions. In some individuals, complete control may be very hard to achieve without the side effects of glucocorticoid therapy becoming apparent. Ciclosporin or topical tacrolimus (not licensed for animals) can be effective and better tolerated. Pentoxifylline (10 mg/kg po q12 h) ameliorated lesions in three dogs sensitised to plants of the Commelinaceae family.[10] Barrier creams, Lycra™ bodysuits and/or prompt washing can be used if some exposure is unavoidable.

Key point

- Allergic contact dermatitis may be refractory to steroid therapy.

References

1   White PD. Contact dermatitis in the dog and the cat. *Semin Vet Med Surg (Small Anim)* 1991; **6**: 303–315.

2   Olivry T, Prelaud P, Heripret D *et al.* Allergic contact dermatitis in the dog: principles and diagnosis. *Vet Clin North Am Small Anim Pract* 1990; **20**: 1443–1456.

3   Thomsen MK, Kristensen F. Contact dermatitis in the dog: a review and clinical study. *Nordisk Veterinaer Medicin* 1986; **38**: 129–134.

4   Kunkle GA, Gross TL. Allergic contact dermatitis to *Tradecantia fluminensis* (Wandering Jew) in a dog. *Compend Cont Educ Pract Vet* 1983; **5**: 925–930.

5   Nesbitt GH, Schmitz JA. Contact dermatitis in dogs: a review of 35 cases. *J Am Anim Hosp Assoc* 1977; **13**: 155–163.

6   Grant DI, Thoday KL. Canine allergic contact dermatitis: clinical review. *J Small Anim Pract* 1980; **21**: 17–27.

7   Kimura T. Contact hypersensitivity to stainless steel cages (chromium metal) in hairless descendants of Mexican hairless dogs. *Environ Toxic* 2007; **22**: 176–184.

8   Nuttall TJ, Cole LK. Ear cleaning: the UK and US perspective. *Vet Dermatol* 2004; **15**: 127–136.

9   Bensignor E. Sensitisation to the contact of prednisolone in a Golden Retriever. *Prat Med Chir Anim* 2002; **37**: 141–146.

10 Marsella R, Kunkle GA, Lewis DT. Use of pentoxifylline in the treatment of allergic contact reactions to plants of the Commelinaceae family in dogs. *Vet Dermatol* 1997; **8**: 121–126.

11 Ho KK, Campbell KL, Lavergne SN. Contact dermatitis: a comparative and translational review of the literature. *Vet Dermatol* 2015; **26**: 314–e67.

EPITHELIOTROPHIC LYMPHOMA
(Mycosis fungoides, cutaneous T-cell lymphoma, Sézary's syndrome)

Definition

Epitheliotrophic lymphoma is an uncommon cutaneous neoplasm of dogs and cats characterised by epidermotrophic T-lymphocytic infiltration of the skin. In Sézary's syndrome these lymphocytes are also found in lymph nodes, blood and sometimes internal organs.

Aetiology and pathogenesis

Epitheliotrophic lymphoma is caused by an infiltration of clonal T lymphocytes into the epidermis, mucosa and adnexa. This infiltrate causes thickening, hyperkeratosis, plaques and ulcerations. The trigger for this cancer is not known, but in cats and humans viruses may possibly play a role.[1]

Clinical features

Older dogs and cats are predisposed, and the disease is very rare in cats. Initially, one or two erythematous patches or plaques may form that resemble a bacterial infection with scaling and hair loss (**Fig. 2.29**), but there is no response to antibiotics. These coalesce and enlarge to cover large areas of the body, eventually becoming generalised, with hair loss, silvery white scaling, plaques and nodules, erythema and ulceration (**Fig. 2.30**). Pruritus may be severe, but is sometimes absent with mild lesions. Lesions may take months to years to progress. Lesions often involve the mucocutaneous junctions (lips, nose, eyelids) and commonly cause depigmentation (**Figs. 2.31, 2.32**). Rarely, lesions may be restricted to the oral mucosa (gingiva, tongue, palate), or may start at the mucocutaneous junctions and spread. It is rare to have this disease spread to internal organs. Most pets are euthanised due to intractable pruritus, side effects from prednisone, or draining, odiferous, infected, ulcerated skin lesions, or lethargy. Oral lesions may cause drooling and inappetence, and foot lesions may cause painful cracked footpads.

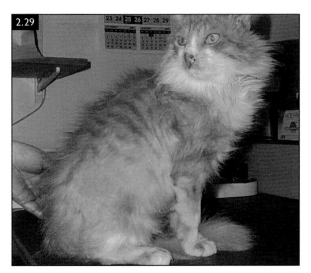

Fig. 2.29 Generalised erythema, exfoliation and pruritus in an affected cat.

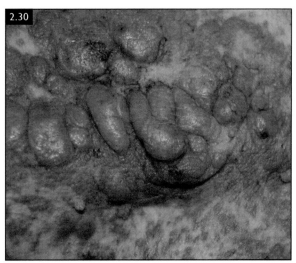

Fig. 2.30 Erythematous and ulcerated papules, plaques and nodules in a Basset Hound.

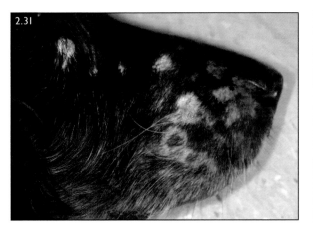

Fig. 2.31 Mucocutaneous depigmentation in a Border Collie.

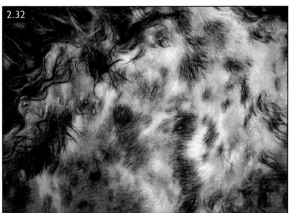

Fig. 2.32 Loss of pigment and ulceration in a Border Collie.

Differential diagnoses
- Atopic dermatitis and/or food allergy.
- Pemphigus foliaceus.
- Dermatophytosis.
- Cutaneous lymphoma without epidermotrophism (lymphocytic lymphoma).
- Superficial necrolytic dermatitis (metabolic epidermal necrosis; hepatocutaneous syndrome).
- Erythema multiforme.
- Severe yeast or bacterial dermatitis.
- Infected generalised demodicosis.
- Infestation with *Sarcoptes*, *Demodex* or *Cheyletiella* spp.

- Discoid lupus erythematosus (if localised to nasal planum) or systemic lupus erythematosus when generalised.
- For the mucocutaneous or oral mucosal forms, rule outs include mucous membrane pemphigoid, bullous pemphigoid, mucocutaneous lupus erythematosus, erythema multiforme and stomatitis.

Diagnosis
There are many diseases to rule out with epitheliotrophic lymphoma because symptoms may be variable and severe; conversely, epitheliotrophic

lymphoma should be considered in a wide range of presentations in older animals. With any severe skin disease in an older animal, a complete blood count and chemistry panel should be performed. A skin cytology, skin scraping and dermatophyte culture should also be obtained. Parasites should be ruled out with treatment trials. Infections should be treated and, if lesions and pruritus remain despite negative cytology for infections, especially in an older dog or cat with no previous history of skin disease, biopsies should be performed. It is best to perform biopsies when the pet is receiving antibiotics. Do not biopsy ulcerated areas because the epidermis must be present for diagnosis.

Treatment in dogs

- The prognosis for this disease in dogs is poor, but if caught early the progress may be slowed slightly and quality of life improved with treatment. The survival time is 3 months to 2 years.
- Prednisone 1 mg/kg per day po and tapered to lowest dose may be helpful to control pruritus and some inflammation.
- The mainstay of chemotherapy is lomustine (CCNU) at 60–70 mg/m^2 po every 3 weeks, with a response rate of around 80%.[1] This should be used with specialist supervision.
- Safflower oil at 3 ml/kg per day reportedly helped six of eight dogs in one study,[2] and safflower oil 3 ml/kg on 2 days per week helped two dogs in another study.[3] Diarrhoea and unwillingness to consume this volume of oil are possible, so the dose should be increased slowly.
- Systemic retinoids such as isotretinoin (3 mg/kg po q24 h) may be helpful.[4]

- Systemic antibiotics may be helpful, but with long-term use resistance is likely to develop.
- Topical antimicrobial baths with hydrocortisone leave-on lotions may be helpful.
- Monoclonal anti-IL-31 antibody therapy may decrease pruritus, but oclacitinib and ciclosporin should be avoided.

Treatment in cats

- The prognosis for this disease in cats is variable, and there is no optimum treatment regimen.[5]

Key point

- Biopsies are necessary for diagnosis, because many other skin conditions have a similar appearance.

References

1 Fontaine J, Bovens C, Bettenay S, Mueller RS. Canine cutaneous epitheliotropic T-cell lymphoma: a review. *Vet Comp Oncol* 2009; **7**: 1–14.

2 Iwamoto KS, Bennett LR, Norman A, Villalobos AE, Hutson CA. Linoleate produces remission in canine mycosis fungoides. *Cancer Lett* 1992; **64**: 17–22.

3 Petersen A, Wood S, Rosser E. The use of safflower oil for the treatment of mycosis fungoides in two dogs. In: *Proceedings of the 15th Annual Meeting of the American Academy of Veterinary Dermatology (concurrent sessions), Maui (HI)*, 1999: pp. 49–50.

4 White SD, Rosychuk RA, Scott KV *et al.* Use of isotretinoin and etretinate for the treatment of benign cutaneous neoplasia and cutaneous lymphoma in dogs. *J Am Vet Med Assoc* 1993; **202**: 387–391.

5 Fontaine J, Heimann M, Day MJ. Cutaneous epitheliotropic T-cell lymphoma in the cat: a review of the literature and five new cases: Feline cutaneous epitheliotropic lymphoma. *Vet Dermatol* 2011; **22**: 454–461.

FELINE HYPERSENSITIVITY DERMATITIS (Feline allergic dermatitis, feline atopic dermatitis)

Definition

Hypersensitivity (allergic) dermatitis comprises a series of reaction patterns associated with environmental allergens (pollens, dusts and moulds) and/or food allergens, resulting in pruritus and/or susceptibility to infections.

Aetiology and pathogenesis

See Canine allergic dermatitis, page 18. Much less is known about this condition in cats compared with dogs. It is likely that it is a result of a complex interaction between genetics and the environment. However, the role of skin barrier function, lymphocytes and allergic sensitisation is as yet unclear.

Clinical features

The clinical features of feline hypersensitivity dermatitis are extremely variable, with no single physical or historical finding that definitively diagnoses the disease. The clinical presentations (see below) are often identical to other conditions.[1,2]

The true incidence of feline hypersensitivity dermatitis is unknown, although it is probably second only to fleas as a cause of skin disease in cats. The age of onset varies dramatically in cats, from 6 months to old age; however, most cats begin showing signs between age 6 and 24 months.[3]

Pollen sensitivities should be associated with seasonal clinical signs or seasonal flares of pruritus and inflammation. Indoor allergens, in contrast, should be associated with perennial clinical signs. Pruritus and inflammation associated with indoor allergens may be worse in winter months. Cats with food allergies would also be expected to have year-round symptoms. Flea exposure may be seasonal, intermittent or continuous, depending on lifestyle, climate and parasite control. Nevertheless, many cats have intermittent symptoms that appear to occur randomly.

Unlike atopic dogs, cats tend to present with well-defined reaction patterns that are poorly specific for any one condition. Most, if not all, affected cats are pruritic but the degree of pruritus varies greatly and is often mistaken for anxiety or other problems.

Symmetrical self-induced alopecia is very common. Affected cats overgroom to the point of alopecia. This is generally symmetrical and most often affects the medial limbs and ventrum. Some cats lick the ventral neck and sides and bottom of the tail. The underlying skin is often normal, but linear excoriations may develop. This overgrooming may lead to trichobezoars. Erythema is often more difficult to see in the skin of cats unless the skin is severely traumatised.

Miliary dermatitis is characterised by erythematous papules and crusts scattered throughout the haircoat, especially the flanks and dorsum. Overgrooming may cause alopecia associated with these lesions. A dorsal distribution is more common with flea-allergic dermatitis.

Eosinophilic complex lesions (see page 256):

- Eosinophilic plaques are well-demarcated, eroded or ulcerated plaques most common on the ventral abdomen and medial thighs.
- Eosinophilic granulomas are well-demarcated, often non-ulcerated, firm, pink to yellow, raised, and often linear lesions commonly present on the caudal aspects of the hindlimbs, but they can also occur in the oral cavity, chin ('fat chin'), interdigital skin and elsewhere.
- Indolent ulcers typically occur on the upper lips where the tongue and/or upper canines contact the mucosa, and are thick ulcers with raised erythematous borders.

Head and neck dermatitis results in variable, but potentially very severe, erythema, papules, crusts, seborrhoea and excoriation of the head and neck (**Figs. 2.33, 2.34**). This distribution is most commonly associated with food allergies.[1]

Secondary otitis (see page 267) is seen in affected cats, but it much less common than in atopic dogs.[2] Otitis may be the only symptom, but the cats should be carefully evaluated for other causes of the otitis (especially inflammatory polyps – see page 267).

Periocular dermatitis is characterised by varying degrees of erythema, alopecia, excoriation of the periocular skin and ocular discharge. Cats will

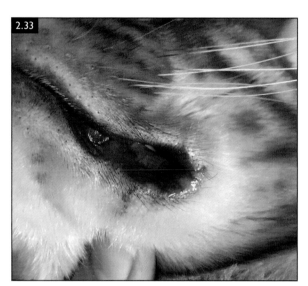

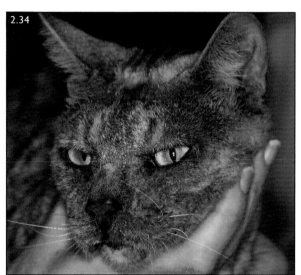

Fig. 2.33 Perioral inflammation and excoriation in a Bengal cat with an adverse food reaction. This cat also had indolent ulcers.

Fig. 2.34 Inflammation, excoriation and alopecia of the face of a cat with an adverse food reaction.

scratch at their eyes and periocular skin with a hind-limb or rub their eyes with the front legs. Again, cats should be carefully evaluated for other causes of conjunctivitis (particularly viral infections).

Other signs include twitching of the skin, shaking the feet, and biting the feet and skin as if trying to remove something. Some cats have sneezing or nasal discharge (50%) and/or asthma (approximately 7%) concurrent with hypersensitivity dermatitis.[4]

Secondary yeast and bacterial infections are less common in cats than in dogs.[4] *Malassezia* spp. may be found in the nailfold, ears and sometimes other skinfolds, but generalised malassezia dermatitis is more commonly associated with metabolic and other conditions (see page 30). Staphylococcal bacteria are common in ulcerated lesions. Their role in skin disease is less clear. However, oral antibiotic treatment may largely resolve eosinophilic plaques and indolent ulcers in some cats.

Differential diagnoses
- Parasites (fleas, mites and lice), especially *Demodex gatoi*, which may be difficult to find.
- Yeast or bacterial infection caused by other internal disease.
- Dermatophytosis (see page 115).
- Feline hyperaesthesia syndrome (see page 15).

- Herpesvirus dermatitis.
- Feline idiopathic ulcerative dermatitis.
- Pemphigus foliaceus (see page 81).
- Feline psychogenic alopecia (which may be concurrent with hypersensitivity dermatitis).
- Hyperthyroidism.
- With excessive scaling: parasitic (especially *Cheyletiella* and *Notoedres* spp.), thymoma-associated exfoliative dermatosis, lymphocytic mural folliculitis and cutaneous lymphoma.
- When affecting the face only: methimazole reaction, trigeminal neuropathy (orofacial pain syndrome), herpesvirus dermatitis, facial dermatitis of Persian cats, *Notoedres* mites.
- When affecting the ears only: ear mites, foreign body, middle-ear disease, inflammatory polyps.
- When affecting periocular skin only: demodicosis, dermatophytosis, staphylococci and herpesvirus keratoconjunctivitis.

Diagnosis
See flow chart (**Fig. 2.35**) for the diagnostic work-up. Hypersensitivity dermatitis is diagnosed by history, clinical findings, ruling out of other diseases and response to therapy. Hair plucks, tape-strips and skin scrapings should be taken from multiple affected locations and a faecal floatation performed

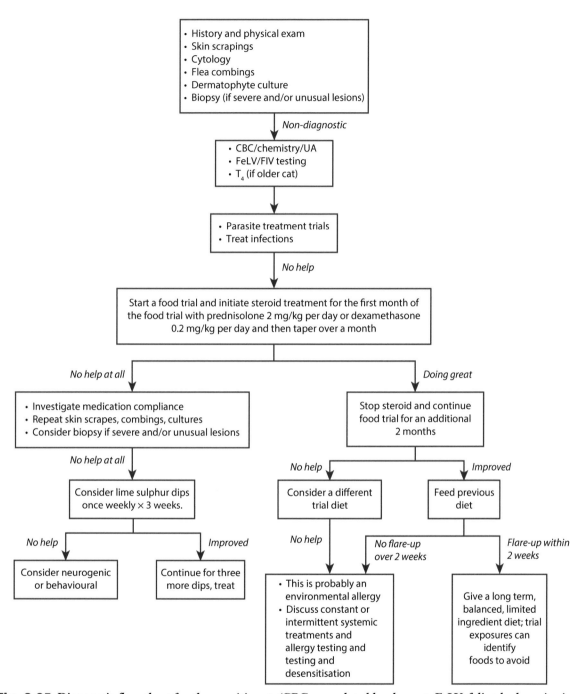

Fig. 2.35 Diagnostic flow chart for the pruritic cat. (CBC, complete blood count; FeLV, feline leukaemia virus; FIV, feline immunodeficiency virus; T₄, thyroxine; UA, urinalysis.)

to look for mites. A fungal culture should be obtained. Cytology for yeast and bacterial infections should be taken from several affected locations, especially the ears and nailbeds (if affected). A thorough treatment trial for fleas, lice and mites should

be performed in all cases, whether or not evidence of parasites is found. At the time of publication, no single parasiticide treats all external parasites in cats, although drugs in the isoxazoline class appear promising. Imidacloprid/moxidectin or selamectin every

2 weeks topically or weekly lime sulphur dip (2–3%) trials can be performed for 6–8 weeks. If pruritus is year-round, a food trial for 8–12 weeks should be performed (see below). If the cat is still affected, intradermal or serological allergen tests can be performed to identify allergens for avoidance and allergen-specific immunotherapy. Flea allergen tests are highly specific and therefore positive tests can be used to convince owners of the need for thorough flea control. However, they are poorly sensitive and there are many false-negative tests.

Diagnosis of adverse reaction to food

The diagnosis of a food allergy is based on the response to a restricted diet, composed of unique ingredients to which the cat has never, or only very rarely, been exposed. It is therefore critically important to obtain a full dietary history including data on commercial diets, treats, human foods, flavoured medicines and any vitamin or mineral supplements. However, this may be difficult where the owner cannot recall which foods have been fed or what the ingredients were. Moreover, undeclared ingredients are common in commercial foods (including 'single' protein diets). Food-specific serum allergen tests have not been validated in cats at the time of writing, and their use to diagnose food allergies cannot be recommended.

General details about diet trials can be found on page 24. However, diet trials in cats are often difficult due to their more finicky dietary behaviour. In addition, anorexia in cats can rapidly cause hepatic lipidosis and death, so owners must be warned and cats monitored. Transitions to new diets should be gradual. Home-cooked diet trials usually employ meat or fish protein only and most cats won't eat unprocessed carbohydrates. These diets are deficient in EFAs and taurine, although this should not affect otherwise healthy cats over the length of the diet trial. Greater care should be taken with cats that have concurrent problems and with longer-term feeding. Diet trials in cats can also be performed using fully supplemented and balanced, commercially prepared, hydrolysed or limited-ingredient prescription diets. However, over-the-counter and even prescription diets may contain ingredients not on the label,[5,6] and

so sometimes more than one diet trial should be performed. The length of a diet trial necessary to confirm an adverse reaction to food is controversial, but most authorities recommend 8–12 weeks for cats.[7] Outdoor cats may have access to other foods and, where possible, should be kept indoors. This may not be feasible if it leads to behavioural problems.

As allergy signs commonly fluctuate, a cat that improves with a restricted diet should be challenged with its original diet, which should include all treats, chews and dietary supplements. If a food allergy is involved, there will be an increase in pruritus within 7–14 days of the dietary challenge. If there is no increase in pruritus after the dietary challenge, then a food allergy can be ruled out. If there is recurrence of pruritus with the dietary challenge, then the restricted diet should be reinstituted. If a diagnosis of food allergy is made, it is helpful to identify the specific foods to avoid. The most accurate method for determining specific food allergies is to introduce one new ingredient into the diet every 2 weeks and monitor for pruritus.

Failure to recognise and treat secondary infections and ectoparasites during a dietary trial are a common cause of problems. Another major reason for poor compliance during a dietary trial is continued pruritus. One solution is to allow the use of short courses of glucocorticoids for the first 4–8 weeks of the trial, and then taper to see if the improvement can be maintained. Alternatively, the owners can give 3- to 7-day courses of glucocorticoids at their discretion to manage unacceptable pruritus during the food trial.

Treatment

It is important to emphasise to the client that hypersensitivity dermatitis cannot be cured, and will need to be managed as a lifelong condition. Treatment must be tailored to the specific signs and secondary changes or complications present in an individual animal. Owners need to be aware that it is not possible to predict initially which animal will respond to a particular therapy. They also need to understand that clinical manifestations frequently change, resulting in the need to adjust the therapy over time.

Parasite prevention

Long-term rigorous flea and parasite prevention should be instituted.

Avoidance of allergens

If a food allergy is deemed to be causing all or part of the clinical signs, the offending foods must be eliminated from the diet. It may be possible to avoid environmental allergens but this is often difficult and of limited efficacy.

Topical therapy

Topical steroids are useful for short-term or intermittent treatment of localised lesions. Combinations of steroids with antibiotics and antifungals are helpful for areas prone to frequent infection. However, cats are more likely to groom medications off the skin. Using potent topical steroids for more than 2 months may cause significant skin thinning and hair loss, which may take years to resolve and long-term treatment should be as infrequent as possible and/or employ less potent glucocorticoids (e.g. hydrocortisone or hydrocortisone aceponate). Despite this, some cats may still experience systemic absorption and subsequent side effects and cats on long-term treatment should be monitored carefully.

Antimicrobial shampoos can helpful in severely affected cases with secondary infections, but most cats will not tolerate bathing and these can be used only on focal lesions. Owners should be discouraged from scrubbing or picking at the skin, and should not rub against the grain of the hair. Lukewarm water should be used, and the skin should be rinsed well. There is no evidence that emollient and antipruritic shampoos, sprays or spot-on products are effective in cats, and any efficacy may be reduced by cats' grooming habits.

Otitis – see page 272 for management of ear infections. Otitis externa typically responds best to topical medications.

Systemic control of infections

Recurrent yeast and bacterial infections indicate that skin inflammation is not controlled if other causes of the infections have been eliminated.

Antibacterial agents effective for secondary staphylococcal infections include: cefpodoxime (5 mg/kg po q24 h), clindamycin (5.5–11 mg/kg po q12 h), cefalexin (20–30 mg/kg po q12 h), clavulanic acid-potentiated amoxicillin (25 mg/kg po q12 h). Cefovecin (8 mg/kg sc q14 days) can be considered where oral medication isn't feasible (see Bacterial dermatitis, page 65).

Antifungal agents that can be used for *Malassezia* infections include: itraconazole (5–10 mg/kg po q48 h) or fluconazole (5–10 mg/kg po q24 h) for 4–6 weeks (see Malassezia dermatitis, page 31).

Systemic allergy therapy

The only treatments with good evidence of high efficacy are glucocorticoids and ciclosporin. Most other treatment options are only partially effective and are typically used as adjunct therapy.

EFA-rich diets and supplements may help coat texture and skin barrier function, although there is less evidence for this than in dogs. The effective products and doses are unclear.

Antihistamines can be tried, but the frequent administration, poor efficacy, bitter taste and sedating qualities make this therapy less desirable in cats. Cetirizine (2 mg/kg po q12–24 h), hydroxyzine (1–2 mg/kg po q12 h) or chlorpheniramine (2 mg/cat po q12 h) may be helpful.

Glucocorticoids rapidly and reliably control symptoms of hypersensitivity dermatitis in cats. Methylprednisolone or prednisolone (1–2 mg/kg po q12 h) may be used until resolution and then the dose should be tapered to the lowest dose necessary to control signs. Some cats respond better to dexamethasone (0.2–0.4 mg/kg po q24 h) or triamcinolone (0.3–0.6 mg/kg po q24 h), although these are longer acting and should be tapered to twice-weekly administration for maintenance. Short-acting injectable dexamethasone solutions can be administered in food with cats that are difficult to pill. Long-acting injectable steroids may be warranted if only one to three injections are needed per year or if the client finds it impossible to administer oral medications to the animal. Some owners can be taught to give twice weekly short acting dexamethasone sc at home, tapered to the lowest dose and frequency needed for maintenance.

Possible adverse effects of continuous steroid use include: congestive heart failure, hypertension, diabetes mellitus, iatrogenic Cushing's syndrome, injection site atrophy, polyphagia, weight gain and behaviour changes (including aggression). The onset of iatrogenic Cushing's syndrome and/or diabetes is dose and duration dependent, and varies among individual cats. Regular urinalysis and monitoring of blood pressure is recommended. As a result of potential adverse effects of glucocorticoids, long-term use is not recommended unless other treatments cannot be used.

Ciclosporin is a calcineurin inhibitor and immunomodulating drug that is useful for lymphocytic and granulomatous inflammation, including hypersensitivity dermatitis. The recommended dose for cats is 7 mg/kg po q24 h. Ciclosporin is best suited for chronic use because it requires 2–6 weeks to observe clinical improvement.[8] Oral steroids can be coadministered for 2–3 weeks to give initial relief. Once the disease is controlled on ciclosporin alone (2–6 weeks), the frequency of dosing can be changed to every other day and, in some cases, to twice weekly. The dose can be tapered in cats that require ongoing daily therapy. Satisfactory control of signs will occur in approximately 70% of the cats treated with ciclosporin.[9] Difficulty in the administration of medications is the biggest problem with ciclosporin. A liquid formulation can be given in canned food or highly flavoured oily foods (e.g. fish, pate, butter, cream and ice cream). Chilling seems to improve palatability, and slowly increasing the dose over 1–2 weeks can also help. Side effects of ciclosporin in cats include: vomiting, diarrhoea, anorexia, weight loss and gingival hyperplasia. There are rare reports of fatal toxoplasmosis in cats exposed to *Toxoplasma* spp. while receiving ciclosporin. To prevent this, cats should (where possible) be kept indoors or antihunting measures implemented (at least two bells and flashing light-emitting diodes [LEDs] on a collar) and not fed raw meat, and ciclosporin should be tapered to the lowest dose possible after clinical improvement. Herpesvirus may relapse in cats receiving ciclosporin. Ciclosporin trough concentrations can be performed 20 h postpill, 1–2 weeks after starting therapy to screen for high absorbing cats, who are at most risk. Ciclosporin is metabolised by the liver, so caution should be used if the animal to be treated has liver disease. Drugs that inhibit cytochrome P450 microsomal enzyme activity (e.g. itraconazole) will increase blood levels of ciclosporin and potentiate possible toxicity or other side effects. Regular urinalysis is recommended but it is not necessary to check complete blood counts (CBCs) or serum biochemistry in the absence of any specific concerns.

Oclacitinib (Apoquel®, Zoetis) is not labelled or EMA/FDA approved for use in cats. There is one small study showing efficacy in 4 of 12 cats.[10] Oclacitinib should be given at 0.4–0.6 mg/kg twice daily for 14 days and then once daily thereafter, although some cats may do better on doses up to 1 mg/kg q12 h. If symptoms are completely controlled, this drug should be further tapered to the lowest dose and frequency needed. It is recommended to check a CBC, serum biochemistry and urinalysis before therapy, at the 2-month and 5-month points, and every 6 months. Side effects associated with long-term use are not known in cats.

Allergen testing and ASIT

In cats, allergen skin testing is a specialised procedure that requires sedation and may be difficult to interpret. Referral is recommended for this.

Serum allergen-specific tests (RAST, ELISA and liquid-phase immunoenzymatic assay) can be performed to detect increased concentrations of allergen-specific IgE. However, very few of these tests have been validated for cats. In dogs, they lack specificity and have moderate intra- and interlaboratory variability of results.[11] Serological testing may be helpful in some cases to select allergens for ASIT but the results must be interpreted with care. Serological testing for food allergens is not accurate and not recommended. Food trials must be performed for diagnosis of food allergy.

ASIT using SCIT has been reported to result in at least a 50% improvement in 60–78% of cats with hypersensitivity dermatitis.[12] It may take animals as long as 6–12 months (and sometimes longer) to respond to immunotherapy and, therefore, critical clinical evaluation should not take place until a year of therapy has been completed.[12] Concurrent therapy is appropriate pending the full effects of immunotherapy. Adverse effects are uncommon. Injection site reactions and anaphylactic shock are very rare. Mild reactions can generally be prevented by pretreating with antihistamines 1–2 h before the injection. Intervals between injections can be individualised to the needs of the animal. SLIT is also available for cats, although the reports of efficacy are largely short term or anecdotal.

Key points

- The diagnosis of hypersensitivity dermatitis depends on recognising cats with pruritus and appropriate cutaneous reaction patterns, ruling out other diseases and the response to therapy.
- Allergy tests are not diagnostic for the disease – food trials and allergy tests are used to determine the food and/or environmental allergens to which each cat could be sensitised.
- Therapy is typically multi-modal and needs to be constantly modified to best suit the individual.
- Proactive therapy that maintains remission is more effective than simply reacting to recurrent flares.

References

1 Hobi S, Linek M, Marignac G *et al*. Clinical characteristics and causes of pruritus in cats: a multicentre study on feline hypersensitivity-associated dermatoses: Feline hypersensitivity dermatitis. *Vet Dermatol* 2011; **22**: 406–413.

2 Ravens PA, Xu BJ, Vogelnest LJ. Feline atopic dermatitis: a retrospective study of 45 cases (2001–2012). *Vet Dermatol* 2014; **25**: 95–e28.

3 Roosje PJ, Thepen TH, Rutten V, Willemse T. Feline atopic dermatitis: a review. *Vet Dermatol* 2000; **11**: 12–12.

4 Miller WH, Griffin CE, Campbell KL, Muller GH. Autoimmune and immune-mediated dermatoses. In: *Muller and Kirk's Small Animal Dermatology*, 7th edn. New York: Elsevier Health Sciences, 2013: pp. 363–431.

5 Ricci R, Granato A, Vascellari M, *et al*. Identification of undeclared sources of animal origin in canine dry foods used in dietary elimination trials. *J Anim Physiol Anim Nutr* 2013; **97**: 32–38.

6 Willis-Mahn C, Remillard R, Tater, K. ELISA testing for soy antigens in dry dog foods used in dietary elimination trials. *J Am Anim Hosp Assoc* 2014; **50**: 383–389.

7 Vogelnest LJ, Cheng KY. Cutaneous adverse food reactions in cats: retrospective evaluation of 17 cases in a dermatology referral population (2001–2011). *Aust Vet J* 2013; **91**: 443–451.

8 Palmeiro BS. Cyclosporine in veterinary dermatology. *Vet Clin North Am Small Anim Pract* 2013; **43**: 153–171.

9 Wisselink MA, Willemse T. The efficacy of cyclosporine A in cats with presumed atopic dermatitis: A double blind, randomised prednisolone-controlled study. *Vet J* 2009; **180**: 55–59.

10 Ortalda C, Noli C, Colombo S, Borio S. Oclacitinib in feline nonflea-, nonfood-induced hypersensitivity dermatitis: results of a small prospective pilot study of client-owned cats. *Vet Dermatol* 2015; **26**: 235–e52.

11 Thom N, Favrot C, Failing K *et al*. Intra- and interlaboratory variability of allergen-specific IgE levels in atopic dogs in three different laboratories using the Fc-ε receptor testing. *Vet. Immunol Immunopathol* 2010; **133**: 183–189.

12 Trimmer AM, Griffin CE, Rosenkrantz WS. Feline immunotherapy. *Clin Tech Small Anim Pract* 2006; **21**: 157–161.

FELINE *DEMODEX GATOI* INFESTATION

Definition
Demodex gatoi infestation is the persistent presence of this mite on the skin.

Aetiology and pathogenesis
D. gatoi is a short-bodied contagious mite that can inhabit the stratum corneum of cats. The number of mites on the skin can vary based on the grooming habits of the individual.

Clinical features
Most affected cats are from multi-cat households. Clinical signs include: pruritus, overgrooming and alopecia of the ventral abdomen, inner thighs and forelimbs (see **Fig. 4.44**).[1,2] The alopecia may be patchy to generalised. Indolent lip ulcers and miliary dermatitis are also reported.[1] Affected housemates may be asymptomatic. *D. gatoi* appears to be uncommon but may be underdiagnosed.

Differential diagnoses
- Hypersensitivity dermatitis (see page 41).
- Dermatophytosis.
- Other parasites – fleas, *Cheyletiella* spp., lice, *Notoedres* and *Sarcoptes* spp.

Diagnosis
Diagnosis may be difficult, because mites are not always found on skin scrapings and tape preparations due to grooming behaviour in cats (**Fig. 2.37**). The mite is sometimes found in faecal examinations[3] or in the stratum corneum of skin biopsies.[2] The mite should be suspected in cases of pruritus that are not or only partially responsive to steroid therapy.

Treatment
All affected and in-contact cats must be quarantined and treated. There is no ideal treatment because therapeutic failures have been reported with all the options.[2] Rechecks should be performed monthly and treatments continued for 2–4 weeks beyond clinical cure and two consecutive negative skin scrapings. If a treatment has not helped clinically and scrapings are still positive after a 2-month trial, a different therapy should be instituted.

- Imidacloprid 10%/moxidectin 2.5% (the canine products) topically every 2 weeks is sometimes effective.[1]
- Imidacloprid 10%/moxidectin 1% spot-on (the feline and ferret products) applied to a focal area on the skin over the neck or shoulders once a week for 8–10 treatments has been demonstrated to be effective.[8]
- Selamectin is usually not effective, even applied every 2 weeks.[2]
- Lime sulphur 2% dips applied weekly for six treatments is historically the most effective therapy[1,4] but is labour intensive, odiferous and stains light-coloured coats. Clinical improvement is usually observed within three dips.
- Ivermectin 0.2–0.3 mg/kg po q24 h or q48 h is often effective.[1] Neurological side effects are possible and should be monitored for.
- Doramectin 0.6 mg/kg sc weekly appears to be effective for *D. cati*[5] and can be attempted for *D. gatoi*. Large studies have not been done to evaluate safety in cats.
- Fluralaner topically every 2–3 months shows promise for treatment of *D. gatoi*.[6]
- If all treatments fail, the use of amitraz dips (0.0125% applied weekly) may be considered. This is half the manufacturer's recommended dose for dogs.[7] Amitraz should be used only as the last treatment option, because there is well-known potential for toxicity in cats and side effects for owners.

Key point
- *D. gatoi* is pruritic, contagious, difficult to diagnose and difficult to treat.

References
1 Beale K. Feline demodicosis: A consideration in the itchy or overgrooming cat. *J Feline Med Surg* 2012; **14**: 209–213.
2 Saari SA, Juuti KH, Palojärvi JH, Väisänen KM, Rajaniemi R-L, Saijonmaa-Koulumies LE. *Demodex gatoi*-associated contagious pruritic dermatosis in cats – a report from six households in Finland. *Acta Vet Scand* 2009; **51**: 40.

3 Silbermayr K, Joachim A, Litschauer B *et al*. The first case of *Demodex gatoi* in Austria, detected with fecal flotation. *Parasitol Res* 2013; **112**: 2805–2810.
4 Mueller RS. Treatment protocols for demodicosis: an evidence-based review. *Vet Dermatol* 2004; **15**: 75–89.
5 Johnstone IP. Doramectin as a treatment for canine and feline demodicosis. *Aust Vet Pract* 2002; **32**: 98–103.

6 Kilp S, Ramirez D, Allan MJ, Roepke RK. Comparative pharmacokinetics of fluralaner in dogs and cats following single topical or intravenous administration. *Parasit Vectors* 2016; **9**: 1.
7 Cowan LA, Campbell K. Generalized demodicosis in a cat responsive to amitraz. *J Am Vet Med Assoc* 1988; **192**: 1442–1444.

NOTOEDRIC MANGE

Definition

A contagious dermatosis of cats due to infection with the psoroptic mite *Notoedres cati*.

Aetiology and pathogenesis

Infection with the mite results in severe pruritus, presumably due to a hypersensitivity, as with canine scabies, although the biology and life cycle of the mite are less well understood.[1]

Clinical features

There is no breed, age or sex predisposition. Affected cats exhibit intense pruritus on the head and pinnae. The initial lesions are an erythematous, papular dermatitis, but a greyish crust soon becomes apparent (**Fig. 2.36**). The anterior edges of the pinnae are often affected. If not treated, the lesions may progress to affect the feet and perineum.[1] Lymphadenopathy may also be present.

Differential diagnoses

- Other parasitic dermatoses – fleas, lice, *Demodex gatoi* or other mites.
- Hypersensitivity dermatitis (especially head and neck dermatitis – see page 41).
- Pemphigus foliaceus.
- Dermatophytosis.

Diagnosis

Skin scrapings usually reveal eggs or mites. A treatment trial may be needed to rule out this mite if scrapings are negative.

Treatment

All in-contact cats, dogs and rabbits should be treated. For dogs, refer to Sarcoptic mange

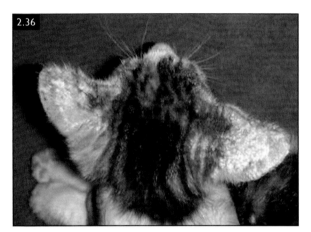

Fig. 2.36 Cat with notoedric mange with severe inflammation, scaling and crusting of the pinnae (photo courtesy of Mike Canfield).

treatments, page 58. The following treatments are for cats only:

- Ivermectin 0.2–0.3 mg/kg sc every 2 weeks for three treatments is curative.
- Imidacloprid 10%/moxidectin 1% (cat and ferret products) topically once may be curative,[2] but at least two doses every 2–4 weeks are recommended.
- Selamectin every 2–4 weeks for three treatments is effective.[3]
- Total body application of 3.1% lime sulphur solution weekly for 6–8 weeks is effective.[1]
- A single injection of doramectin (0.2–0.3 mg/kg sc) has been reported as curative.[4]
- A single application of a product containing fipronil 8.3%, (*S*)-methoprene 10%, eprinomectin 0.4% and praziquantel 8.3% was effective.[5]

Key point

• Pruritus in cats that markedly affects the ear margins should raise suspicion of *Notoedres* spp.

References

1   Ghubash R. Parasitic miticidal therapy. *Clin Tech Small Anim Pract* 2006; **21**: 135–144.
2   Hellmann K, Petry G, Capari B, Cvejic D, Krämer F. Treatment of naturally *Notoedres cati*-infested cats with a combination of imidacloprid 10%/moxidectin 1% Spot-on (Advocate/Advantage Multi, Bayer). *Parasitol Res* 2013; **112**(suppl 1): 57–66.
3   Beale KM, Fujioka C. Effectiveness of selamectin in the treatment of *Notoedres cati* infestation in cats. *Vet Dermatol* 2001; **12**: 13–18.
4   Delucchi L, Castro E. Use of doramectin for treatment of notoedric mange in five cats. *J Am Vet Med Assoc* 2000; **216**: 215–216.
5   Knaus M, Capári B, Visser M. Therapeutic efficacy of Broadline against notoedric mange in cats. *Parasitol Res* 2014; **113**: 4303–4306.

CHEYLETIELLA MITE INFESTATION

Definition

Cheyletiellosis is an infestation of *Cheyletiella* spp. mites on the surface of the skin.

Aetiology and pathogenesis

Three species of mites are responsible for most clinical cases in dogs, cats and rabbits. Although none is host specific, *C. yasguri* is found more frequently in dogs, *C. blakei* in cats and *C. parasitovorax* in rabbits. The mites live on the skin surface and the eggs are attached to the hair shafts. The mites are characterised by prominent hooks at the end of the accessory mouthparts (**Fig. 2.37**). The life cycle is approximately 35 days and is completed on one host. Adult mites may live 1 month off the host.[1] The mites are transmitted from one animal to another via direct contact, fomites or the environment.

Clinical features

Diffuse scaling over the dorsum of the animal is the characteristic feature of infestation in dogs (**Fig. 2.38**).[1,2] Pruritus in dogs varies from absent to severe. Although variably pruritic scaling may be a feature in cats, small (0.2–0.4 cm) pruritic crusted papules over the dorsum are more common (**Fig. 2.39**),[3] particularly in long-haired cats.[4] Both dogs and cats can be asymptomatic carriers. People in contact with infested animals show signs in 30–40% of cases.[3] The typical signs are small, pruritic, erythematous papules in groups of two or three, usually on the arms and trunk (i.e. the parts in contact with infested animals) (**Fig. 2.40**).[5]

Differential diagnoses

• Other parasitic dermatoses – fleas, lice, *Demodex gatoi* (cats) or other mites.
• Atopic and other hypersensitivity dermatitis.
• Sebaceous adenitis.
• Primary keratinisation defects.
• Bacterial or yeast dermatitis.

Diagnosis

Skin scrapings, tape-strips and fine-toothed combings taken from scaling or crusted areas may demonstrate the mites or eggs attached to the hair.[1,2] Mites cannot be demonstrated in all animals and trial therapy may be necessary in some cases to confirm a diagnosis.[2]

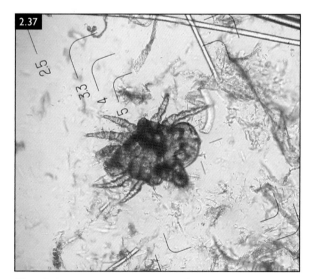

Fig. 2.37 A *Cheyletiella* mite (photo courtesy of Boerhinger Ingelheim Animal Health).

Treatment

All in-contact animals must be treated, even if not symptomatic. Environmental cleaning involves laundering all bedding weekly and disinfecting all fomites, but extensive environmental treatment is not needed as mites do not survive long off the host and (unlike fleas) there is no environmental reservoir of immature forms.

Dogs

* Fipronil spray 0.25% – 3–6 ml/kg topically every 2 weeks for four treatments.[3]
* Fipronil 10% spot-on solution every 4 weeks for two treatments.[4]
* Selamectin – 6.2–20 mg/kg topically every 2 weeks for four treatments.[6]
* Imidacloprid 10%/moxidectin 2.5% – 0.1 ml/kg topically every 4 weeks for two treatments.[7]
* Milbemycin – 2 mg/kg po once weekly for nine treatments.[8]
* Ivermectin or doramectin – 0.3 mg/kg sc every 2 weeks for three treatments (do not use in sensitive breeds or test for the *MDR-1* gene mutation before use).
* Three to four weekly dips of lime sulphur or pyrethrin.
* Three 0.025% amitraz dips given at 2-week intervals are appropriate for adult dogs.
* Isoxazoline ectoparasitics (fluralaner, afoxolaner and sarolaner) used as per label instructions are very likely to eliminate this parasite, but no studies have been performed.

Cats

* Fipronil 10% spot-on every 4 weeks for two treatments (may be effective with only one application).[9]
* Selamectin 45 mg/cat topically every 4 weeks for three treatments.[10]
* Imidacloprid 10%/moxidectin 1% topically once monthly for three treatments.
* Ivermectin at 0.3 mg/kg sc every 2 weeks for four treatments.[11]
* Lime sulphur dips at 3.1% concentration once weekly for 6 treatments.[12]

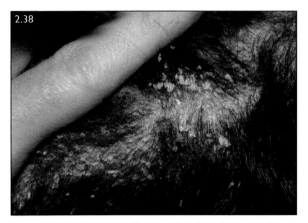

Fig. 2.38 Profuse scaling on the dorsal trunk of a Russian Terrier.

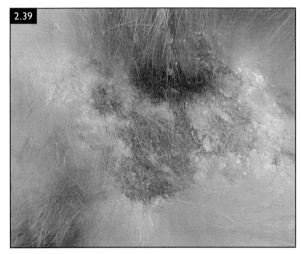

Fig. 2.39 Profuse scaling and erythema on the dorsal trunk of a cat.

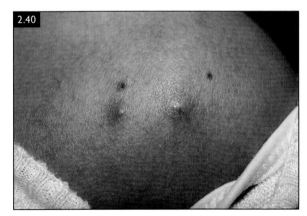

Fig. 2.40 Zoonotic lesions on the shoulder of an owner with affected pet.

Key point

- Mites may not always be demonstrated and a treatment trial may be needed.

References

1 Arther RG. Mites and lice: biology and control. *Vet. Clin North Am Small Anim Pract* 2009; **39**: 1159–1171.

2 Paradis M, Villeneuve A. Efficacy of ivermectin against *Cheyletiella yasguri* infestation in dogs. *Can Vet J* 1988; **29**: 633.

3 Chadwick AJ. Use of a 0.25 per cent fipronil pump spray formulation to treat canine cheyletiellosis. *J Small Anim Pract* 1997; **38**: 261–262.

4 Bourdeau P, Lecanu JM. Treatment of multiple infestations with *Otodectes cynotis*, *Cheyletiella yasguri* and *Trichodectes canis* with fipronil (Frontline Spot-on; Merial) in the dog. In: *Proceedings of the Autumn Meeting of the British Veterinary Dermatology Study Group, Bristol, United Kingdom*, British Veterinary Dermatology Study Group, 1999: pp. 35–36.

5 August JR, Loar AS, Scott DW, Horn RT. Zoonotic dermatoses of dogs and cats. *Vet Clin North Am Small Anim Pract* 1987; **17**: 117–144.

6 Mueller RS, Bettenay SV. Efficacy of selamectin in the treatment of canine cheyletiellosis. *Vet Rec* 2002; **151**: 773–773.

7 Loft KE, Willesen JL. Efficacy of imidacloprid 10 per cent/moxidectin 2·5 per cent spot-on in the treatment of cheyletiellosis in dogs. *Vet Rec* 2007; **160**: 528–529.

8 White SD, Rosychuk RA, Fieseler KV. Clinicopathologic findings, sensitivity to house dust mites and efficacy of milbemycin oxime treatment of dogs with *Cheyletiella* sp. infestation. *Vet Dermatol* 2001; **12**: 13–18.

9 Scarampella F, Pollmeier M, Visser M, Boeckh A, Jeannin P. Efficacy of fipronil in the treatment of feline cheyletiellosis. *Vet Parasitol* 2005; **129**: 333–339.

10 Chailleux N, Paradis, M. Efficacy of selamectin in the treatment of naturally acquired cheyletiellosis in cats. *Can Vet J* 2002; **43**: 767.

11 Paradis M. Ivermectin in small animal dermatology. II. Extralabel applications. *Compend Contin Educ Vet* 1998; **20**: 193.

12 Ghubash R. Parasitic miticidal therapy. *Clin Tech Small Anim Pract* 2006; **21**: 135–144.

FLEAS AND FLEA ALLERGIC DERMATITIS (Flea bite hypersensitivity)

Definition

Flea allergic dermatitis (FAD) is caused by a hypersensitivity to flea salivary allergens in allergy-prone animals, causing severe pruritus and a papular dermatitis. Very low numbers of fleas can cause dermatitis.

Aetiology and pathogenesis

Most flea infestations are associated with the cat flea (*Ctenocephalides felis*). In most households, the life cycle takes 21–30 days, with a range of 12–174 days.[1] Fleas feed within minutes of landing on a host, and females produce eggs in 1–2 days. The pupal stage, which is very resistant to chemicals and drying, can remain viable for 140 days. Unfed adult fleas die in 12 days. On the host, fleas can live for more than 100 days. Fleas are vectors for *Bartonella* sp. (cat scratch fever), *Rickettsia felis*, *Haemoplasma* sp. (feline infectious anaemia), *Yersinia pestis* (plague) and *Dipylidium caninum* (tapeworm).[2]

Other fleas are occasionally seen. These may include the sedentary flea *Spilopsyllus cuniculi* from wild rabbits, which is most commonly found on the head and ears, and fleas from bird nests, hedgehogs, rodents and other wild animals.

Clinical features

Flea-allergic dogs develop severe pruritus and papular dermatitis. The caudal dorsum, perineal and umbilical areas are typically affected (**Figs. 2.41, 2.42**), although lesions can also be found around the neck. The primary lesion is a crusted papule, but self-trauma quickly results in excoriation, crusting, alopecia and secondary bacterial or *Malassezia* infections. Chronic inflammation leads to lichenification and hyperpigmentation. Flea-allergic dogs often have concurrent atopic or food allergic dermatitis (see page 18).

Flea-allergic cats most commonly develop a crusted papular dermatitis along the caudal–dorsal midline, but can also present with more generalised miliary dermatitis (**Fig. 2.43**), symmetrical self-induced alopecia (**Fig. 2.44**), eosinophilic plaques (**Fig. 2.45**) and granulomas, indolent lip ulcers and

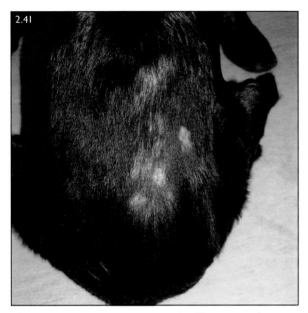

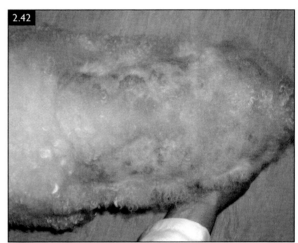

Figs. 2.41, 2.42 Symmetrical self-trauma, alopecia, erosions and crusts in two dogs with flea bite hypersensitvity/flea allergic dermatitis.

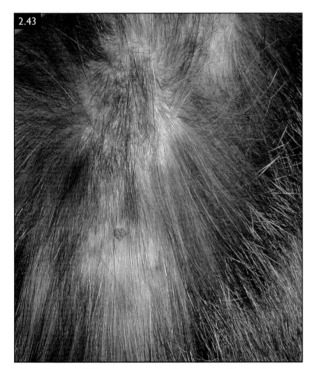

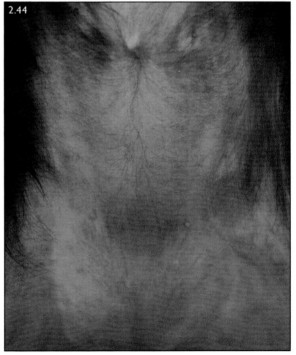

Fig. 2.43 Miliary dermatitis in a cat with flea bite hypersensitvity/flea allergic dermatitis.

Fig. 2.44 Self-induced alopecia of the ventral abdomen in a cat with flea bite hypersensitivity. There is little to no inflammation of the underlying skin.

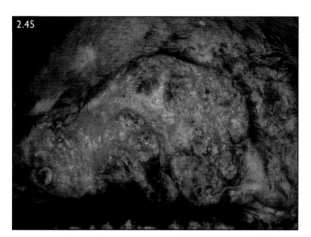

Fig. 2.45 Extensive eosinophilic plaque on the lateral hindlimb of a cat with chronic flea bite hypersensitvity.

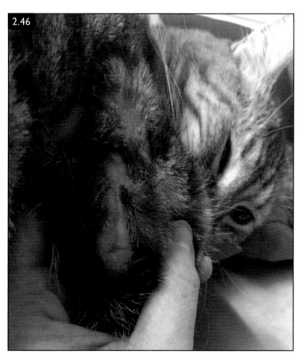

Fig. 2.46 A linear granuloma on the limb of a cat.

linear granulomas (**Fig. 2.46**). Fleas should therefore be considered in all cases of suspected hypersensitivity dermatitis (see page 41).

Flea bites on humans are typically located around the lower legs and ankles, waist, groin, skinfolds and lower back. Some family members may appear to be unaffected whereas others are intensely pruritic.

Differential diagnoses
- Other ectoparasites: mites or lice.
- Dermatophytosis.
- Food-allergic dermatitis.
- Atopic dermatitis.
- Feline hypersensitivity dermatitis and/or eosinophilic granuloma syndrome.
- Pemphigus foliaceus.
- Epitheliotrophic lymphoma.
- Staphylococcal pyoderma.
- Malassezia dermatitis.

Diagnosis
A diagnosis of flea-allergic dermatitis is highly likely when fleas or flea dirt is present on an animal with appropriate clinical signs (**Figs. 2.47–2.49**), and can be confirmed with resolution of the signs by aggressive flea control. Diagnosis can be difficult because often animals have concurrent allergies and, especially in cats, fleas may be difficult to find due to grooming behaviour. Tape-strips can be used to find microscopic fragments of flea dirt that would otherwise be invisible on combings and wet paper tests (**Fig. 2.50**).

Treatment
Aggressive flea control includes treatment of all in-contact animals (cats, dogs, ferrets and rabbits, including any neighbours' pets) and the environment (indoor and potentially outdoor, depending on the climate). Full elimination of fleas may take months, and pruritus may persist beyond flea extermination. Antipruritic treatments should be considered to provide some relief for itchy animals (see Canine atopic dermatitis, page 26, and Feline hypersensitivity dermatitis, page 41).

Animals
There are many safe and effective flea products available. It is best to use an insect growth regulator (IGR) in combination with a long-acting adulticide. There are a variety of oral and topical treatments available that also cover additional ecto- and endoparasites in addition to fleas. All have advantages and disadvantages, and it is worth spending time with clients to select the products that best suit their household animals, aims and lifestyle. For example, bathing (especially with degreasing shampoos) or

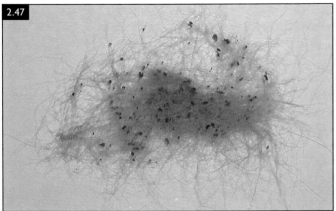

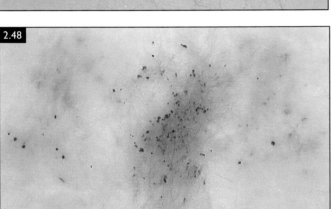

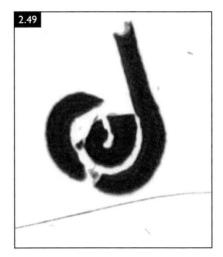

Figs. 2.47–2.49 Flea faeces demonstrated in coat combings (Fig. 2.47), tape-strip cytology ×40 (Fig. 2.48 [photo courtesy of P Forsythe]), and red staining on wet cotton wool (Fig. 2.49).

swimming will necessitate a systemic or waterproof topical product,[4] and additional tick control will be important for outdoor animals in tick endemic areas. Products labelled for dogs only should not be used in cats, and great care should be taken when using permethrin products on dogs if there are cats in the household.

The main aim of treatment is to reduce flea exposure to tolerable levels. This can be achieved by population control and it is not always necessary to prevent fleas biting. Ingredients that repel fleas and prevent biting can be useful in severely affected animals, but these often have a short duration of effect and are more toxic in cats. Fleas in endemic areas often develop insecticide resistance,[3] and so combinations of products or rotation of products may be needed.

The most common reason for treatment failure is not resistance but failure to follow label directions

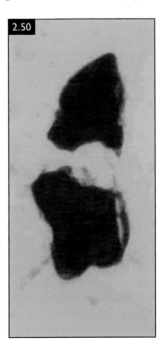

Fig. 2.50 Microscopic fragment of flea faeces from a self-traumatising cat (adhesive tape-strip ×40).

and recommendations.[3] It is vital to work with clients to select the most suitable products for their animals, to fully explain treatment and demonstrate application. Clipping small patches on the dorsum may facilitate application of spot-on products. It is particularly important to explain that the pupal stage is resistant to pesticides and adults may continue to emerge and bite pets over 4–5 months despite effective treatments – this does not equate to insecticide resistance, and highlights the need for long-term on-animal and environmental therapy to eliminate an infestation.

Environment

Vacuum cleaning will help remove adult fleas from the flooring, reduce the numbers of eggs and larvae within the carpet, elevate the carpet pile and so enhance penetration of the insecticide, and stimulate emergence of pupated adults. Carpet cleaning with hot water may, however, create a very favourable moist environment for fleas. Environmental products are usually aerosol sprays consisting of a permethrin/pyrethroid combined with an insect growth regulator such as methoprene, pyriproxifen or cyromazine. The insecticide provides a rapid kill of larvae and adults that can be effective for up to 2–3 months. IGRs prevent normal development of the eggs, larvae and pupae, with residual activity for up to 12 months. Foggers are easy to apply, but often miss protected sites under furniture and may not penetrate carpets or rugs very well. Great care must be taken when using environmental treatments in homes with small rodents, birds and fish. Fleas are susceptible to sunlight and extremes of temperatures, but shaded and mild outdoor areas can be treated with insecticides and/or the parasitic nematode *Steinernema carpocapsa*.[4] Treatment of sheds, garages, outhouses, cars and homes of neighbours, family and friends may be needed if fleas are persistent.

Key points
- Flea allergic dermatitis is common.
- All in-contact animals and the environment must be treated.
- Regular preventive therapy is recommended.

References
1 Blagburn BL, Dryden MW. Biology, treatment and control of flea and tick infestations. *Vet Clin North Am Small Anim Pract* 2009; **39**: 1173–1200.
2 Otranto D, Wall R. New strategies for the control of arthropod vectors of disease in dogs and cats. *Med Vet Entomol* 2008; **22**: 291–302.
3 Rust MK. Insecticide resistance in fleas. *Insects* 2016; **7**: 10.
4 Marsella R. Advances in flea control. *Vet Clin Small Anim Pract* 1999; **29**: 1407–1424.

SARCOPTIC MANGE

Definition

Sarcoptic mange is caused by the mite *Sarcoptes scabiei*.

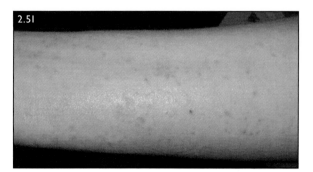

Fig. 2.51 Zoonotic lesions of scabies on the forearm of an owner.

Aetiology and pathogenesis

Sarcoptic mange is common in dogs, and is very rare in cats. *Sarcoptes scabiei* mites are highly contagious through direct contact, fur, crusts and fomites. They will infest a variety of species including humans (**Fig. 2.51**), although different varieties are relatively species specific. The mites tunnel through the epidermis, laying eggs that hatch into six-legged larvae, which then moult into eight-legged nymphs. Finally adults emerge on to the surface. The life cycle takes 14–21 days to complete.[1] Adult females can survive off the host for up to 19 days, but 2–6 days is more typical in normal household conditions.[2] Signs of infestation occur 3 days to 8 weeks after exposure.[3] The pruritus is associated with a hypersensitivity response to mites and mite products. It may be severe even with low numbers of mites and can persist for 1–6 months after eliminating the mites.

Clinical features

The primary clinical signs can vary from asymptomatic to intensely pruritic. Mites cause papules that eventually coalesce to form large areas of erythema and crust, complicated by secondary bacterial infections. The pruritus from sarcoptic mange is only partially responsive to glucocorticoids and oclacitinib. Dogs typically are affected on the ear margins with alopecia, erythema, crusting and ear margin hyperkeratosis (**Fig. 2.52**). Scratching the ear margin will often cause the hindlimb to twitch or thump (pinnal–pedal scratch reflex) and when this is seen a treatment trial for sarcoptic mange should be performed. Other affected areas are caudal–lateral aspects of the legs (elbows, hocks and feet), face, ventral chest and abdomen (**Figs. 2.53–2.55**). Focal to multi-focal dermatitis can also be seen. Long-standing disease may be severe and generalised with malaise, weight loss and lymphadenopathy (**Fig. 2.56**). Large numbers of mites and profuse crusting are often seen after treatment with glucocorticoids, ciclosporin, oclacitinib or chemotherapy.

Differential diagnoses

- Atopic dermatitis and food allergies.
- Other parasitic dermatoses – fleas, lice or other mites.
- Epitheliotrophic lymphoma.
- Pemphigus foliaceus.
- Bacterial or yeast dermatitis.

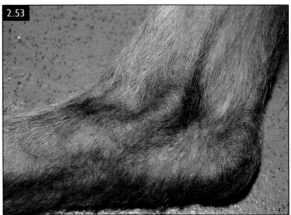

Fig. 2.53 Erythema, excoriation, alopecia and lichenification of the hock in a dog with scabies.

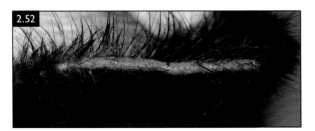

Fig. 2.52 Erythema, excoriation, and alopecia of the pinna margin.

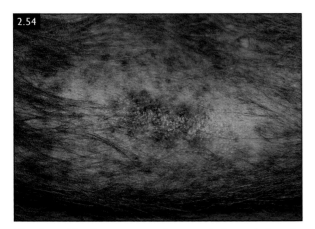

Fig. 2.54 Erythematous papules, excoriation and alopecia of the ventral chest.

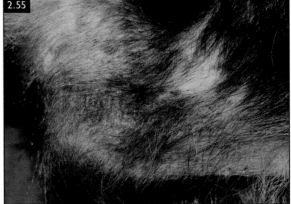

Fig. 2.55 Erythematous papules, excoriation, alopecia and lichenification of the elbow.

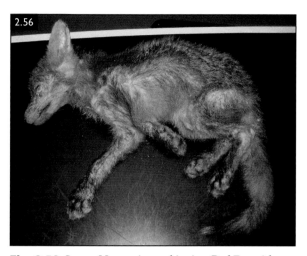

Fig. 2.56 Severe Norwegian scabies in a Red Fox with generalised scaling, crusting, excoriation and alopecia (photo courtesy of M Allington).

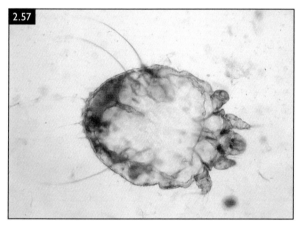

Fig. 2.57 Adult female *Sarcoptes scabiei*.

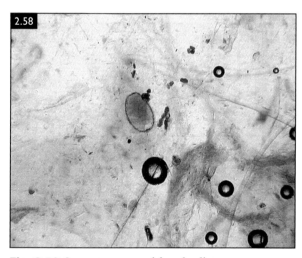

Fig. 2.58 Sarcoptes eggs and faecal pellets.

Diagnosis

The history and clinical signs will often allow a tentative diagnosis of scabies. A positive pinnal scratch reflex is highly suggestive of scabies.[4] Multiple deep skin scrapings may reveal mites, faecal pellets or eggs (**Figs. 2.57, 2.58**). Scrapings are only positive 50% of the time, so ruling out this mite requires a well-performed treatment trial. Several ELISA tests for *Sarcoptes*-specific IgG are available, but their use is limited by false-positive and -negative results.[5]

Treatment

All in-contact dogs, cats and rabbits must be treated, even if not symptomatic. Environmental cleaning involves laundering all bedding weekly and disinfecting all fomites, but extensive environmental treatment is not needed because mites do not survive long off the host, as long as the premises are quarantined until all animals have no symptoms of the disease. This requires 4 weeks in most cases. Affected humans should seek medical attention for treatment. Dogs often need systemic antibiotic therapy for secondary infections. There are no consistently helpful treatments for pruritus caused by mites other than eliminating the mite; oclacitinib 0.6 mg/kg po q12 h for 14 days, prednisolone 1 mg/kg per day tapered over 2 weeks and antihistamines may be variably helpful. Soaks with warm water, peppermint, tea tree and/or witch hazel may provide short-term relief. Longer-term treatment may be needed to manage residual pruritus after elimination of the mites in some dogs.

The following treatments are for dogs only – for treatments for cats, see Notoedric mange, page 49.

- Isoxazoline ectoparasitics (fluralaner, afoxolaner, sarolaner), used as per label instructions (for fleas and ticks), eliminate ectoparasites rapidly.[6,7]
- Lime sulphur 2.5% applied weekly for 4–6 weeks is also effective and well tolerated, but rotten eggs odour and staining of light-coloured coats make it less desirable in some dogs.[8]
- Fipronil spray 0.25% – 3–6 ml/kg q7–21 days for 3–6 weeks in young, pregnant or nursing dogs, where more potent treatments may be contraindicated.[8]

- Selamectin – topically q2 weeks for four treatments.
- Imidacloprid 10%/moxidectin 2.5% – topically once monthly for two treatments has been effective,[9] although every 2 weeks for four treatments is probably better.
- Pyriprole 12.5% topically once monthly for three treatments has been effective.[9]
- Ivermectin or doramectin – 0.3 mg/kg sc q2 weeks for three treatments (do not use in sensitive breeds or test for the *MDR-1* gene mutation before use).
- Amitraz dip 0.025% is effective applied q7–14 days for 4–6 weeks.[8]

Key point

- Sarcoptic mange is difficult to find on scrapings but easy to cure in most cases.

References

1 Arther RG. Mites and lice: biology and control. *Vet Clin North Am Small Anim Pract* 2009; **39**: 1159–1171.
2 Arlian LG, Runyan RA, Achar S, Estes SA. Survival and infectivity of *Sarcoptes scabiei* var. *canis* and var. *hominis. J Am Acad Dermatol* 1984; **11**: 210–215.
3 Bornstein, S. Experimental infection of dogs with *Sarcoptes scabiei* derived from naturally infected wild red foxes (*Vulpes vulpes*): clinical observations. *Vet Dermatol* 1991; **2**: 151–159.
4 Mueller R, Bettenay SV, Shipstone M. Value of the pinnal–pedal reflex in the diagnosis of canine scabies. *Vet Rec* 2001; **148**: 621–623.
5 Lower KS, Medleau LM, Hnilica K, Bigler B. Evaluation of an enzyme-linked immunosorbent assay (ELISA) for the serological diagnosis of sarcoptic mange in dogs. *Vet Dermatol* 2001; **12**: 315–320.
6 Becskei C, De Bock F, Illambas J *et al.* Efficacy and safety of a novel oral isoxazoline, sarolaner (Simparica), for the treatment of sarcoptic mange in dogs. *Vet Parasitol* 2016; **222**: 56–61.
7 Romero C, Heredia R, Pineda J *et al.* Efficacy of fluralaner in 17 dogs with sarcoptic mange. *Vet Dermatol* 2016; **27**: 353.
8 Curtis CF. Current trends in the treatment of *Sarcoptes*, *Cheyletiella* and *Otodectes* mite infestations in dogs and cats. *Vet Dermatol* 2004; **15**: 108–114.
9 Fourie JJ, Horak IG, de la Puente Redondo V. Efficacy of a spot-on formulation of pyriprole on dogs infested with *Sarcoptes scabiei*. *Vet Rec* 2010; **167**: 442–445.

HARVEST MITE INFESTATION
(Trombiculiasis, chiggers)

Definition

A seasonal dermatosis associated with infestation of the parasitic larvae of harvest mites such as *Neotrombicula autumnalis* and *Eutrombicula alfredugesi*. A related burrowing mite, *Straelensia cynotis*, causes a papular-to-nodular dermatitis.

Aetiology and pathogenesis

Adult harvest mites are free living and non-parasitic. Eggs are laid in batches on vegetation in the late summer. The parasitic larvae (**Fig. 2.59**) infest the host in groups of up to several hundred, often clustering on the head, ears, feet or ventrum. The larvae feed for a few days and then leave. As infestation may be non-pruritic in some cases, it is probable that those individuals displaying pruritus develop a hypersensitivity to the mite or its products.

Clinical features

The infestation is a seasonal threat to the free-ranging dog or cat. However, infestations may occur all year round in warmer climates and changing weather patterns appear to be extending the season in northern Europe. Infested animals may be asymptomatic. Those displaying signs are pruritic. Examination of the affected area reveals clusters of orange–red larvae (**Fig. 2.60**), sometimes associated with a papular or crusting dermatitis.[1]

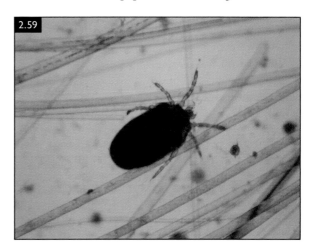

Fig. 2.59 Six-legged orange-red larva of *Neotrombicula autumnalis*.

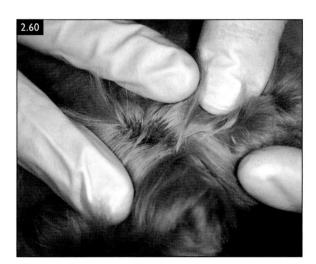

Fig. 2.60 Clusters of bright orange *Trombicula autumnalis* larvae in the interdigital skin of a Cocker Spaniel.

Most commonly, the mites are found in the interdigital regions, on the ventral abdomen, in the folds at the base of the pinnae or, in cats especially, the tip of the tail. Very heavy infestations have been associated with seasonal canine illness in the UK. This causes acute collapse and can be fatal. *Straelensia cynotis* is endemic to the Mediterranean area. Infestations in dogs are most common in hunting breeds that may go into the dens of foxes and other wild animals. The parasitic larvae burrow into the skin, forming pouches that result in a papular-to-nodular pruritic to painful dermatitis. The larvae may persist for several weeks to months.

Differential diagnoses
- Other parasites.
- Atopic dermatitis.
- Contact dermatitis.

Diagnosis
Careful examination of the affected areas will reveal tiny orange–red patches, which are clusters of larvae. In some cases, the mites have left the host before it is presented to the veterinarian and, in these cases, local knowledge of the disease is important, because summer seasonal pedal pruritus may suggest atopic dermatitis. Skin scrapes or skin biopsies are necessary to diagnose straelensia infestations.

Treatment
- As the larvae are a seasonal threat and associated with rough vegetation, the logical approach is to restrict access during periods of risk.
- There are not many studies on effectiveness of the newer parasiticides for treatment or prevention of these mites, although the isoxazolines have anecdotally shown some promise.
- Fipronil spray 0.25% is effective in treating infested dogs. When applied monthly it is effective in preventing infestations in dogs.[2,3] In a few cases local treatment may be necessary every 14 days.[2] Although fipronil spray is effective for treating infestations in cats, it will prevent reinfestation only for 7–10 days after application.[2]
- If mites are found on an affected animal, they may also be removed with a topical ectoparasitic aerosol, wash or dip.
- The pruritus usually abates quickly, but in some cases a short course of prednisolone (0.5–1.1 mg/kg po q12–24 h) may be necessary.
- Prompt removal of all mites, intravenous fluids and supportive care should be used for dogs with seasonal canine illness.
- *Straelensia* spp. may be difficult to treat.

Key point
- Trombiculiasis can cause a seasonal pruritic dermatitis that can mimic allergic dermatitis.

References
1 Greene RT, Scheidt VJ, Moncol DJ. Trombiculiasis in a cat. *J Am Vet Med Assoc* 1986; **188**: 1054–1055.
2 Nuttall TJ, French AT, Cheetman HC *et al.* Treatment of *Trombicula autmnalis* infestation in dogs and cats with 0.25 per cent fipronil pump spray. *J Small Anim Pract* 1998; **39**: 237–239.
3 Famose F. Efficacy of fipronil (Frontline) spray in the prevention of natural infestation by *Trombicula autumnalis* in dogs. In: *Proceedings of the Royal Veterinary College Seminar – Ectoparasites and Their Control, London*, 1995: pp. 28–30.

PEDICULOSIS
(Lice)

Definition
Pediculosis is a parasitic infestation with lice.

Aetiology and pathogenesis
Pediculosis infestations are predominantly seen in animals housed together, especially if they are young or debilitated. The most common species that infest dogs is the biting louse *Trichodectes canis*. Other species seen in warmer climates are the sucking lice *Linognathus setosus* and *Heterodoxus spineger*. The only species that infests cats is the biting louse *Felicola subrostratus*.

The entire life cycle is completed on the host within 3 weeks. Eggs ('nits') are laid on hairs and hatch into nymphs, which undergo several moults to become adults. Transmission occurs by direct contact or by grooming with contaminated brushes or combs. Lice are host specific, but transient contamination of other in-contact hosts, including humans, may be seen.

Clinical features
The clinical appearance is quite variable, from asymptomatic to severely pruritic with self-induced trauma and alopecia. Nits firmly attached to hair shafts and lice can be seen with the naked eye (**Fig. 2.61**), most commonly along the neck and dorsum of dogs, and the face, ears and dorsum of cats.[1] Lice also infest the heavily haired ears, ventrum and legs of some dog breeds. Heavy infestations with sucking lice may result in anaemia, especially in young animals.[1]

Differential diagnoses
- Other parasitic dermatoses – fleas, *Demodex gatoi* (cats) or other mites.
- Atopic or hypersensitivity dermatitis.
- Bacterial or yeast dermatitis.

Diagnosis
Diagnosis is based on finding lice or nits on the skin or hair. Lice are wingless, dorsoventrally flattened 1- to 2-mm insects with strong, gripping claws. Biting lice have broad heads, whereas sucking lice

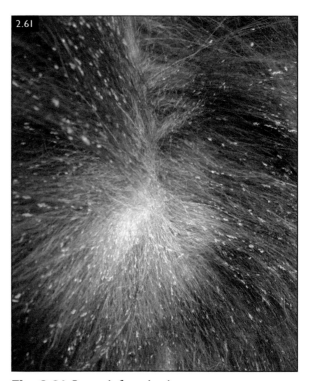

Fig. 2.61 Louse infestation in a cat.

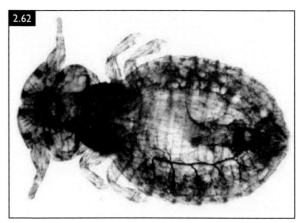

Fig. 2.62 *Trichodectes canis* (photo courtesy of Boerhinger Ingelheim Animal Health).

have narrow heads (**Figs. 2.62, 2.63**). Their eggs ('nits') are large, operculated and cemented to the hair shaft (**Fig. 2.64**).

Treatment
All pets in the household should be treated. Two treatments 14 days apart using pyrethrin sprays, shampoos or dips are effective in most cases; many

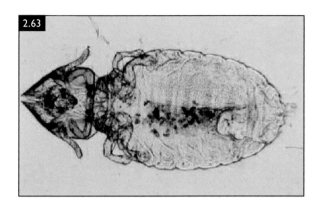

Fig. 2.63 *Felicola subrostratus* (photo courtesy of Boerhinger Ingelheim Animal Health).

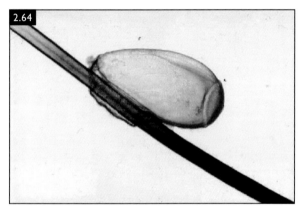

Fig. 2.64 Operculated louse egg tightly cemented to the hair shaft. In comparison, *Cheyletiella* eggs are smaller, bound to the hair shaft at the distal end by silken fibres, and are non-operculated (photo courtesy of Boerhinger Ingelheim Animal Health).

of these treatments may not be safe for use in cats. In cats, selamectin topically is very effective with a single application.[2] In dogs, single or multiple treatments with fipronil, selamectin, 65% permethrin and imidacloprid are also effective.[1-7] A single ivermectin injection (0.2 mg/kg sc) has been reported to be effective, but this is not licensed for dogs and cats, and is contraindicated in *MDR-1* gene mutant breeds. Fomites and bedding should be disinfected, although lice do not live long off the host.

Key point
• Lice are easily found and treated.

References
1 Arther RG. Mites and lice: biology and control. *Vet Clin North Am Small Anim Pract* 2009; **39**: 1159–1171.

2 Shanks DJ, Gautier P, McTier TL *et al*. Efficacy of selamectin against biting lice on dogs and cats. *Vet Rec* 2003; **152**: 234–237.

3 Endris RG, Reuter VE, Nelson J, Nelson JA. Efficacy of a topical spot-on containing 65% permethrin against the dog louse, *Trichodectes canis* (Mallophaga: Trichodectidae). *Vet Ther Res Appl Vet Med* 2000; **2**: 135–139.

4 Gunnarsson L, Christensson D, Palmér E. Clinical efficacy of selamectin in the treatment of naturally acquired infection of sucking lice (*Linognathus setosus*) in dogs. *J Am Anim Hosp Assoc* 2005; **41**: 388–394.

5 Kužner J, Turk S, Grace S *et al*. Confirmation of the efficacy of a novel fipronil spot-on for the treatment and control of fleas, ticks and chewing lice on dogs. *Vet Parasitol* 2013; **193**: 245–251.

6 Pollmeier M, Pengo G, Longo M, Jeannin P. Effective treatment and control of biting lice, *Felicola subrostratus* (Nitzsch in Burmeister, 1838), on cats using fipronil formulations. *Vet Parasitol* 2004; **121**: 157–165.

7 Pollmeier M, Pengo G, Jeannin P, Soll M. Evaluation of the efficacy of fipronil formulations in the treatment and control of biting lice, *Trichodectes canis* (De Geer, 1778) on dogs. *Vet Parasitol* **107**: 2002; 127–136.

NEUROGENIC DERMATOSES
(Including feline orofacial pain
syndrome, trigeminal neuropathy,
feline idiopathic ulcerative dermatosis,
syringomyelia, sensory neuropathy
and tail dock neuroma)

Feline orofacial pain syndrome is most commonly seen as oral discomfort and tongue mutilation in Burmese cats. These cats most commonly present for pawing at the mouth or making exaggerated licking and chewing movements. There do not appear to be sensory defects, and it is proposed that this condition is similar to trigeminal neuralgia in humans.[1] The mean age of cats at first appearance is 7 years (range 1 month–19 years); 26 of 113 cats had one episode or responded to treatments, 75 of 113 had ongoing symptoms, although many years apart in many cats.[1] Stress or oral pain seemed to play a role in many of the cats' onset of symptoms; 12 of 113 cats were euthanised due to symptoms. Treatments include the elimination of any oral/dental pain, nonsteroidal anti-inflammatory drugs, corticosteroids, antibiotics, opioids, phenobarbital, megoestrol and others, including combination therapies. It appeared from the study that phenobarbital (2–3 mg/kg po or im q12 h) worked better than other therapies. Carbamazepine, oxcarbazepine, pregabalin and topiramate are used in humans for trigeminal neuralgia or nerve pain, and may prove useful in cats. Topiramate and gabapentin have anecdotally been used successfully in a few cats. Anecdotally, the antiviral famciclovir may also be helpful if this condition is triggered by herpesvirus.

Trigeminal neuropathy due to a schwannoma of the trigeminal nerve has been reported in a dog, which presented for masticatory muscle atrophy and scratching at one side of the face.[2]

Feline idiopathic ulcerative dermatosis is thought to be caused by neuropathic pruritus.[3] The condition starts out as a small pruritic ulcer, caused by scratching between the cat's scapulae or on the dorsal neck (**Fig. 2.65**). Violent scratching episodes progressively widen the ulcer and cause fibrosis of the ulcer margins. Differentials would include any other pruritic dermatosis, and all would need to be ruled out with cytology, skin scrapings, treatment trials

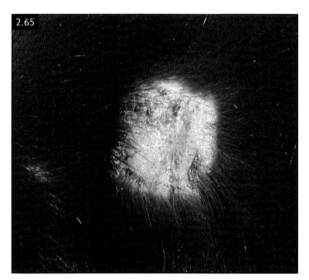

Fig. 2.65 Feline ulcerative dermatitis with a well-circumscribed, severe, deep and crusted ulcer on the dorsal neck of a domestic short-haired cat.

and biopsy. This disease is visually quite characteristic when it is the only abnormality on the cat's skin, and includes episodic violent pruritus resulting in a deep lesion. Many of these lesions respond to bandaging (to prevent further trauma) and glucocorticoids until the lesion has completely healed. Surgery to remove the affected skin may be curative in some cases. There is one report of successful management using topiramate 5 mg/kg po q12 h.[3] (See page 157.)

Syringomyelia is a condition most commonly described in Cavalier King Charles Spaniels associated with abnormal atlantoaxial morphology (Chiari-like malformation), altered cerebrospinal fluid dynamics and damage to the spinal cord. This can result in neurogenic pain and pruritus, often manifesting as scratching and rubbing of the cranial shoulder and lateral neck. Syringomyelia is best diagnosed and managed by a neurologist, because it may involve neurological tests, radiography and MRI. Surgery is rarely performed, because in dogs it is not as helpful as in humans, so treatments are generally medical.[4] Treatment options include cyclooxygenase 2 (COX-2) inhibitors, glucocorticoids, opioids and specific drugs for nerve pain such as gabapentin or pregabalin.[4,5] In one study in which dogs were treated intermittently with gabapentin, pregabalin and/or carprofen, 7 of 48 dogs were euthanised due to disease, 12 were the same or improved over time and 24 worsened with their symptoms.[5] Most owners felt the quality of their dog's life was acceptable. Care should be taken to recognise and manage concurrent atopic dermatitis and primary secretory otitis media, which are also common in Cavalier King Charles Spaniels and may present with similar clinical signs.

Acral mutilation syndrome in puppies is a sensory neuropathic condition in which dogs start, at a very young age, to lick and chew at the feet to the point of severe trauma, including self-amputation of digits. Dogs with this condition appear to feel no pain (see page 242).

Tail dock neuroma is caused by abnormal healing of the tail tip after docking. Dogs repeatedly self-traumatise the tail tip and the tail is very painful on light palpation. The treatment is surgical removal of the neuroma tissue, including the distal vertebra, which is curative in most cases.[6]

References

1   Rusbridge C, Heath S, Gunn-Moore DA, Knowler SP, Johnston N, McFadyen AK. Feline orofacial pain syndrome (FOPS): a retrospective study of 113 cases. *J Feline Med Surg* 2010; **12**: 498–508.

2   Saunders JH, Poncelet L, Clercx C *et al*. Probable trigeminal nerve schwannoma in a dog. *Vet Radiol Ultrasound* 1998; **39**: 539–542.

3   Grant D, Rusbridge C. Topiramate in the management of feline idiopathic ulcerative dermatitis in a two-year-old cat. *Vet Dermatol* 2014; **25**: 226–e60.

4   Rusbridge C, Jeffery ND. Pathophysiology and treatment of neuropathic pain associated with syringomyelia. *Vet J* 2008; **175**: 164–172.

5   Plessas IN, Rushbridge C, Driver CJ *et al*. Long-term outcome of Cavalier King Charles spaniel dogs with clinical signs associated with Chiari-like malformation and syringomyelia. *Vet Rec* 2012; **171**: 501.

6   Gross TL, Carr SH. Amputation neuroma of docked tails in dogs. *Vet Pathol Online* 1990; **27**: 61–62.

GENERAL APPROACH TO PAPULES, PUSTULES AND CRUSTS

The most common differentials include demodicosis, ectoparasites, pyoderma, dermatophytosis and pemphigus foliaceus. Pruritus may or may not be present with any of these differentials.

The following diagnostics should be performed when seeking a diagnosis for papules, pustules and crusts:

- Hair plucks, tape-strips and/or deep skin scrapings to rule demodicosis in or out.
- Tape preparations and impression smears to rule pyoderma in or out.

- Wood's lamp, hair plucks and fungal culture to rule dermatophytosis in or out.
- Treatment trial with a parasiticide to rule ectoparasites in or out.
- Cytology and biopsies of crusts and/or pustules to rule pemphigus foliaceus in or out, or diagnose a less common dermatosis. Biopsies are most diagnostic when secondary infections are controlled first.

SURFACE AND SUPERFICIAL PYODERMA

Definition
Superficial pyoderma describes cutaneous bacterial infection that is confined to the surface, stratum corneum or superficial epidermis of the skin and hair follicles.

Aetiology and pathogenesis
Normal canine and feline skin is colonised by a variety of resident bacterial and fungal organisms. These are not normally pathogenic and may help prevent colonisation by pathogenic species through niche competition. Potential pathogens such as coagulase-positive staphylococci frequently colonise mucocutaneous junctions and may spread to the skin by licking and grooming. Mucosal reservoirs are, therefore, an important source of transient contamination and potential infection. The vast majority of skin and ear infections involve opportunistic commensal organisms.

Primary or idiopathic recurrent superficial pyoderma is rare, and virtually all recurrent pyodermas are secondary to underlying cutaneous or systemic disorders such as ectoparasites, hypersensitivities, endocrinopathies and keratinisation defects (*Table 3.1*).

The vast majority of canine pyodermas are associated with coagulase-positive staphylococci. The most common species is *Staphylococcus pseudintermedius*[1,2], although *S. aureus*, *S. hyicus* and *S. schleiferi* have also been isolated, particularly in North America.

Superficial pyoderma is much less common in cats, and is associated with a wider range of organisms including *S. pseudintermedius*, *S. felis*, *S. aureus*, *Pasteurella multocida* and anaerobes (although the last are more common in abscesses).[1]

Antimicrobial-resistant (AMR) bacteria, including meticillin-resistant *S. pseudintermedius* (MRSP), *S. aureus* (MRSA) and *S. schleiferi* (MRSS), have been

Table 3.1 **Primary causes of superficial pyoderma**	
UNDERLYING CAUSE	**AETIOLOGY**
Allergic, pruritic and inflammatory dermatoses	Self-trauma and skin barrier abnormalities allow for proliferation of bacteria
Keratinisation defects	Disordered desquamation and abnormal skin barrier; altered sebum, follicular hyperkeratosis and obstruction
Endocrinopathies and metabolic diseases	Immunosuppression; keratinisation defects
Immunosuppression	Congenital or acquired immunodeficiency impact cutaneous immune system
Anatomy	Body folds and thick coats increase temperature and moisture and lead to break down of the skin barrier
Iatrogenic	Overbathing, poor nutrition and dirty environment

isolated from dogs and cats. Systemic antimicrobials are critically important in veterinary healthcare and resistance is a major concern. Clinicians must exercise antimicrobial stewardship to maintain clinical efficacy and reduce the development and spread of AMR. Appropriate management of bacterial infections is therefore crucial in any policy for responsible antimicrobial use. The goals of therapy are to confirm that an infection is present, identify the causative bacteria, select the most appropriate antimicrobial, ensure that the infection is treated correctly and identify and manage any underlying conditions to avoid recurrent antimicrobial treatment.

Clinical features

In general, surface and superficial pyodermas are associated with pruritus, erythema, papules, pustules, epidermal collarettes and multi-focal alopecia. Pain, swelling, sinus tracts and haemorrhage are not features of surface and superficial infections, and are associated with deep infections (see page 195). Usually, lesions occur on the groin and axillae; however, any part of the skin may be affected including the dorsum and muzzle. The various clinical phenotypes of pyoderma are described below.

Seborrhoeic pyoderma: erythema, erosion and exudation without pustules and collarettes

Bacterial overgrowth syndrome

Bacterial overgrowth syndrome is characterised by diffuse erythema, scales, a greasy keratoseborrhoeic exudate, pruritus and odour. The abdomen, interdigital skin and pinnae are most commonly affected.

Cytology reveals an excessive number of bacteria with few to no neutrophils.

Intertrigo (Figs. 3.1–3.4)

Intertrigo is infection of skinfolds caused by friction, irritation and lack of ventilation. It is common in axillary, facial (especially in brachycephalic breeds), tail, vulval and other body folds. The affected skin is moist, greasy, erythematous and hyperpigmented, and may harbour a whitish malodorous exudate.

Papules, pustules, scaling and focal alopecia

Impetigo

Impetigo (**Fig. 3.5**) causes non-follicular pustules, with secondary epidermal collarettes and scaling. Impetigo occurs in young animals, particularly if they are poorly cared for. Older animals that are immunosuppressed (e.g. hypothyroidism, hyperadrenocorticism, diabetes mellitus and chemotherapy) may also be affected. Impetigo is not typically pruritic.

Folliculitis

Folliculitis (**Fig. 3.6**) is the most common form of pyoderma. The papules and pustules are small and associated with a hair follicle. Short-haired dogs often present with patchy tufting of the hairs, which are shed, leaving small oval patches of alopecia and hyperpigmentation with a scaly rim (**Fig. 3.7**). Epidermal collarettes are common. The muzzle, dorsum, legs and groin are commonly affected areas. Bacterial folliculitis is an uncommon cause of miliary dermatitis in cats. See Canine acne, page 75.

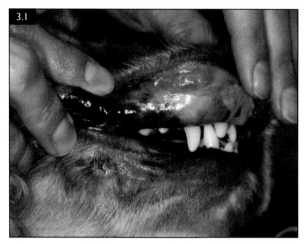

Fig. 3.1 Lip fold dermatitis with alopecia, erythema and ulceration of the lower lip fold in a Cocker Spaniel. There is a corresponding lesion on the upper buccal mucosa.

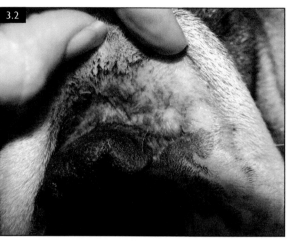

Fig. 3.2 Facial fold dermatitis in an English Bulldog – the fold must be lifted to reveal the lesions.

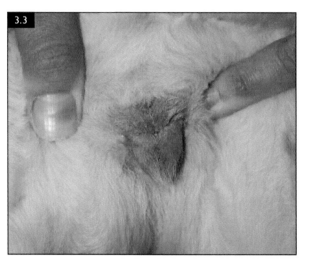

Fig. 3.3 Vulval fold dermatitis in a dog with a small and recessed vulva. This must be manually everted to see the extent of the lesions.

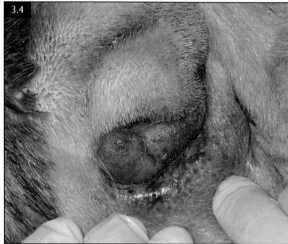

Fig. 3.4 Erythema, seborrhoea and ulceration around a pronounced screwtail in an English Bulldog.

Fig. 3.5 Bullous impetigo in a dog with hyperadrenocorticism.

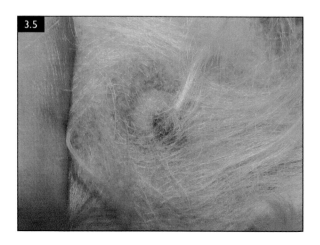

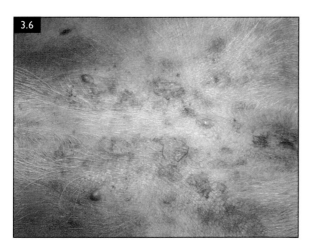

Fig. 3.6 Erythematous papules, pustules and epidermal collarettes in a dog with bacterial folliculitis.

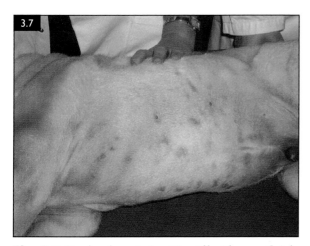

Fig. 3.7 Patchy alopecia in a Mastiff with superficial pyoderma.

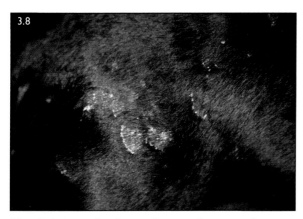

Fig. 3.8 Superficial spreading pyoderma on the lateral flank of a Dachshund.

Superficial spreading pyoderma

Superficial spreading pyoderma (**Fig. 3.8**) is characterised by large, spreading and coalescing epidermal collarettes, with an erythematous, moist, leading edge. Pustules are generally not observed. Some forms result in large areas of erythema and exfoliation. This is most common on the ventral abdomen.

Erosions and/or ulcers
Intertrigo
In severe cases of skinfold pyoderma, the skin may be eroded or ulcerated, and very painful.

Pyotraumatic dermatitis (acute moist dermatitis or 'hot spots')
Pyotraumatic dermatitis is an acute superficial, exudative, highly pruritic and possibly painful bacterial infection caused by repeated self-trauma. Initially there is a rapid well-defined area of moist skin and coat with mild surface erosion (**Fig. 3.9**). This may evolve into a superficial folliculitis or a deep furunculosis with alopecia, erythema, papules, erosion, exudation and ulceration (**Fig. 3.10**). The affected skin becomes thickened and painful, especially if there are deep lesions. Clinically mild erosions may be associated with folliculitis or furunculosis hidden in the surrounding haired skin ('satellite lesions') (**Fig. 3.11**). These lesions can be seen in heavily haired moist areas and near areas of focal itch or pain (especially the ears and tail head). Mild lesions respond to cleaning and topical steroids.

Mucocutaneous pyoderma
Mucocutaneous pyoderma is characterised by erythema, exudation, ulceration and crusting of the lips and other mucocutaneous junctions. It can be mistaken for autoimmune diseases or epitheliotrophic lymphoma but, unlike these, responds completely to antibiotic therapy. Mucocutaneous pyoderma can occur in any breed, but German Shepherd dogs may be predisposed.

Differential diagnoses
- Demodicosis.
- Dermatophytosis.
- Malassezia dermatitis.
- Pemphigus foliaceus.
- Zinc-responsive dermatosis.
- Dermatophilosis.

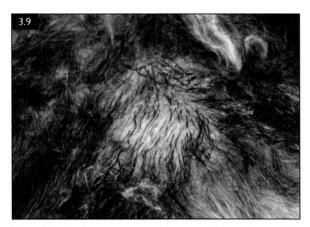

Fig. 3.9 Early pyotraumatic dermatitis in a dog with a well-demarcated area of erythema, matted hair and a moist exudate.

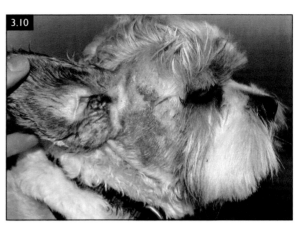

Fig. 3.10 Pyotraumatic dermatitis secondary to otitis externa with a well-demarcated area of erythema, erosion, alopecia and exudation.

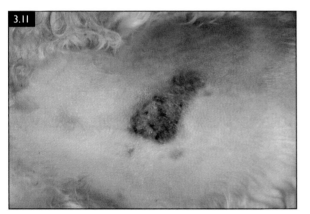

Fig. 3.11 Pyotraumatic furunculosis with deep trauma and infection at a venepuncture site.

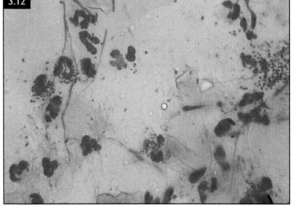

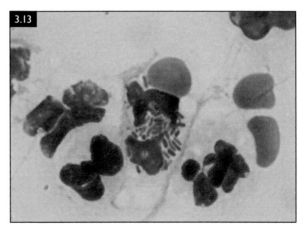

Note: many of these conditions may trigger a secondary pyoderma.

Diagnosis

The clinical signs are highly suggestive, although not specific. Impression smear, adhesive tape-strip and aspirate cytology may reveal degenerate neutrophils and intracellular cocci (**Fig. 3.12**) or rods (**Fig. 3.13**). DiffQuik®-type stains are convenient to use in practice, and stain most microorganisms dark blue–purple (they do not differentiate between gram-positive and gram-negative bacteria). Biopsy and histopathology can also identify infections and help to confirm or rule out underlying conditions.

Figs. 3.12, 3.13 Degenerate neutrophils with extra- and intracellular cocci (Fig. 3.12) and rods (Fig. 3.13) (Diff-Quik®-stained impression smears, ×1000.)

Histopathology is a less sensitive method of detecting pyoderma compared with surface cytology. Bacterial culture is not necessary in all cases, as most staphylococci have a predictable antibiotic sensitivity pattern (*Table 3.2*).

Samples for culture can be obtained by swabbing the underside of crusts, the margin of epidermal collarettes or ruptured pustules. Antibiotic withdrawal is not necessary before obtaining a culture but inform the lab about recent or ongoing antimicrobial therapy. Surface cytology should be performed at the time of the culture, and the cytology results should be compared with the culture results.

The clinician should suspect an inaccurate test result if the cytology and culture do not correlate. It is important to interpret antibiotic susceptibility results carefully (*Tables 3.3–3.5*). In particular, in-vitro susceptibility tests are poorly predictive of the response to topical therapy, which delivers concentrations in milligram per millilitre far in excess of most MICs (which are in microgram per millilitre ranges).

Treatment

Overly long courses of treatment should be avoided wherever possible. In general, superficial pyoderma

---

Table 3.2 When to use empirical antimicrobial therapy and when to consider bacterial culture and antimicrobial susceptibility testing

EMPIRICAL THERAPY	PERFORM CULTURE	WHEN TO SUSPECT ANTIMICROBIAL RESISTANCE
• Surface or superficial pyoderma • First episode of pyoderma • No systemic antimicrobial treatment within 3 months • Topical therapy • Cytology consistent with staphylococci • Non-life threatening infection • No reason to suspect antimicrobial resistance	• Deep pyoderma • After multiple courses of antimicrobials • Systemic antimicrobial use within 3 months • Cytology reveals rods • Inconsistent clinical signs and cytology • Life threatening infection • Any reason to suspect antimicrobial resistance • Treatment failure	• Treatment failure • Nosocomial (i.e. clinic-associated) infection • Intensive care with catheters and/or other implants • Postoperative infection • Non-healing wounds (especially postoperative)

Table 3.3 Interpreting bacterial culture and susceptibility results

Testing methods	
Kirby–Bauer disc diffusion	Report sensitive, resistant or intermediate based on the zone of inhibition around the antibiotic discs
Minimum inhibitory concentration (MIC)	Report sensitive, resistant or intermediate based on the MIC compared with the predicted tissue levels after systemic administration
Results	
Sensitive	It is likely that tissue levels of the antibiotic will exceed the MIC after systemic dosing and the infection should respond to treatment
Resistant	Tissue levels of the antibiotic are unlikely to exceed the MIC after systemic dosing and the infection is not likely to respond to treatment
Intermediate	In most cases tissue levels of the antibiotic will not exceed the MIC after systemic dosing; however, the infection may respond to treatment if high doses can be used and/or the drug concentrates in the infected tissues
MIC range	Drugs with an MIC several dilutions below the breakpoint are more effective as they attain a higher effective concentration in the infected tissue and are less affected by variation in pharmacokinetics, tissue penetration and bacterial populations

---

Table 3.4 Mismatches between antimicrobial susceptibility tests and the clinical response

- In-vitro versus in-vivo environment (inflammation and immunity, tissue responses, underlying diseases, blood flow, pharmacokinetics, drug penetration, etc.)
- Compliance and administration
- Laboratory variation and error
- Course of treatment too short
- Culture is not representative of the infection
- Skin lesions are not caused by a bacterial agent
- Apparent in-vitro susceptibility to β-lactam drugs with some MRSA and MRSP and extended spectrum β-lactamase (ESBL)-producing *Escherichia coli* should be checked – speak to your lab about tests for penicillin-binding protein 2a (PBP2a) or PCR for *mec*A and ESBL genes (especially AmpC)
- MRSA and MRSP isolates showing apparent in-vitro susceptibility to clindamycin should be checked for inducible clindamycin resistance (*erm* genes or an erythromycin D-zone test) to ensure that this drug will be effective
- Enrofloxacin is a prodrug that is part metabolised into ciprofloxacin – tests based on enrofloxacin or ciprofloxacin may not accurately reflect tissue levels of the two drugs in combination

AmpC, ampC beta-lactamases; MRSA, meticillin-resistant *Staphylococcus aureus*; MRSP, meticillin-resistant *Staphylococcus pseudintermedius*; PCR, polymerase chain reaction.

Table 3.5 Predicting drug–specific antimicrobial susceptibility patterns using in-vitro sensitivity tests

ANTIMICROBIAL	SUSCEPTIBILITY PATTERNS AND PREDICTIONS
Amikacin	Predicts resistance to other aminoglycosides; susceptibility does not imply susceptibility to gentamicin (see below)
Amoxicillin–clavulanate	ESBL-producing isolates sensitive to amoxicillin–clavulanate but resistant to cephalosporins AmpC-producing isolates are resistant to amoxicillin–clavulanate and cephalosporins
Ampicillin	Predicts susceptibility to amoxicillin in all bacteria and to penicillin in gram-positive bacteria
Cephalexin	Predicts susceptibility to first and second-generation cephalosporins (including cefovecin) ESBL- and AmpC-producing isolates are resistant (see note above for amoxicillin–clavulanate)
Cefoxitin	MRSA and MRSP are resistant EBSL-producing isolates are susceptible AmpC-producing isolates are resistant
Cefotaxime	Predicts susceptibility to all third-generation cephalosporins (not cefovecin)
Chloramphenicol	Predicts susceptibility to florfenicol
Clindamycin	Predicts susceptibility to all lincosamides (lincomycin) in gram-positive bacteria; inducible resistance should be ruled out by susceptibility to erythromycin (see below) or PCR
Doxycycline	Predicts susceptibility to tetracyclines in gram-positive bacteria (including MRSA/MRSP) Specific susceptibility should be used with gram-negative bacteria
Enrofloxacin or marbofloxacin	Predicts susceptibility to other fluoroquinolones in all bacteria except anaerobes (extended spectrum with pradofloxacin); enrofloxacin is part metabolised into ciprofloxacin so in-vitro susceptibility may not predict in-vivo efficacy
Erythromycin	Predicts inducible resistance to lincosamides (lincomycin and clindamycin); do not use these drugs if the isolate is resistant to erythromycin
Gentamicin	Predicts susceptibility to other aminoglycosides; resistant isolates may still be susceptible to amikacin
Nitrofurantoin	Can be used to treat multi-drug-resistant urinary tract infections
Sulfamethoxazole	Predicts susceptibility or resistance to all sulphonamides
Tetracycline	Predicts susceptibility to doxycycline in gram-positive bacteria (including MRSA/MRSP) Specific susceptibility should be used with gram-negative bacteria

AmpC, ampC beta-lactamases; ESBL, extended spectrum β-lactamase; MRSA, meticillin-resistant *Staphylococcus aureus*; MRSP, meticillin-resistant *Staphylococcus pseudintermedius*; PCR, polymerase chain reaction.

should be treated to a complete clinical cure (i.e. complete resolution of clinical signs and normal cytology). If in doubt, treatment can be continued for a further week beyond apparent clinical resolution.

Topical therapy[1,3]

Topical treatments (*Table 3.6*) should be employed whenever possible to reduce or avoid use of antibiotics. Minimising systemic antibiotic use decreases risk of multi-drug resistant (MDR) and meticillin-resistant staphylococci. Topical therapy softens and removes crusts ameliorates pain and pruritus and induces peripheral vasodilatation, which promotes healing and antibiotic distribution to the skin. Benzoyl peroxide, chlorhexidine, povidone–iodine, hydrogen peroxide, silver compounds, medical honey and sodium hypochlorite dilutions all have the potential to effectively resolve superficial pyoderma. Chlorhexidine products appear to be the most effective; studies have shown that bathing two to three times weekly with chlorhexidine shampoos was as effective as systemic amoxicillin–clavulanate in canine superficial pyoderma. Effectiveness increases if the topical treatment has a contact time of at least 5 minutes, with whirlpool baths and if treatments are repeated daily. Pyodermas typically need at least 2 weeks of treatment for resolution, but some may require up to 8 weeks of topical treatment. The length of time required often depends on what the underlying cause of the pyoderma is, and how quickly it can be brought under control.[1] Regular use of topical antimicrobials can also help prevent recurrent colonisation and infection of the skin.

Staphage lysate injections

Immunostimulants such as staphage lysate are useful for the treatment and prevention of recurrent pyoderma. This treatment is effective for dogs with atopic dermatitis as the underlying cause of pyoderma, and pyoderma recurs at least four times a year. Injections are generally given subcutaneously once or twice weekly for 10–12 weeks, then every 7–30 days for maintenance. Adverse effects are rare, but can include injection site reactions, pyrexia, malaise and anaphylaxis.

Topical antibiotics

Topical antibiotics can be useful in focal lesions, although patients should be carefully checked for more generalised disease. It may also be necessary to treat the ears, mucocutaneous junctions and feet, because these are probably reservoirs of staphylococcal organisms.

Gentamicin is a commonly available topical antibiotic that is found in ointments labelled for treatment of otitis externa. Otic ointments containing gentamicin can be applied twice daily to focal pyoderma lesions. Fusidic acid or fusidate is also effective. Mupirocin 2% has excellent antistaphylococcal activity. However, it should be reserved for cases of meticillin-resistant staphylococci or cases with hyperplastic lesions (i.e. interdigital furunculosis). Mupirocin should be applied twice daily until the pyoderma has resolved.

Systemic antibiotics[4]

It is beyond the scope of this book to provide a complete overview of available antibiotics. The choice

Table 3.6 **Useful shampoos**		
PREPARATION	**ADVANTAGES**	**OTHER CONSIDERATIONS**
2.5% benzoyl peroxide	Excellent antibacterial activity, degreasing, keratolytic, follicular flushing, residual activity	May be drying or irritating, may bleach dark coats, contact sensitiser, toxic to cats
10% ethyl lactate	Excellent antibacterial activity, keratoplastic	Much less drying, safe in cats
2%–4% chlorhexidine	Excellent antibacterial activity, residual activity	Higher concentrations may be irritating, safe in cats
2%sulphur/2%salicylic acid	Antibacterial, residual activity	Safe in cats
Triclosan	Antibacterial	
1% selenium sulphide	Antibacterial, keratolytic	May be drying or irritating, may bleach dark coats, safe in cats

will depend on the species, age and breed of the patient, the target organism and the type of lesion, as well as the owner's commitment, drug availability and licensing regulations. Before using systemic antibiotics, it is important to ensure that a firm diagnosis of infection, using clinical signs and cytology, has been made. Remember also that mild, localised infections may not always need treatment. For example, mild focal pyoderma in an atopic dog will probably resolve once the atopic inflammation has been controlled (particularly if topical antimicrobials are used).

The general principles in choosing an antibiotic include the following:

- It should have activity against staphylococci. Most strains produce β-lactamase, conferring resistance to penicillins. Resistance to tetracyclines is also widespread and resistance to macrolides can be frequent in some countries and areas.
- It should reach the skin at an adequate concentration.
- The frequency of administration depends on whether the drug is concentration (e.g. fluoroquinolones) or time (e.g. penicillins) dependent. The efficacy of concentration-dependent drugs is reliant on delivering pulses 8–10 × MIC once daily. Time-dependent drugs require concentrations above the MIC for at least 70% of the dosing interval; these must be administered every 8–12 hours depending on the half-life. Compliance with the dosing regimen is therefore very important in ensuring clinical efficacy and avoiding resistance.
- Ideally, bactericidal antibiotics should be used, although bacteriostatic drugs are equally effective provided that the immune system is competent.
- Drugs that accumulate in phagocytes (e.g. fluoroquinolones, lincosamides and macrolides) kill intracellular bacteria and penetrate inflamed tissues. Purulent exudate and necrotic debris can inactivate trimethoprim-potentiated sulphonamides (TMPSs), macrolides, lincosamides and aminoglycosides. Lipid-soluble antibiotics with a high volume of distribution

(e.g. fluoroquinolones and rifampin) penetrate well into chronically inflamed and fibrosed skin. In contrast, penetration of water-soluble antibiotics with a low volume of distribution (e.g. penicillins) may be limited.
- Narrow-spectrum antibiotics (e.g. erythromycin, lincomycin, clindamycin, oxacillin and cloxacillin) are preferable, because broad-spectrum drugs are more likely to upset the gut flora and select for resistance among *Escherichia coli*. However, few narrow-spectrum drugs have a veterinary licence.
- Consider any potential interaction with underlying conditions and concurrent treatment, and adverse effects (e.g. sulphonamides in Dobermans).
- Regular exams and cytology are necessary to ensure that the infection has resolved before stopping therapy. Most superficial pyodermas resolve within 2–3 weeks; deep pyodermas may require 4–6 weeks or longer.

Table 3.7 gives useful antibiotics for superficial pyoderma.

Meticillin-resistant staphylococci (MRS)

These are resistant to most antibiotics, and antibiotic selection should be based on culture. Topical antiseptics and antibiotics are especially important in aiding resolution of MRS pyoderma. In addition, the underlying cause of the infection must be addressed, great care must be taken when handling these cases in the clinic and appropriate healthcare advice must be given to the owners. The complex management of these cases often requires referral to a specialist centre.

Antibiotic resistance

Antibiotic use inevitably selects for resistance. Macrolides and lincosamides (e.g. lincomycin, erythromycin, clindamycin and clarithromycin) tend to induce cross-resistance and should not be used for long-term treatment. Rifampin must be administered with a bactericidal antibiotic (except fluoroquinolones) to avoid the rapid development of resistance. Inducible clindamycin resistance is common in MRS, and repeated courses of broad-spectrum antibiotics

Table 3.7 **Useful antibiotics for superficial pyoderma**

ANTIBIOTIC	DOSAGE	ADVERSE EFFECTS
TMPS (also ormetoprim and baquiloprim-potentiated drugs)	15–30 mg/kg po q12 h	Can cause keratoconjunctivitis sicca, sick euthyroid syndrome and cutaneous drug reactions (especially in Dobermans)
Erythromycin*	10–20 mg/kg po q8 h	Can cause gastrointestinal upset
Lincomycin	15–30 mg/kg po q8–12 h	
Clindamycin	5.5–11 mg/kg po q12 h or 11 mg/kg po q24 h	
Cephalexin	22–30 mg/kg po q12 h	Can cause gastrointestinal upset
Cefadroxil	10–20 mg/kg po q12 h	
Cefpodoxime proxetil	5–10 mg/kg po q24 h	
Cefovecin	8 mg/kg sc q14d	
Clavulanate-potentiated amoxicillin	12.5 mg/kg po q8–12 h or 22 mg/kg po q12 h	
Oxacilin, cloxacillin*	20 mg/kg po q8 h	
Enrofloxacin	5–20 mg/kg po q24 h	Can cause cartilage damage in dogs <12 months of age (18 months in giant breeds), neurological signs at high doses and blindness in cats; may also cause gastrointestinal upset; reserve use for resistant bacteria
Marbofloxacin	2–5.5 mg/kg po q24 h	
Difloxacin	5–10 mg/kg po q24 h	
Orbifloxacin	2.5–7.5 mg/kg po q24 h	
Pradofloxacin	3 mg/kg q24 h	Extended spectrum activity against some anaerobic bacteria

* Not licensed for use in animals. po, by mouth; sc, subcutaneous; TMPS, trimethoprim-potentiated sulphonamide.

are risk factors for the acquisition of MRS colonisation and/or infection.

Good practice to limit antibiotic resistance
The factors that influence prevalence of resistance are listed below:

- Inappropriate case selection.
- Inappropriate drug.
- Poor compliance.
- Low dose.
- Infrequent treatment.
- Short treatment periods.
- Low efficacy.

Fluoroquinolones and drugs licensed for humans such as anti-*Pseudomonas* penicillins and ceftazidime are very important to humans and animals, particularly against MDR gram-negative organisms. They should be used only where culture and sensitivity indicate that they are necessary. Drugs vitally important to human health (e.g. vancomycin, teicoplanin and carbapenems) should probably never be used in animals.

Treatment of recurrent pyoderma[1,3]
Recurrent pyoderma typically decreases in frequency and severity if the underlying cause (e.g. atopic dermatitis, adverse reaction to food, demodicosis, endocrine disease) can be corrected. If the underlying disease cannot be corrected, then the individual must have antiseptic applied to the skin regularly to avoid frequent courses of antibiotics. Staphage lysate may also be helpful.

Key points
- Topical therapy speeds resolution of infection, decreases antibiotic use and helps prevent MRS.
- If meticillin resistance is encountered, attempts should be made to resolve the pyoderma without

using antibiotics. Discontinuing antibiotic use may cause resistant bacteria to revert to normal antibiotic susceptibilities.

- Pyoderma is almost always secondary to another problem. Pyoderma will recur until the underlying problem has been addressed.
- Resolution of lesions may take 2–8 weeks depending on the underlying cause and comorbidities.

WARNING

These guidelines are the opinions of the authors based on published evidence and guidelines as well as their personal experience. The treatment options include off-label or off-cascade suggestions. Any decision on treatment protocols for a particular case remains the complete responsibility of the prescribing veterinarian. In particular, veterinarians must be aware of relevant medicines legislation and whether it is legal to administer certain antimicrobials in their country of work.

References

1 Mueller RS, Bergvall K, Bensignor E, Bond R. A review of topical therapy for skin infections with bacteria and yeast. *Vet Dermatol* 2012; **23**: 330–e62.
2 Yu HW, Vogelnest LJ. Feline superficial pyoderma: a retrospective study of 52 cases (2001–2011). *Vet Dermatol* 2012; **23**: 448–e86.
3 Borio S, Colombo S, La Rosa G, De Lucia M, Damborg P, Guardabassi L. Effectiveness of a combined (4% chlorhexidine digluconate shampoo and solution) protocol in MRS and non-MRS canine superficial pyoderma: a randomised, blinded, antibiotic-controlled study. *Vet Dermatol* 2015; **26**: 339–e72.
4 Summers JF, Brodbelt DC, Forsythe PJ, Loeffler A, Hendricks A. The effectiveness of systemic antimicrobial treatment in canine superficial and deep pyoderma: a systematic review. *Vet Dermatol* 2012; **23**: 305–e61.

Further reading

Beco L, Guaguère E, Lorente Mendez C, Noli C, Nuttall TJ, Vroom M. Suggested guidelines for using systemic antimicrobials in bacterial skin infections: part one – diagnosis based on clinical presentation, cytology and culture. *Vet Rec* 2013; **172**: 72–78.
Beco L, Guaguère E, Lorente Mendez C, Noli C, Nuttall TJ, Vroom M. Suggested guidelines for using systemic antimicrobials in bacterial skin infections: part two – antimicrobial choice, treatment regimens and compliance. *Vet Rec* 2013; **172**: 156–160.
Brissot H, Cervantes S, Guardabassi L *et al. Guidance for the Rational Use of Antimicrobials* (GRAM). France: Ceva Sante Animale, 2016.
Hillier A, Lloyd DH, Weese JS *et al.* (2014) Guidelines for the diagnosis and antimicrobial therapy of canine superficial bacterial folliculitis (Antimicrobial Guidelines Working Group of the International Society for Companion Animal Infectious Diseases). *Vet Dermatol* **25**: 163–75.
Morris DO, Loeffler A, Davis MF, Guardabassi L, Weese JS. Recommendations for approaches to meticillin resistant staphylococcal infections of small animals: diagnosis, therapeutic considerations, and preventative considerations and preventative measures. Clinical Consensus Guidelines of the World Association for Veterinary Dermatology. *Vet Dermatol* 2017; **28**: 304–e69.

CANINE ACNE
(Chin and muzzle folliculitis and furunculosis)

Definition
Canine acne is a papular and/or pustular dermatosis associated with folliculitis and furunculosis.

Aetiology and pathogenesis
Follicular plugging and parafollicular inflammation may predispose to follicular rupture. This results in a foreign body reaction and secondary bacterial infection. The condition resolves spontaneously in many animals when they reach adulthood, although some individuals remain affected for life. In many dogs the lesions are associated with underlying diseases such as hypothyroidism, atopic dermatitis, adverse food reactions or lifestyles that result in trauma to the affected skin. *Trichophyton mentagrophytes* should be considered (see page 85).

Clinical features
Canine acne occurs most commonly over the chin and lips of young, short-coated breeds of dogs such

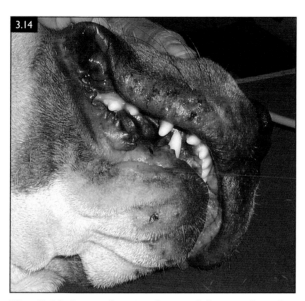

Fig. 3.14 Severe deep pyoderma of the muzzle and lips in a Bullmastiff.

as the Doberman Pinscher, English Bulldog, Great Dane, Weimaraner, Rottweiler, Boxer and German Short-haired Pointer. Lesions consist of follicular papules and/or pustules that may ulcerate and fistulate, draining a serosanguineous-to-seropurulent material (**Fig. 3.14**). Follicles may rupture (furunculosis) and, if the accompanying foreign body inflammation is extensive, small fibrous nodules may develop. Animals may suffer no discomfort if the lesions are minimal, although extensively affected areas may be sensitive or painful and mildly pruritic. Affected dogs should be examined carefully for any signs of primary disease.

Differential diagnoses
- Demodicosis.
- Dermatophytosis.
- Foreign body reaction.
- Mild juvenile cellulitis.
- Mild eosinophilic furunculosis associated with insect bite.

Diagnosis
The physical description and clinical signs are very suggestive. Surface cytology or cytology from an area of furunculosis will reveal bacteria and mixed inflammation. Skin scrapings should be taken to rule out demodicosis. Bacterial and dermatophyte culture and antibiotic sensitivity testing are indicated in cases that do not respond to empirical treatment. Additional appropriate diagnostics may be necessary for any suspected primary disease.

Treatment[1]
Affected areas may be cleaned daily with a benzoyl peroxide shampoo or gel to enhance removal of debris from the hair follicle and decrease the number of bacteria on the skin surface. The shampoo should be carefully rinsed from the affected area, because benzoyl peroxide can be irritating in some cases and will bleach fabrics. Chlorhexidine also has good antibacterial activity. Mild infections may respond to cleansing and a topical antibacterial such as mupirocin, fusidic acid, polymyxin B or gentamicin ointment applied twice daily. More severely affected cases may benefit from topical glucocorticoids (betamethasone or fluocinolone/dimethyl sulphoxide [DMSO] preparations) applied twice daily. If lesions are extensive, systemic antibiotics for 3–6 weeks would be appropriate (see Superficial pyoderma, page 70). Deep pyoderma may develop in severe cases and requires up to 6 weeks of antibiotic therapy (see page 197). Underlying diseases should be addressed and lifestyle changes implemented as necessary to prevent recurrence. A small number of cases require either continuous or episodic treatment for life.

Key point
- Often secondary to an underlying disease.

Reference
1 Mueller RS, Bergvall K, Bensignor E, Bond R. A review of topical therapy for skin infections with bacteria and yeast. *Vet Dermatol* 2012; **23**: 330–e62.

FELINE ACNE

Definition

Feline acne is a multi-factorial skin disease characterised by comedone formation on the chin and lips.

Aetiology and pathogenesis

Feline acne may result from demodicosis, dermatophytosis, contact dermatitis, keratinisation defects, atopic dermatitis or food allergy. However, excessive rubbing and scent marking seem to be the most consistent cause. The hair follicles become distended with lipid and keratin debris, resulting in the classic comedones (blackheads) of acne. If these follicles rupture and release keratin and sebaceous material into the dermis, a foreign body reaction with inflammation will develop. Secondary pyoderma or yeast dermatitis is a common sequela to feline acne.

Clinical features

Feline acne can occur in cats of any age and there is no breed or sex predisposition. Lesions generally occur on the lower lips, the chin and, occasionally, the upper lips. Comedones, especially around the chin, lateral commissures of the mouth and the lower lip, are the predominant findings (**Figs. 3.15, 3.16**). If the condition progresses, erythematous crusted papules, folliculitis and furunculosis may develop, which can result in pruritus and scarring. Alopecia, erythema and swelling of the chin are seen in severe cases. In Persian cats the lesions may affect the face as well as the chin, which may merge into the facial dermatitis seen in this breed (see page 90). Excoriations from scratching may occur in cases with severe inflammation. When secondary bacterial infections are present, *Pasteurella multocida*, β-haemolytic streptococci and coagulase-positive staphylococci have been isolated.[1]

Differential diagnoses

- Contact dermatitis.
- Eosinophilic granuloma.
- Pyoderma.
- Dermatophytosis.
- Demodicosis.
- Food allergy.
- Atopic dermatitis.

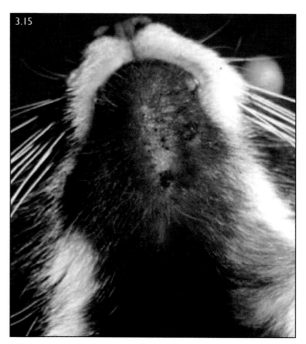

Fig. 3.15 Feline acne: characteristic appearance of multiple comedones on the rostral aspect of the mandible.

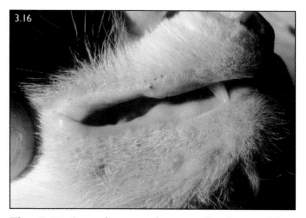

Fig. 3.16 Comedones on the upper lip of a cat with feline acne (photo courtesy of Pat McKeever).

Diagnosis

The history and clinical signs are characteristic. Microscopic examination of skin scrapings and impression smears of follicular plugs, dermatophyte culture and bacterial culture and sensitivity will rule out infectious causes. Histopathological examination of biopsy samples will confirm the diagnosis. Often the lesions are so characteristic that skin biopsies are not necessary. The difficulty can be in determining the underlying cause, which requires a good history and thorough clinical examination.

Treatment

Clients should be forewarned that feline acne is a condition that generally is not cured, but just controlled with periodic or continuous treatment. If there is an underlying predisposing condition (e.g. demodicosis, allergy or dermatophytosis), it should be addressed with specific treatment.

Treatment for idiopathic feline acne will vary with the type and severity of lesions. Small numbers of asymptomatic comedones may not require any treatment. Larger numbers of comedones with seborrhoea and some swelling of the chin will benefit from the antibacterial and follicular flushing actions of alternate-day or twice-weekly benzoyl peroxide gel or shampoo. Benzoyl peroxide may be irritating to some cats and should be discontinued if erythema develops; this is less likely to happen if the concentration is kept to 3% or less. Cats cannot detoxify benzoyl products as readily as humans or dogs, but toxicity is unlikely if the products are used in small quantities on small areas, treated skin is rinsed and cats are prevented from ingesting the products as much as possible. Alternative shampoos would be those containing ethyl lactate, sulphur, salicylic acid and chlorhexidine. A product containing phytosphingosine, which is antibacterial and decreases sebaceous secretions when applied weekly, is also beneficial.

If bacteria are found on impression smears, topical antibacterial preparations containing mupirocin,[2] fusidic acid or polymyxin B may be helpful. Topical therapy with otic preparations containing betamethasone, gentamicin and clotrimazole are also quite effective to clear infection and decrease inflammation.

The comedolytic activity of topical vitamin A products (0.05% retinoic acid cream), applied daily at first and then on alternate days or twice weekly, has been beneficial in some cases. This product may also cause irritation and its use should be monitored closely because cats are very susceptible to vitamin A toxicity.

If deep bacterial folliculitis or furunculosis is present, systemic antibiotics (e.g. clavulanated amoxicillin or cephalosporins) for 2–6 weeks would be appropriate.

If there is severe inflammation resulting from a foreign body reaction to keratin and sebum of ruptured hair follicles, a course of systemic corticosteroids (prednisone, prednisolone or methylprednisolone 1–2 mg/kg po q24 h for 10–14 days) is indicated. Isotretinoin (2 mg/kg po q24 h) has been advocated for the treatment and control of refractory cases. It acts by decreasing the activity of sebaceous glands and normalising keratinisation within hair follicles; therapeutic benefits have been observed in 30% of treated cases. Clinical response should occur within 1 month. Once improvement is seen, the isotretinoin dose may be reduced to twice weekly for control. Side effects of its use in cats include conjunctivitis, periocular crusting, vomiting and diarrhoea. Monthly laboratory screenings are suggested when it is used over prolonged periods. Isotretinoin is extremely teratogenic and appropriate caution should be observed for both animals and humans. As the commercial availability of this drug is limited, the alternative would be acitretin (0.5–2 mg/kg po q24 h).

Key points

- Although pathognomonic, the clinical signs may also reflect demodicosis or dermatophytosis. All cases should be subjected to skin scrapings and fungal culture.
- Resolution of lesions may take 2–8 weeks depending on severity and underlying cause.

References

1 Jazic E, Coyner KS, Loeffler DG, Lewis TP. An evaluation of the clinical, cytological, infectious and histopathological features of feline acne. *Vet Dermatol* 2006; **17**: 134–140.
2 White SD, Bordeau PB, Blumstein P *et al*. Feline acne and results of treatment with mupirocin in an open clinical trial: 25 cases (1994–96). *Vet Dermatol* 1997; **8**: 157–164.

FLY AND MOSQUITO BITE DERMATITIS

Definition
A papular or papulocrustous reaction to the bites of flies and mosquitoes.

Aetiology and pathogenesis
Fly bite dermatitis is usually caused by the stable fly *Stomoxys calcitrans* and is a non-specific reaction to the pain and injury caused by the bite. Similarly, the clinical signs of insect bite dermatosis in dogs are thought to be caused by bites of the mosquito, bush fly, sand fly, deer fly, horse fly, midge or buffalo gnat (black fly). Other biting insects may also be involved. Feline mosquito bite hypersensitivity is a specific form of eosinophilic granuloma, caused by a type 1 reaction to substances within saliva that are injected into the skin when the mosquito bites.

Clinical features
Fly bite dermatitis is a crusting, pruritic dermatosis affecting the pinnae, muzzle and other sites in dogs during the summer months. In Rough Collies, Shetland Sheepdogs and other breeds in which the tips of the pinnae bend over, the bites occur on the dorsal aspect of the earfold, whereas in those breeds with erect ears the lesions occur at the tips of the pinnae. Lesions consist of erythema, alopecia and haemorrhagic crusting, resulting from oozing of blood and serum (**Fig. 3.17**).

Insect bite dermatitis is most commonly seen in short-coated dogs such as Weimaraners, Doberman Pinschers, German Short-haired Pointers and Bull Terriers, which are kept outdoors, especially in warm climates. Papules and crusted papules are followed by focal alopecia (**Fig. 3.18**). The lesions are usually confined to the head, dorsal and lateral surfaces of the trunk and upper limbs. Buffalo gnat bites will result in circular 1-cm areas of erythema on the non-haired areas of the ventral abdomen (**Fig. 3.19**). Midge bites are similar but smaller. Fly and mosquito bites may trigger eosinophilic folliculitis and furunculosis in some dogs (**Fig. 3.20**).

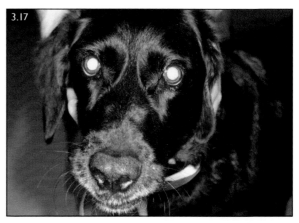

Fig. 3.17 Acute oedema, swelling and draining tracts in a Labrador cross with eosinophilic folliculitis and furunculosis.

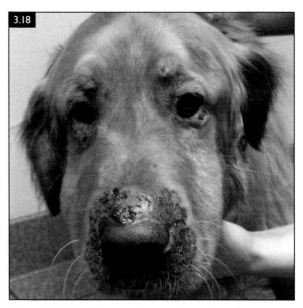

Fig. 3.18 Swelling, erythema, alopecia, erosions and exudation on the muzzle and around the eyes of a dog.

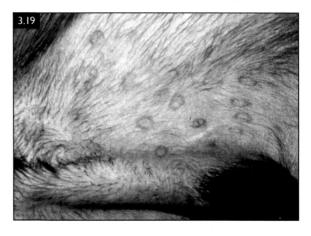

Fig. 3.19 Erythematous target lesions due to gnat bites on the abdomen of a dog (photo courtesy of Pat McKeever).

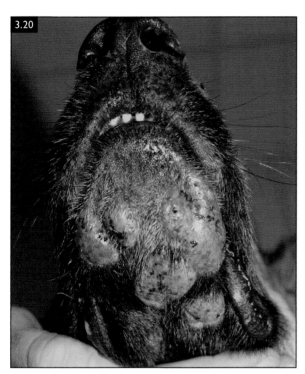

Fig. 3.20 Well-demarcated eosinophilic granulomas following insect bites in a German Shepherd dog.

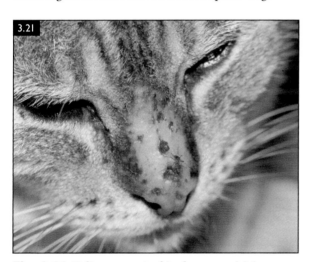

Fig. 3.21 Feline mosquito bite hypersensitivity (photo courtesy of K Mason).

of all four feet, preceded by swelling, tenderness, erythema and, sometimes, fissuring, may be seen. There is peripheral lymphadenopathy. Rarely, the condition will be accompanied by a corneal eosinophilic granuloma.

Differential diagnoses
- Squamous cell carcinoma.
- Scabies.
- Superficial pyoderma.
- Demodicosis.
- Urticaria.
- Pemphigus foliaceus.
- Feline eosinophilic granuloma complex.
- Notoedric mange.
- Pemphigus erythematosus.
- Systemic lupus erythematosus.
- Atopic dermatitis.

Diagnosis
The seasonal and environmental nature of the dermatosis means that many individuals are affected year after year. A history of exposure is often known, particularly for fly bite dermatosis of the pinnae. Microscopic examination of skin scrapes will eliminate demodicosis from the differential of insect bite dermatitis. Superficial pyoderma is characterised by papules, pustules and epidermal collarettes. The combination of the clinical signs described for the cat is pathognomonic. An impression smear from under a crust may reveal mixed inflammatory cells, including eosinophils. Acanthocytes will not be present.

Treatment
Ideally, these dermatoses are managed by preventing animals being exposed to the insects, although it is often impossible to enforce. A 10% imidacloprid/50% permethrin topical flea and tick preventive for dogs also has mosquito repellent efficacy.[1] In addition, various other pyrethrin products that repel mosquitoes are available for dogs. Cats are sensitive to most repellents, although there is a licensed flumethrin/imidacloprid collar, so avoidance of exposure to mosquitoes is best.

Flies and mosquitoes may be excluded from closed areas by fine mesh. Most cases resolve spontaneously when exposure to the insects is prevented, although in some instances it may be necessary to use systemic glucocorticoids to induce remission.

Key points

- Control of the condition is difficult unless exposure to insects is minimised.
- Resolution of lesions generally occurs within a few days, provided that secondary infection is not present and re-exposure has been prevented.

Reference

1 Tiawsirisup S, Nithiuthai S, Kaewthamasorn M. Repellent and adulticide efficacy of a combination containing 10% imidacloprid and 50% permethrin against *Aedes aegypti* mosquitoes on dogs. *Parasitol Res* 2007; **101**: 527–531.

PEMPHIGUS FOLIACEUS

Definition

Pemphigus foliaceus (PF) is an autoimmune disease in which autoantibodies are directed against components of the epidermis, resulting in acantholysis and subcorneal vesicle formation.

Aetiology and pathogenesis

Autoantibody (IgG) is formed against desmocollin-1,[1] a component of desmosomes, which are responsible for cell-to-cell cohesion. Most cases of PF are idiopathic, although the disease may also be drug induced. Drugs associated with PF in dogs include: topical metaflumizone/amitraz products, topical fipronil/amitraz/S-methoprene products, topical dinotefuran/pyriproxyfen/permethrin products[2,3] and antibiotics. Antibiotics, methimazole and vaccines can trigger PF in cats. Drug-triggered PF usually resolves after the drug is withdrawn; drug-induced PF, in contrast, will persist after drug withdrawal.

Clinical features

PF most commonly affects middle-aged to older animals, but young animals and puppies have been reported. Collies, Spaniels, Chows, Newfoundlands and Akitas are predisposed. No sex predilection has been recognised.

Dogs may develop large pustules, erosions and crusts on the face (particularly the concave aspect of the pinnae, periocular region and nasal planum), paw pads and/or trunk. Pruritus may or may not be present, but may be severe in some cases (**Figs. 3.22–3.25**).

PF in cats is characterised by pustules, erosions and crusting on the pinnae, face and/or nailbeds (**Fig. 3.26**). Caseous debris may also be present around the nails (**Fig. 3.27**). There is often

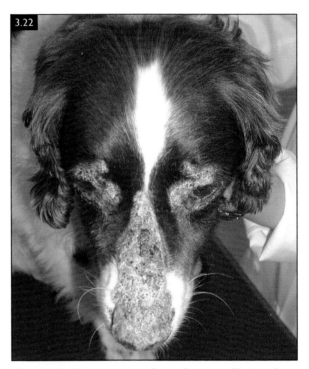

Fig. 3.22 Extensive pustules and crusts affecting the nose and periocular skin in an English Springer Spaniel.

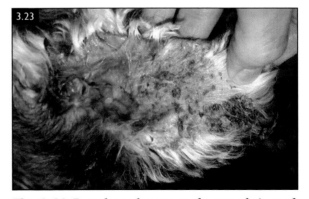

Fig. 3.23 Pustules and crusts on the ventral pinna of a Miniature Schnauzer; this dog also had a suppurative otitis externa secondary to lesions in the ear canals.

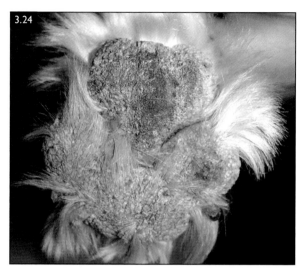

Fig. 3.24 Severe hyperkeratosis, scaling and crusting of the footpads in a Cavalier King Charles Spaniel.

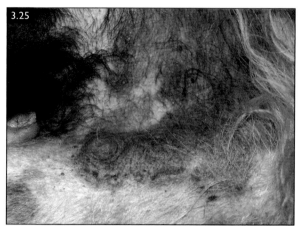

Fig. 3.25 Irregular and coalescing pustules in a Newfoundland; unlike staphylococcal pyoderma the pustules do not expand and there are no epidermal collarettes.

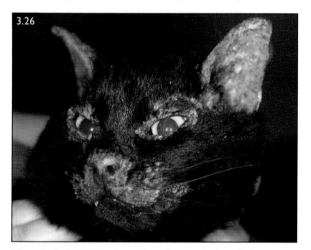

Fig. 3.26 Perioral, periocular and pinnal alopecia and crusts in a domestic short-haired cat; the pemphigus foliaceus was triggered by a multi-valent vaccine.

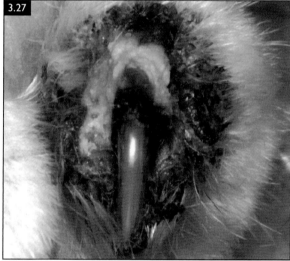

Fig. 3.27 Caseous purulent exudate from the claw sheath – this is highly suggestive of pemphigus foliaceus in cats, and cytology of the exudate will reveal numerous neutrophils and acantholytic keratinocytes.

mild-to-moderate scaling on the pads (**Fig. 3.28**). Pruritus is usually absent, but lesions of the claw fold may be painful.

Lesions on the nasal planum, oral cavity and mucocutaneous junctions, and nail loss and dystrophy are rare.

Complications include fever, weight loss, lethargy and anorexia in pets that have widespread lesions. Concurrent dermatophytosis, demodicosis and secondary pyoderma may also be present.

Differential diagnoses
- Superficial pyoderma.
- *Trichophyton* spp. dermatophytosis.
- Zinc-responsive dermatosis.
- Actinic dermatosis.
- Epitheliotrophic lymphoma.
- Drug eruption.
- Discoid lupus erythematosus.
- Systemic lupus erythematosus.
- Superficial necrolytic dermatitis.

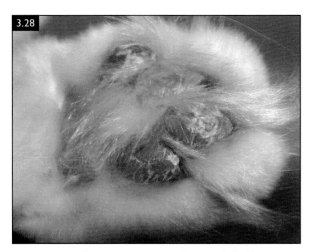

Fig. 3.28 Characteristic round-to-oval shallow erosions and scaling on the footpads of a Himalayan cat with pemphigus foliaceus.

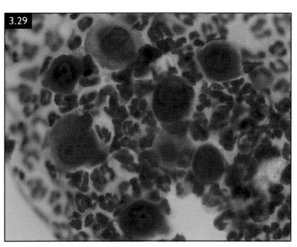

Fig. 3.29 Neutrophils, eosinophils and acantholytic keratinocytes in an impression smear from an intact pustule (Diff-Quik®; ×400). Similar findings are seen in impression smears from the underside of fresh crusts or from erosions.

Diagnosis

The hallmark of PF is acantholytic keratinocytes and these can be identified on cytology (**Fig. 3.29**) and on histology. *Trichophyton mentagrophytes* and exfoliative staphylococcal pyoderma are the primary differentials for PF because acantholytic keratinocytes can also occur in these conditions.

A direct impression smear from under a moist crust or a pustule will reveal numerous nondegenerate neutrophils, acantholytic keratinocytes and sometimes eosinophils. Bacteria may be present, but there are generally many more neutrophils than are present in the typical pyoderma. Careful consideration of the clinical signs will help differentiate exfoliative staphylococcal pyoderma from PF[4] (*Table 3.8*).

The punch biopsy technique is appropriate for diagnosing PF. The skin should not be shaved or cleaned before obtaining the biopsy, and crusts should not be removed. Skin devoid of epithelium should not be biopsied because epithelium is required for a histological diagnosis. Moist, tightly adhered crusts or intact pustules are the ideal lesions to biopsy. Periodic acid–Schiff (PAS) or Grocott–Gomori silver stains should be requested to evaluate the sample for fungal elements.

Table 3.8 **Differentiating exfoliative staphylococcal pyoderma from pemphigus foliaceus (PF)**

FEATURE	PF	PYODERMA
Symmetrical facial and periocular lesions	+	−
Medial pinna affected	+	−
Footpads affected	+	−
Trunk initially affected	±	+
Irregular, polycyclic or annular pustules	+	−
Coalescing pustules	+	−
Non-follicular pustules	+	±
Flaccid pustules	+	±
Turgid pustules	−	±
Epidermal collarettes	−	+
Expanding collarettes and lesions	−	+
Pallisading crusts	+	−
Moist erosions	+	−

Treatment[5]

The first step in treatment should be to discontinue topical flea/tick preventives that have been associated with PF. Other suspect drugs should also be stopped – where treatment is necessary a different class of drug should be used. Secondary infections should be treated when starting immunosuppressive therapy.

Treatment has two aims: the rapid induction of remission and then maintenance of clinical remission. Aggressive steroid therapy to achieve remission is warranted in severe cases. Prednisolone at 2.2 mg/kg po per day until remission and then slowly tapering to maintenance over several months is the traditional therapy. Many dogs with PF will respond favourably to glucocorticoids combined with azathioprine (azathioprine should not be used in cats). Azathioprine may take several weeks to reach maximum effect, so the glucocorticoid should be tapered slowly over the course of 2 months. The maintenance dose of glucocorticoid should be administered every other day to decrease risk of long-term side effects. Methylprednisolone may cause less polyuria and polydipsia than prednisone, and should be considered in affected patients. Topical steroids can be used as adjunct and maintenance therapy in some animals. Glucocorticoids can also be combined with other steroid-sparing drugs such as ciclosporin, chlorambucil, mycophenolate mofetil or tetracycline-class drugs, and niacinamide. (See Immunosuppressive Drug Therapy Table, page 289.)

High-dose pulse therapy of glucocorticoids[4] for one to three cycles is highly effective. In dogs, this involves 10 mg/kg of prednisolone q24 h for 3 days, followed by 1 mg/kg q24 h for 4 days. An alternative in cats is to use 1 mg/kg of dexamethasone for 3 days followed by 0.1 mg/kg for 4 days. Some patients will have long periods of remission and can be maintained with infrequent glucocorticoid pulses.

Feline PF should be treated with prednisolone or methylprednisolone. Dexamethasone can be used for refractory cases. The clinician should bear in mind that dexamethasone is the most diabetogenic steroid in cats and maintenance therapy should be given once to twice weekly. Ciclosporin is an effective steroid-sparing drug in most cases, although it may take 2–8 weeks to reach maximum effect, and so should be started together with steroids and the steroids tapered. Ciclosporin alone may effectively control PF in some cats. Chlorambucil is effective and well tolerated in cats, and can be used as sole therapy.

The prognosis is guarded for patients that do not respond to or cannot tolerate initial therapy with glucocorticoids. The prognosis is good for patients that respond easily to therapy and that can be controlled with low doses of medication.

Key points

- Most patients require life-long management of PF.
- Pyoderma can occur in dogs with PF. The clinical signs, cytology and/or culture id required to differentiate pyoderma from a PF flare.
- Significant improvement of lesions should be observed within 2 weeks.

References

1　Bizikova P, Dean GA, Hashimoto T, Olivry T. Cloning and establishment of canine desmocollin-1 as a major autoantigen in canine pemphigus foliaceus. *Vet Immunol Immunopathol* 2012; **149**: 197–207.

2　Bizikova P, Moriello KA, Linder KE, Sauber L. Dinotefuran/pyriproxyfen/permethrin pemphigus-like drug reaction in three dogs. *Vet Dermatol* 2015; **26**: 206–e46.

3　Bizikova P, Linder KE, Olivry T. Fipronil–amitraz–S-methoprene-triggered pemphigus foliaceus in 21 dogs: clinical, histological and immunological characteristics. *Vet Dermatol* 2014; **25**: 103–e30.

4　Banovic F, Linder KE, Olivry T. Clinical, microscopic and microbial characterization of exfoliative superficial pyoderma-associated epidermal collarettes in dogs. *Vet Dermatol* 2017; **28**: 107–e23.

5　Bizikova P, Olivry T. Oral glucocorticoid pulse therapy for induction of treatment of canine pemphigus foliaceus–a comparative study. *Vet Dermatol* 2015; **26**: 354–e77.

TRICHOPHYTON MENTAGROPHYTES DERMATOPHYTOSIS

Definition
Trichophyton mentagrophytes is a fungus found in soil that can cause a superficial pustular dermatophytosis in mammals.

Aetiology and pathogenesis
T. mentagrophytes is contracted through contact with infected soil or mammals (especially rodents). *T. mentagrophytes* invades the epidermis and hair follicle. The fungus releases proteolytic enzymes that recruit neutrophils and induce acantholysis of epithelial cells.[1]

Clinical features
T. mentagrophytes results in a crusting, pustular dermatosis. Any area of the skin may be affected, but the ears, face and trunk are especially prone. Paronychia can be seen in dogs that dig in contaminated soil. Lesions may appear identical to canine PF, and dogs with pemphigus may have concurrent dermatophytosis. Pruritus varies, but many cases are strongly pruritic.

Differential diagnoses
- Pemphigus foliaceus.
- Pyoderma (note that a secondary pyoderma can complicate the dermatophytosis).

Diagnosis
T. mentagrophytes may be diagnosed via fungal culture of hairs on dermatophyte test medium (DTM). *T. mentagrophytes* does not fluoresce with a Wood's lamp. Fungal elements may be observed among hairs and skin cells on hair plucks and skin scrapes. Acantholytic keratinocytes may also be observed on impression smears obtained from under crusts or pustules. In addition fungal hyphae may be observed on skin biopsy, and will be highlighted if special stains are requested.

Treatment
See Dermatophytosis, page 115.

Key points
- May appear clinically identical to pemphigus foliaceus.
- Lesions should resolve within 2–6 weeks depending on severity and comorbidities.

Reference
1 Olivry T, Linder KE. Dermatoses affecting desmosomes in animals: a mechanistic review of acantholytic blistering skin diseases. *Vet Dermatol* 2009; **20**: 313–326.

IDIOPATHIC EAR MARGIN VASCULITIS
(Proliferative thrombovascular necrosis of the pinna)

Definition
Idiopathic ear margin vasculitis is a rare disease characterised by ulcerative lesions localised to the tips and margins of the pinnae.

Aetiology and pathogenesis
The pathogenesis of this disease is unknown. However, it is probably an immune-mediated vasculitis caused by immune-complex disease (type III hypersensitivity). Triggers may include drugs, supplements, adverse reaction to food, tick-borne disease and vaccination.

Clinical features
Dachshunds and Chihuahuas are predisposed to this condition, but other breeds may also be affected. Too few cases have been documented to determine whether there is an age or sex predisposition. Affected animals first develop alopecia along the margins of the pinna. Then, skin in focal areas (0.2–2.0 cm) along the very edge of the pinna becomes darkened and slightly thickened, and undergoes necrosis resulting in ulcers (**Figs. 3.30, 3.31**).[1] Typically, both ears are involved and each will have from one lesion to eight lesions. Occasionally, 0.2- to 0.5-cm

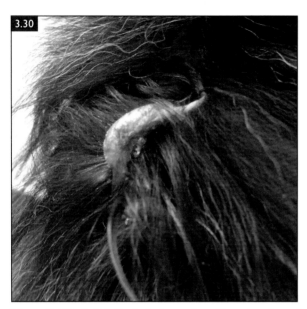 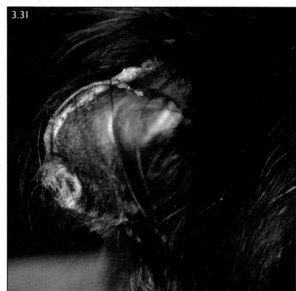

Figs. 3.30, 3.31 Early lesions of proliferative thrombovascular necrosis of the pinna in a Papillion with alopecia, swelling and purpura of the pinna margins (Fig. 3.30). Later lesions of proliferative thrombovascular necrosis of the pinna in a Papillion with necrosis, eschar and sloughing of the tip of the pinna (Fig. 3.31).

ulcers will be noted on the inner aspects of the pinna. No other skin lesions or systemic signs are present. The ulcers will slowly enlarge if left untreated. Often the necrotic skin will slough and result in an irregular, punched-out appearance to the ear margin. In severe cases, chondritis also occurs.

Differential diagnoses

- Immune-mediated vasculitis secondary to other diseases.
- Frostbite.
- Cold agglutinin disease.
- Cryoglobulinaemia.
- Trauma from shaking the head due to chronic otitis.
- Sarcoptic mange.

Diagnosis

The presence of vasculitis in other body organs must be ruled out with a thorough physical exam, complete blood count, serum biochemistry and urinalysis. Underlying causes of vasculitis such as drugs, supplements, adverse reaction to food, tick-borne disease and vaccination should also be investigated.[2]

Once systemic vasculitis and underlying causes have been ruled out, a diagnosis of idiopathic ear margin vasculitis can be made. In atypical cases, the diagnosis can be confirmed with biopsy. Several biopsies may be necessary to demonstrate the classic leukocytoclastic pattern of vasculitis, and often biopsies are not diagnostic.

Treatment

Ear margin vasculitis is a condition that is controlled rather than cured.

The following drugs have been advocated for the treatment of ear margin vasculitis (see Immunosuppressive Drug Therapy Table, page 289).

- Sulfasalazine (10–20 mg/kg po q8 h). Once controlled the dose can be reduced to q12 h or q24 h. Side effects of this drug include keratoconjunctivitis sicca and hepatotoxicity, so animals should be monitored using Schirmer's tear test and liver enzyme tests. Improvement should be observed within 2–4 weeks. The dose frequency should be reduced to the least amount that prevents recurrence of lesions.

- Tetracycline and niacinamide (250 mg of each drug po q8 h in dogs <10 kg and 500 mg of each drug po q8 h in dogs >10 kg; doxycycline or minocycline 5–10 mg/kg po q12 h may be used instead of tetracycline). Improvement may take 8–12 weeks to occur. Side effects are minimal and typically limited to gastrointestinal upsets.
- Pentoxifylline (15–25 mg/kg po q8–12 h). Improvement may take 8 weeks to occur. Side effects are minimal and typically limited to gastrointestinal upsets.
- Prednisone, prednisolone or methylprednisolone (1.0–4.0 mg/kg po q12 h) may also result in resolution of lesions. Steroids may be used temporarily while waiting for another treatment to take effect. Improvement should be observed within 10 days.
- Ciclosporin (5–10 mg/kg po q24 h). Improvement should be observed within 4 weeks and may take 8 weeks to reach maximum effect. The dose frequency should be reduced to the lowest that prevents recurrence of lesions. Side effects are minimal and typically limited to gastrointestinal upsets, gingival hyperplasia, hirsutism and rarely papillomatosis.

Tissues do not fill back in after undergoing necrosis, so the ear margins will still have punched-out areas present even with successful treatment. In most cases the condition is controlled rather than cured. Surgery may be necessary to remove necrotic tissue.

Key points
- The clinician must rule out systemic vasculitis.
- Resolution of lesions generally occurs within 2–4 weeks, although cartilage that has necrosed will not regrow.

References
1 Morris DO. Ischemic dermatopathies. *Vet Clin North Am Small Anim Pract* 2013; **43**: 99–111.
2 Innerå M. Cutaneous vasculitis in small animals. *Vet Clin North Am Small Anim Pract* 2013; **43**: 113–134.

SOLAR DERMATITIS
(Actinic keratosis)

Definition
Solar dermatitis results from prolonged exposure to ultraviolet (UV) light.

Aetiology and pathogenesis
Prolonged exposure to UV light results in epithelial cell apoptosis and inflammation. Lesions vary in severity but may progress to include haemangiomas, squamous cell carcinomas and basal cell carcinomas.[1]

Clinical features
Both dogs and cats are affected, especially those that have lightly coloured sparse hair and spend extended time in the sun. Variable degrees of pruritus, erythema, fibrosis and alopecia may develop.

In cats, the margins of the pinnae are particularly susceptible and often become thickened with fine scaling (**Fig. 3.32**). Scarring, curling, crusting and cutaneous horns of the distal pinnae may be noted. The eyelids and nose are also commonly affected. Squamous cell carcinoma may develop in chronic lesions.[2]

In dogs the most common site of sun damage is the rostral face, immediately caudal to the planum nasale (**Fig. 3.33**). In dogs that habitually sleep in the sun, lesions may develop on the lower flank, ventrum, scrotum and limbs. The affected skin is characterised by erythema, fibrosis, macules, fine scale and progressive alopecia. Comedones, furunculosis, pruritus and vasculopathy may also develop.

Many cases become secondarily infected with staphylococcal bacteria.

Differential diagnoses
- Demodicosis (when comedones are present).
- Dermatophytosis.
- Superficial pyoderma.
- Pemphigus foliaceus or erythematosus (when crusts are present).
- Discoid lupus erythematosus.
- Atopic dermatitis when pruritic.
- Cutaneous neoplasia (squamous cell carcinoma).

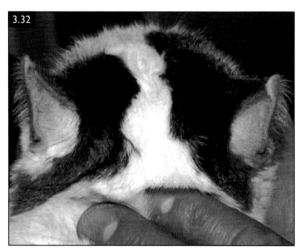

Fig. 3.32 Actinic keratosis in a cat with erythema, scaling, thickening and curling of the pinnae.

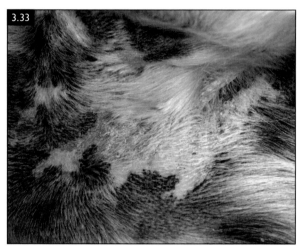

Fig. 3.33 Chronic UV light damage on the ventral abdomen of a Collie cross with erythema, lichenification and scaling.

Diagnosis

Observation that lightly pigmented skin is affected whereas adjacent pigmented skin is unaffected is very suggestive of an actinic dermatosis. Microscopic examination of skin scrapings will rule out demodicosis. Fungal culture will rule out dermatophytosis. Skin biopsy samples will reveal changes consistent with actinic dermatitis (e.g. superficial dermal fibrosis and follicular keratosis).

Treatment

Early lesions may resolve spontaneously when exposure to sunlight is prevented. Chronic or severe lesions should be surgically removed to alleviate pruritus and prevent malignant transformation. A CO_2 laser or cautery is an effective way to remove multiple, small lesions.

Firocoxib administered 5 mg/kg po q24 h improves and even resolves lesions in some dogs, and should be used when removal of lesions is not possible.[3]

Secondary pyoderma is often present and contributes significantly to crusting, inflammation and pruritus (see Pyoderma, page 65).

Sun avoidance must be instituted to prevent further lesions from developing. Solar suits and sunscreen are useful when sun exposure is unavoidable. High-factor (SPF 50+), water- and sweat-resistant products should be used.

Key points

- Neoplastic transformation may occur.
- White-haired cats and dogs and are particularly susceptible.
- Pyoderma is often present.

References

1　Saridomichelakis MN, Day MJ, Apostolidis KN, Tsioli V, Athanasiou LV, Koutinas AF. Basal cell carcinoma in a dog with chronic solar dermatitis. *J Small Anim Pract* 2013; **54**: 108–111.

2　Friberg C. Feline facial dermatoses. *Vet Clin North Am Small Anim Pract* 2006; **36**: 115–140.

3　Albanese F, Abramo F, Caporali C, Vichi G, Millanta F. Clinical outcome and cyclo-oxygenase-2 expression in five dogs with solar dermatitis/actinic keratosis treated with firocoxib. *Vet Dermatol* 2013; **24**: 606–e147.

FELINE SQUAMOUS CELL CARCINOMA *IN SITU*

Bowen's disease, bowenoid in-situ carcinoma, feline papillomaviral plaques

Definition

Feline Bowen's disease is a preneoplastic lesion associated with papillomavirus (see page 255).

Aetiology and pathogenesis

Many cats have papillomavirus present within normal skin.[1] In some cats, the papillomavirus causes formation of crusts and plaques. Sun exposure may also be a factor in the development of lesions. Lesions generally do not resolve spontaneously and may eventually progress to squamous cell carcinoma. The lesion is defined histologically as Bowen's disease if it is confined to the epidermis. Squamous cell carcinoma is diagnosed if the lesion extends into the dermis. Most cases do not progress to squamous cell carcinoma.[2]

Clinical features

Lesions occur in middle-aged to older adult cats.[3] Lesions are characterised by tightly adherent, multifocal, variably sized, variably pruritic, scaly plaques and crusts. Lesions tend to occur on the head, neck and trunk. The pruritus is poorly responsive to glucocorticoids.

Differential diagnoses

- Hypersensitivity dermatitis.
- Eosinophilic plaques.
- Feline ulcerative dermatitis.
- Ectoparasites.
- Dermatophytosis.
- Pemphigus foliaceus.
- Squamous cell carcinoma.

Diagnosis

The typical history is acute onset of pruritic plaques and crusts in an older cat. Skin cytology, skin scrapings, fungal culture and mite trials are useful to rule out differentials. Diagnosis is achieved with a skin biopsy.

Treatment

Imiquimod cream applied every other day until resolution of lesions, then as needed to prevent recurrence, is effective in many cases. An Elizabethan collar should be used to prevent ingestion of the medication. Some cats develop cutaneous irritation when imiquimod is applied, which can be managed by reducing the volume and frequency of application. Resolution of lesions should be achieved within a month. Some cats do not respond to or do not tolerate imiquimod. An alternative treatment is surgical removal, cautery or CO_2 laser ablation of lesions. Although this is an effective treatment for lesions that are visible at the time of the procedure, additional lesions develop in other areas of the skin as time goes on. Some affected cats require treatment of lesions every 6–12 months. Drugs with the potential to exacerbate the progression to neoplasia (e.g. ciclosporin and oclacitinib) should be avoided.

Key points

- This condition can be confused with hypersensitivity dermatitis. Histopathology is important for diagnosis.
- Concern for squamous cell carcinoma should arise if lesions become erythematous, ulcerated or swollen.

References

1 Egberink H, Thiry E, Möstl K *et al.* Feline viral papillomatosis. *J Feline Med Surg* 2013; **15**: 560–562.
2 Munday JS, Benfell MW, French A, Orbell G, Thomson N. Bowenoid in situ carcinomas in two Devon Rex cats: evidence of unusually aggressive neoplasm behavior in this breed and detection of papillomaviral gene expression in primary and metastatic lesions. *Vet Dermatol* 2016; **27**: 215–e55.

FACIAL DERMATITIS OF PERSIAN AND HIMALAYAN CATS

Dirty face syndrome

Definition

Facial dermatitis of Persian and Himalayan cats is characterised by the accumulation of dark waxy debris around the eyes, facial folds and chin.

Aetiology and pathogenesis

This is an inflammatory condition with an unknown pathogenesis. The waxy debris is thought to originate from the sebaceous glands.[1]

Clinical features

Lesions are characterised by the accumulation of a black, waxy, tightly adherent material that mats the hair of the chin, perioral and periocular facial fold areas (**Figs. 3.34, 3.35**). Affected areas may have varying degrees of erythema, which may be associated with pruritus when it becomes severe.[1] A bilateral erythematous otitis with accumulation of black waxy debris is seen in many cases.[1] *Malassezia* spp. and bacteria are frequently found in impression smears from affected areas, although these are most likely to be secondary to the underlying scaling. Submandibular lymphadenopathy may develop in some cats.[1] The age of onset varies from 10 months to 6 years.[1] Persian and Himalayan cats are predisposed but it may also occur in other breeds.

Differential diagnoses

- Demodicosis.
- Feline acne.
- Dermatophytosis.
- Hypersensitivity dermatitis.
- Herpesvirus dermatitis.

Diagnosis

Diagnosis is based on history and clinical findings. Surface cytology, skin scrapings and dermatophyte culture are necessary to determine if secondary infection is present and to rule out other diseases. If pruritus is present, the patient should be worked up for hypersensitivity dermatitis (see page 41) before assuming a diagnosis of idiopathic facial dermatitis.

Treatment

Treatment and prevention of bacterial and yeast infections may be sufficient to control signs in some patients. Cleaners and ointments designed for ear infections can often be used to clean and treat the face, facial folds and chin. The selection of such a product should be based on surface cytology findings. Ciclosporin (5–7 mg/kg po q24–48 h) is effective in some cats. Tacrolimus 0.1% ointment applied q12 h and then tapered to lowest effective frequency can also be effective.[2]

Key point

- This is a condition that is generally controlled, but not cured.

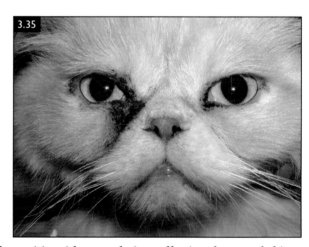

Figs. 3.34, 3.35 A Persian cat suffering from facial dermatitis, with severe lesions affecting the rostral chin (Fig. 3.34) and face (Fig. 3.35).

References

1 Bond R, Curtis CV, Ferguson EA *et al*. An idiopathic facial dermatitis of Persian cats. *Vet Dermatol* 2000; **11**: 35–41.

2 Chung TH, Ryu MH, Kim DY, Yoon HY, Hwang CY. Topical tacrolimus (FK506) for the treatment of feline idiopathic facial dermatitis. *Aust Vet J* 2009; **87**: 417–420.

FELINE THYMOMA-ASSOCIATED DERMATOSIS

Definition

Thymoma-associated dermatitis is a rare paraneoplastic condition in cats.

Aetiology and pathogenesis

This is a paraneoplastic condition associated with a primary tumour of the thymus gland.

Clinical features

Thymoma-associated dermatitis occurs in older adult cats and is characterised by generalised, nonpruritic, scaling dermatitis and alopecia. Crusts may or may not be present. There may be a secondary malassezia dermatitis. Affected cats may also experience systemic signs such as lethargy, anorexia and weight loss.[1]

Differential diagnoses

- Ectoparasites.
- Dermatophytosis.
- Sebaceous adenitis.
- Mural folliculitis.
- Feline leukaemia virus (FeLV) or feline immunodeficiency virus (FIV) dermatitis.
- Drug eruption.
- Paraneoplastic alopecia.

Diagnosis

Surface cytology, skin scrapings, mite trials and fungal cultures are useful for ruling out ectoparasites and dermatophytosis. Skin biopsy[2] combined with thoracic radiographs or other mediastinal imaging is diagnostic for thymoma-associated dermatitis.

Treatment

Surgical excision of the thymoma is the most widely described treatment. The prognosis is guarded, but many cats can be cured with surgery.[3]

Key point

- A rare skin disease that should be considered when other more common differentials have been excluded.

References

1 Cavalcanti JVJ, Moura MP, Monteiro FO. Thymoma associated with exfoliative dermatitis in a cat. *J Feline Med Surg* 2014; **16**: 1020–1023.

2 Rottenberg S, Von Tscharner C, Roosje PJ. Thymoma-associated exfoliative dermatitis in cats. *Vet Pathol Online* 2004; **41**: 429–433.

3 Zitz JC, Birchard SJ, Couto GC, Samii VF, Weisbrode SE, Young GS. Results of excision of thymoma in cats and dogs: 20 cases (1984–2005). *J Am Vet Med Assoc* 2008; **232**: 1186–1192.

CHAPTER 4

ALOPECIC DERMATOSES

NON-PRURITIC ALOPECIA

Non-pruritic alopecias can be divided into focal/multi-focal alopecia or symmetrical/diffuse alopecia (for the clinical features associated with these alopecias see *Tables 4.1* and *4.2*).

The general approach to non-pruritic alopecia is illustrated in **Fig. 4.1**. A trichogram should always be performed to assess the relative amounts of anagen and telogen hairs, shaft abnormalities and broken hairs. Hair plucks, adhesive tape-strips, deep skin scrapings and/or faecal examination can be used to confirm demodicosis. Cytology should be performed to detect *Malassezia* spp.

and bacteria, and Wood's lamp examinations, hair plucks and fungal cultures can be used to rule out dermatophytosis.

Screening tests can be used to look for evidence of endocrinopathies and metabolic conditions. In dogs the most common endocrinopathies are hypothyroidism and hyperadrenocorticism, but these are much less frequent in cats. Specific endocrine tests and/or diagnostic imaging (e.g. for Sertoli cell tumours and paraneoplastic alopecia) can be used to confirm the diagnosis.

Skin biopsies can be used to diagnose hair cycle disorders, vasculopathies, follicular dysplasias and immune-mediated conditions.

Table 4.1 **Clinical features of alopecias**	
FOCAL-TO-MULTI-FOCAL ALOPECIA	**SYMMETRICAL TO DIFFUSE ALOPECIA**
Single or multiple non-symmetrical lesions	Multiple symmetrical, diffuse or generalised lesions
Well demarcated	Often poorly demarcated with the alopecia merging into the normal coat
Usually complete alopecia	Usually partial to diffuse hair loss; areas of complete alopecia are surrounded by areas of partial hair loss
Underlying skin normal to inflamed (scarring atrophy can be seen in vasculitis)	Underlying skin normal to atrophic
Lace-like postinflammatory hyperpigmentation	Macular to complete hyperpigmentation
Rest of the coat usually normal	Rest of the coat usually dry, dull and scaling

Table 4.2 Differential diagnosis of alopecia

FOCAL-TO-MULTI-FOCAL ALOPECIA	SYMMETRICAL OR DIFFUSE ALOPECIA
INFECTIOUS/PARASITIC	
Staphylococcal pyoderma	
Demodex spp.	
Dermatophytosis	
Leishmania spp.	
IMMUNE MEDIATED	
Dermatomyositis	
Alopecia areata	
Vasculitis	
Lymphocytic mural folliculitis (cats)	Lymphocytic mural folliculitis (cats)
ENDOCRINE/METABOLIC	
Steroid injection site	Hyperadrenocorticism
	Hypothyroidism
	Sex hormone dermatoses
	Telogen effluvium/anagen defluxion
Paraneoplastic alopecia	Paraneoplastic alopecia
NEOPLASIA	
Epitheliotrophic cutaneous T-cell lymphoma	Epitheliotrophic cutaneous T-cell lymphoma
CONGENITAL/HEREDITARY	
Keratinisation defects	
Sebaceous adenitis	
Follicular dysplasias (including colour dilute and black hair follicular dysplasia)	Follicular dysplasias (including colour dilute and black hair follicular dysplasia)
Congenital alopecias (including pattern baldness)	Congenital alopecias (including pattern baldness)
MISCELLANEOUS	
Postclipping alopecia	Cyclical flank alopecia
Scars	Alopecia X
Traction alopecia (e.g. rubber bands, ties)	

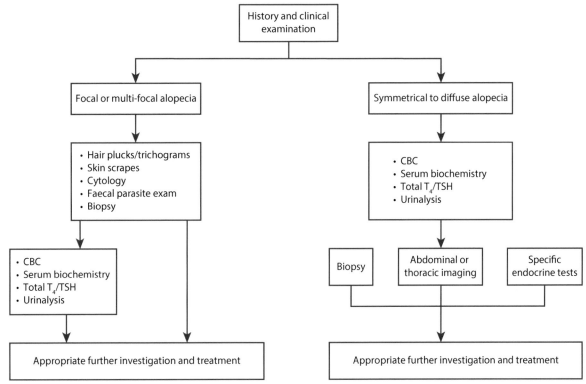

Fig. 4.1 General approach to non-pruritic alopecia. (CBC, complete blood count; TSH, thyroid-stimulating hormone.)

ALOPECIA X

Definition
Alopecia X is a hair cycle disorder of dogs characterised by non-pruritic alopecia and hyperpigmentation on characteristic areas of the body in breeds with dense undercoats.

Aetiology and pathogenesis
Alopecia X is a hair cycle disorder that occurs because of a hormone abnormality. The exact type of abnormality remains unclear, but androgen hormones appear to play a role.[1] The abnormality may be with either circulating hormones or the hormone receptors that reside on the hair follicle.[1]

Clinical features
Pomeranians, Chow Chows, Siberian Huskies, Keeshonds, Samoyeds, Alaskan Malamutes and Miniature Poodles are predisposed. Most dogs are affected between 1 and 2 years of age, although it may also affect older dogs. Either sex may be affected and the dermatosis may occur before or after neutering. The clinical signs include symmetrical, non-pruritic alopecia and eventual hyperpigmentation of the trunk, caudal thighs and neck (**Figs. 4.2, 4.3**). Occasionally, mild secondary seborrhoea and superficial pyoderma are present. Affected dogs do not have systemic signs.

Differential diagnoses
- Hypothyroidism.
- Hyperadrenocorticism.
- Sex hormone endocrinopathies.
- Follicular dysplasia.
- Cyclic flank alopecia.
- Telogen or anagen defluxion.

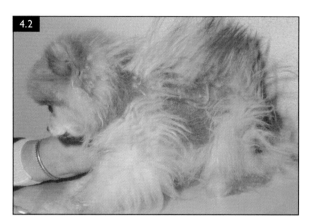

Fig. 4.2 Alopecia and hyperpigmentation of the neck, trunk and tail of a Pomeranian with alopecia X (photo courtesy of Pat McKeever).

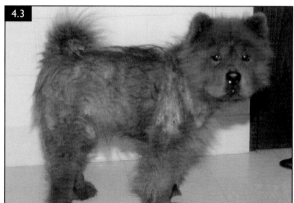

Fig. 4.3 Alopecia and hyperpigmentation over the trunk of a Chow with alopecia X (photo courtesy of Pat McKeever).

Diagnostic tests

The diagnosis of alopecia X is based on the history and physical examination, and ruling out other endocrinopathies and follicular dysplasias. A complete blood count, serum chemistry, urinalysis and, if necessary, endocrine testing should be performed to rule out hypothyroidism and hyperadrenocorticism. Skin scrapings and surface cytology should be performed to rule out demodicosis and secondary pyoderma in appropriate cases.

Skin biopsies reveal many telogen hairs, epidermal pigmentation and trichilemmal keratinisation.[2] These findings can be found to a certain degree in other hair cycle disorders so must be interpreted in light of clinical signs and blood work. Regrowth of hair at the biopsy sites is fairly consistent in alopecia X.

Measurement of sex hormones is of limited value because no consistent abnormality has been documented, and some affected dogs have normal levels.[3]

Treatment

Various treatment modalities are available, but none is effective in all cases. As alopecia X is purely cosmetic and the health of affected dogs is not impaired, monitoring without treatment is a reasonable treatment option. Nevertheless, many owners find the condition distressing and will seek treatment.

Melatonin is a common treatment for affected dogs. It is widely available, generally inexpensive, and dogs tolerate it very well. Melatonin induces hair growth in approximately 40% of affected dogs. Responders will grow hair within 3–4 months of starting treatment. Treatment can be continued indefinitely. The dose is generally 1–2 mg/kg po q12 h,[4] although higher doses have been used.

Castration leads to hair regrowth in at least 40% of affected dogs,[5] but is irreversible and not acceptable to some owners. Deslorelin (4.7 mg per dog) subcutaneous implants have been shown to regrow hair in 75% of intact male dogs.[5] Implants should be administered to male dogs only, because it has not proven efficacious in female dogs. Responders will grow hair within 2–3 months of receiving the implant.[5] Treatment can be repeated after 6 months if needed to promote further hair growth.

Microneedling was effective in two dogs in a recent case report.[6] The dogs were anaesthetised and 1.5- to 2.5-mm Dermaroller® devices were used to abrade the alopecic skin to the point of slight capillary bleeding. Hair regrowth occurred 5 weeks after treatment in both cases.[6] Microneedling should not be recommended as a routine treatment for alopecia X until more evidence for efficacy has been documented.

Oral trilostane was found to result in hair regrowth within 4–8 weeks in 85% of cases in one study.[7] Trilostane can be administered at a dose of 1.25–2.75 mg/kg po with food q12 h.[8] If no hair regrows after 4–6 months, the dose can be doubled.[7] The dose can be decreased to two or three times per week in some cases once the desired hair coat has been achieved.[7] Frequent monitoring and caution are necessary when using trilostane because it may result in adrenal insufficiency. Owners should be instructed to stop treatment and administer prednisone if depression, inappetence, vomiting or diarrhoea occurs. Pre- and post-ACTH cortisol concentrations should be obtained periodically to monitor the dog.[8] Cortisol levels return rapidly once trilostane administration has been stopped, and the drug can be reinstituted at a lower dose in 5–7 days. (See Hyperadrenocorticism, page 104.)

Key points

- As alopecia X is purely cosmetic, and the health of affected dogs is not impaired, monitoring without treatment is a reasonable option.
- There is no one successful treatment option.
- The prognosis for hair regrowth can be guarded.

References

1 Bernardi de Souza L, Paradis M, Zamberlam G, Benoit-Biancamano MO, Price C. Identification of 5α-reductase isoenzymes in canine skin. *Vet Dermatol* 2015; **26**: 363–e81.

2 Müntener T, Schuepbach-Regula G, Frank L, Rüfenacht S, Welle MM. Canine noninflammatory alopecia: a comprehensive evaluation of common and distinguishing histological characteristics. *Vet Dermatol* 2012; **23**: 206–e44.

3 Frank LA, Hnilica KA, Rohrbach BW, Oliver JW. Retrospective evaluation of sex hormones and steroid hormone intermediates in dogs with alopecia. *Vet Dermatol* 2003; **14**: 91–97.

4 Frank LA, Donnell RL, Kania SA. Estrogen receptor evaluation in Pomeranian dogs with hair cycle arrest (alopecia X) on melatonin supplementation. *Vet Dermatol* 2006; **17**: 252–258.

5 Albanese F, Malerba E, Abramo F, Miragliotta V, Fracassi F. Deslorelin for the treatment of hair cycle arrest in intact male dogs. *Vet Dermatol* 2014; **25**: 519–e88.

6 Stoll S, Dietlin C, Nett-Mettler CS. Microneedling as a successful treatment for alopecia X in two Pomeranian siblings. *Vet Dermatol* 2015; **26**: 387–e88.

7 Cerundolo R, Lloyd DH, Persechino A, Evans H, Cauvin A. Treatment of canine Alopecia X with trilostane. *Vet Dermatol* 2004; **15**: 285–293.

8 Arenas C, Melian C, Pérez-Alenza MD. Evaluation of 2 trilostane protocols for the treatment of canine pituitary-dependent hyperadrenocorticism: twice daily versus once daily. *J Vet Intern Med* 2013; **27**: 1478–1485.

CYCLICAL FLANK ALOPECIA
(Seasonal flank alopecia, flank alopecia, recurrent flank alopecia)

Definition

Cyclical flank alopecia is a follicular dysplasia of dogs resulting in alopecia and hyperpigmentation in the flank regions.

Aetiology and pathogenesis

It is likely that there is some genetic predisposition to cyclical flank alopecia, because it is quite common in some breeds (e.g. Boxers, Bulldogs, Airedales and Schnauzers) but rare in others (including German Shepherd dogs, Spaniels and Arctic breeds). There is no age predisposition, although the mean age of onset is about 4 years.[1,2] The seasonal nature of the condition and the fact that it is more common north of the 45° latitude suggest that light exposure and changing photoperiod are important. Onset in most cases is associated with short photoperiod seasons, which are opposite in the northern and southern hemispheres. Paradoxically, lesions may develop during prolonged photoperiods, with partial or complete resolution during shorter photoperiods. In other cases, lesions develop and there is no resolution with changes in photoperiod. This latter scenario is more likely to occur in areas of the world that do not have well-defined seasons.[1] Infrequently, multi-focal areas of interface dermatitis affecting alopecic skin may be observed, and the aetiology of this finding is unknown.

Clinical features

Lesions are typically characterised by the onset of well-demarcated, irregular-to-serpiginous areas of alopecia in the thoracolumbar areas (**Fig. 4.4**). Occasionally, other areas such as the nose, ears, tail, back, cranial ribcage and perineum can be affected. The underlying skin is usually hyperpigmented but otherwise normal. Airedale Terriers can have widespread involvement of the back, with lesions extending down to the trunk. Dogs with interface dermatitis may exhibit small, circular to arcuate, multi-focal patches of scaling, erosions and crusting. These lesions may be mildly painful or pruritic.

Hair regrowth usually occurs in 3–8 months as the photoperiod lengthens. However, the extent of alopecia can vary from year to year. Regrowth can be complete or partial and may be lighter or darker in colour and have a different texture. Hyperpigmentation and/or alopecia may eventually become permanent.

Affected dogs have no systemic clinical signs and the rest of the skin and coat appears normal.

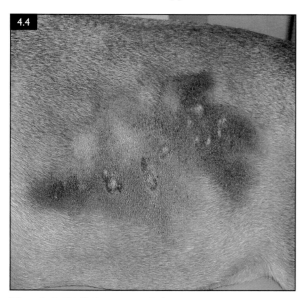

Fig. 4.4 Well-demarcated alopecia, hyperpigmentation and focal scaling over the flanks of an English Bulldog with cyclical flank alopecia.

Differential diagnoses

- Demodicosis.
- Dermatophytosis.
- Hypothyroidism.
- Injection site alopecia.
- Alopecia areata.
- Follicular dysplasia.

Diagnosis

Diagnosis is based on history, clinical findings and ruling out other differentials. The history and clinical appearance are often diagnostic. Dermatohistopathology can be supportive, with follicular atrophy, dysplastic follicles (which have infundibular hyperkeratosis extending into the secondary follicles) and sebaceous ducts giving an 'octopus'- or 'witches' foot'-like appearance. Infrequently, a multi-focal interface dermatitis may be seen.

Treatment

As lesions are cosmetic and hair may regrow on its own, observation only is reasonable. Melatonin (3–12 mg/dog po q12 h for 4–6 weeks and then as needed) may stimulate hair regrowth in some dogs. Some dogs will not regrow hair despite receiving melatonin, and in others giving the melatonin 4–6 weeks before the expected season seems to prevent hair loss.

Key points

- The alopecia may recur annually or be permanent.
- This condition is cosmetic only.

References

1 Gross TL, Ihrke PJ, Walder EJ, Affolter VK. Cyclical flank alopecia. In: *Skin Diseases of the Dog and Cat: Clinical and Histopathologic Diagnosis*, 2nd edn. Blackwell Publishing, Oxford, 2005: pp. 525–528.

2 Miller MA, Dunstan RW. Seasonal flank alopecia in Boxers and Airedale Terriers: 24 cases (1985–1992). *J Am Vet Med Assoc* 1993; **203**:1567–1572.

TELOGEN AND ANAGEN DEFLUXION

Definition
These are conditions of diffuse alopecia that occur because of a disruption in the normal hair cycle.

Aetiology and pathogenesis
The normal hair growth cycle follows exogen (expulsion of the old hair), anagen (active growth phase), catagen (transition phase) and telogen (resting phase).[1] A normal coat has hairs that are slightly offset from each other, so that they do not all shed at the same time. Growth therefore takes place in a mosaic pattern throughout the coat. Most dogs and cats have relatively short anagen phases and longer telogen phases (which is why they moult but do not need haircuts). Poodles and similar breeds have longer anagen phases, which is why they moult less but need haircuts. Some Arctic breeds can have very long telogen phases.

Anagen defluxion is associated with an abrupt disruption in the anagen phase of the hair cycle. This is typically caused by a sudden and severe illness, often involving pyrexia or chemotherapy. The hair loss occurs within days of the stressful event. The disruption of anagen is so acute that the microscopic morphology of the hair changes, rendering them vulnerable to breaking and loss.

Telogen defluxion is a slower process. An illness, such as hypothyroidism or hyperadrenocorticism, malnutrition or stress (including pregnancy, parturition and lactation) causes hairs to stay in telogen. Glucocorticoid administration can also synchronise the hairs into telogen. The hairs may be gradually lost through grooming and wear and tear, and are not replaced. More typically, there is a synchronous wave of exogen and hair loss when underlying diseases are treated and follicular activity begins again (typically within 1–3 months).

Clinical features
Telogen and anagen defluxion result in diffuse, symmetrical, partial-to-complete alopecia, especially of the trunk. Telogen defluxion may also be particularly marked in areas prone to wear and trauma. The coat can sometimes be 'peeled' off the skin in anagen defluxion. The underlying skin is usually normal (**Fig. 4.5**).

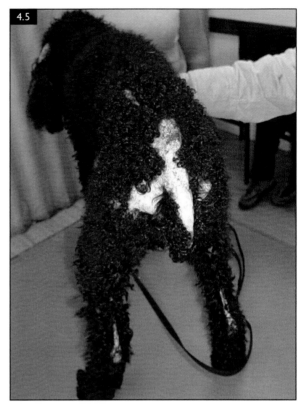

Fig. 4.5 Anagen defluxion after azathioprine treatment in a Miniature Poodle.

Differential diagnoses
• Hypothyroidism.
• Hyperadrenocorticism.
• Other metabolic and endocrine disorders.
• Follicular dysplasia.

Diagnosis
Diagnosis is based on history and clinical findings (**Figs. 4.6, 4.7**). Appropriate diagnostics to rule out a systemic insult should be performed as indicated. Hair plucks reveal normal telogenised hairs or, with anagen defluxion, twisted and fractured dysplastic hairs that often have prominent pinch points. Histopathological examination of skin biopsy samples will reveal dysplastic telogen hair follicles or new hairs in the hair shafts, but are not always diagnostic.

Treatment
Anagen and telogen defluxion self-cure in 1–6 months after the insult has been resolved.

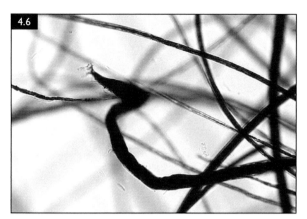

Fig. 4.6 Hair pluck from the dog in Fig. 4.5 with broken and distorted hairs.

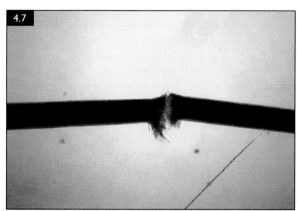

Fig. 4.7 Trichorrhexis nodosa in a hair pluck from a cat with anagen defluxion.

Key points

- The prognosis is generally good.
- Owners of Poodles and similar breeds should be warned that chemotherapy and cytotoxic drugs may induce hair loss.

Reference

1 Diaz SF, Torres SM, Dunstan RW, Lekcharoensuk C. An analysis of canine hair re-growth after clipping for a surgical procedure. *Vet Dermatol* 2004; **15**: 25–30.

HYPOTHYROIDISM

Definition

Hypothyroidism is a clinical syndrome associated with a failure of the thyroid glands to produce and release thyroid hormones. It is classified as primary, secondary or tertiary if the abnormality affects the thyroid gland, pituitary gland or hypothalamus, respectively.

Aetiology and pathogenesis

Most cases of hypothyroidism in dogs are due to lymphocytic thyroiditis or idiopathic follicular atrophy. Less commonly, hypothyroidism can be caused by pituitary neoplasia, which results in a thyroid-stimulating hormone (TSH) deficiency. Rarely, congenital hypothyroidism may occur secondary to an iodine deficiency.[1] Iatrogenic hypothyroidism can be caused by abruptly stopping prolonged inappropriate administration of levothyroxine, prolonged therapy with sulphonamides[2] or thyroidectomy.

Hypothyroidism is very rare in cats, but naturally occurring congenital cases in kittens and iatrogenic cases after surgical or radioactive treatment for hyperthyroidism may be seen.

Clinical features

The clinical signs of canine hypothyroidism are extremely variable and may include both systemic signs and dermatological signs.[1] The classic presentation is a bilaterally symmetrical truncal alopecia with thickened, hyperpigmented and cool skin (**Figs. 4.8–4.10**). Myxoedema is unusual except in advanced cases. Common dermatological problems include a dry, brittle coat, seborrhoea, scaling, postclipping alopecia, hyperpigmentation and recurrent pyoderma (**Figs. 4.11, 4.12**). In others, alopecia may be restricted to the tail and dorsal nose (**Figs. 4.13, 4.14**). Some dogs have abnormally retained hair (hypertrichosis) rather than alopecia. Clinical hypothyroidism is rarely seen in dogs under 2 years old. Congenital hypothyroidism is a rare condition that is also associated with disproportionate dwarfism, dental abnormalities and cretinism.

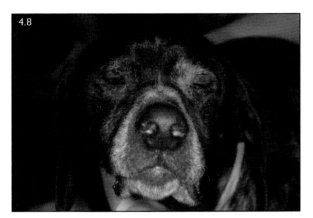

Fig. 4.8 Lethargy, tragic expression, periocular alopecia and fading of the coat in a hypothyroid cross-bred dog.

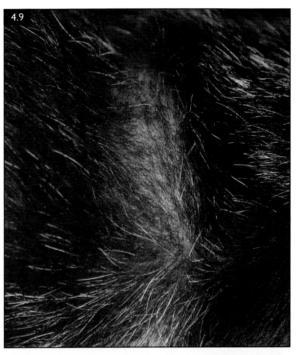

Fig. 4.9 Alopecia and reddening of the coat on the neck of a hypothyroid cross-bred dog.

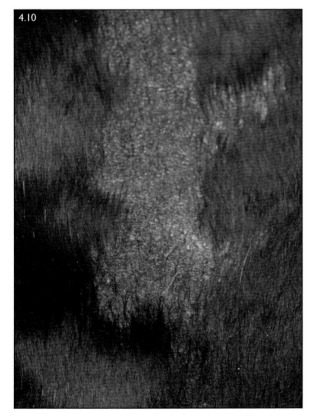

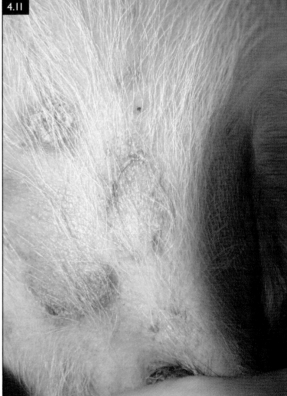

Fig. 4.10 Alopecia, hyperpigmentation and scaling on the flank of a hypothyroid Boxer.

Fig. 4.11 Acantholytic and exfoliative pyoderma with bullous impetigo and epidermal collarettes in a hypothyroid dog.

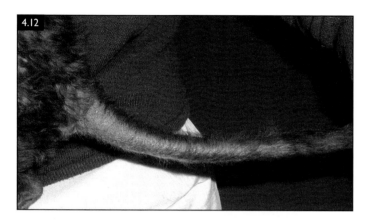

Fig. 4.12 Alopecia of the tail in a Devon Rex cat with congenital hypothyroidism.

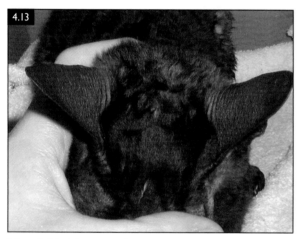

Fig. 4.13 Alopecia of the ears in this hypothyroid Devon Rex cat.

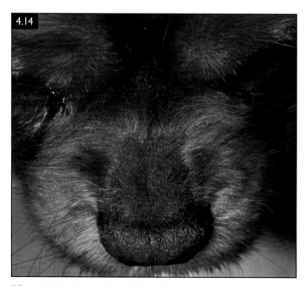

Fig. 4.14 Hypothyroidism: focal alopecia of the dorsal nose in a Cavalier King Charles Spaniel.

Hypothyroidism can also be a component of pituitary dwarfism. The clinical signs of hypothyroidism are as follows:

- Common signs: thin, poor quality coat; alopecia (including postclipping alopecia); scaling; secondary pyoderma; demodicosis; lethargy; and weight gain.
- Uncommon signs: neuromuscular disease; cretinism; ocular disorders; bradycardia; facial myxoedema ('tragic face') and hypothermia ('heat-seeking').

Differential diagnoses
- Hyperadrenocorticism.
- Alopecia X.
- Sex hormone disorders including Sertoli cell tumour.
- Sebaceous adenitis.
- Colour-dilution alopecia.
- Seasonal flank alopecia.
- Telogen effluvium/anagen defluxion.
- Pattern baldness.

Hypothyroidism may cause susceptibility to infections of the skin (e.g. superficial pyoderma, demodicosis and dermatophytosis).

Diagnosis
Hypothyroidism is commonly overdiagnosed in dogs. The diagnosis of hypothyroidism is achieved with appropriate clinical signs (dermatological and systemic), supportive blood work and response to therapy. Screening tests are usually non-specific,

but there may be anaemia, hypercholesterolaemia, hypertriglyceridaemia, hyperlipidaemia and elevated aspartate aminotransferase, alanine aminotransferase (ALT), alkaline phosphatase (ALP), creatinine kinase and fructosamine. A thyroid panels should demonstrate a low total thyroxine (T_4), a low free T_4 and a high TSH.

A low normal total T_4 is indicative of a euthyroid dog. A low total T_4 has relatively poor specificity as dogs with a non-thyroidal illness may have a transient low total T_4 (euthyroid sick syndrome). Thyroid supplementation is not beneficial and may be harmful in these cases. There are many drugs and diseases that interfere with the diagnosis of hypothyroidism. Commonly used drugs that may influence thyroid testing include: glucocorticoids, phenobarbital, sulphonamides and carprofen. Free T_4 tests are more specific and less prone to interference by drugs and concurrent conditions. Nevertheless, pyoderma and other conditions should be treated before assessing thyroid function.

Low total or free T_4 levels should be accompanied by elevated TSH in primary hypothyroidism. However, TSH will be normal in up to 20% of cases. Thyroglobulin autoantibodies (TGAAs) may also be increased, particularly in lymphocytic thyroiditis.[3] However, not all dogs with elevated TGAAs will subsequently develop the disease.

Treatment

Therapy involves lifelong administration of levothyroxine (L-thyroxine). The initial dose is 0.02 mg/kg or 0.5 mg/m^2 body surface area po twice daily. Dosing based on body surface area minimises underdosing of small dogs and overdosing of large dogs. The dose should be adjusted following the results of 4- to 6-hour post-thyroxine dosing T_4 levels. The T_4 post-treatment sample should be near the upper end of the range. T_4 testing and dose adjustments should be performed at 1, 2 and 3 months, and then every 3–6 months or as necessary in the long term. It is possible to switch many dogs to once-daily medication once the clinical signs have resolved. Signs of overdose include anxiety, restlessness, polyphagia, polydipsia, polyuria, weight loss and tachycardia. It may be necessary to use appropriate systemic and/or topical treatment to control secondary infections or demodicosis initially.

The timeline for resolution of lesions is as follows:

- Mentation and activity: 2–7 days.
- Serum biochemical abnormalities: 2–4 weeks.
- Dermatological abnormalities: 2–4 months.
- Neurological abnormalities: 1–3 months.
- Cardiac abnormalities: 1–2 months.
- Reproduction abnormalities: 3–10 months.

Some dogs experience a massive shedding of hair and skin cells 1–2 months after initiation of thyroid supplementation. This represents the hair re-entering the active growth (anagen) phase as the dog becomes euthyroid. Old, resting (telogen) hairs are expelled (exogen) before the new anagen hairs become apparent. The shedding is normal and will resolve with time.

Key points

- Some drugs and disease may have an impact on thyroid testing.
- Low normal total T_4 does not indicate hypothyroidism.
- A common cause of recurrent pyoderma.

References

1 Parry N. Hypothyroidism in dogs: pathophysiology, causes and clinical presentation. *Companion Animal* 2013; **18**(2): 34–38.
2 Daminet S, Ferguson DC. Influence of drugs on thyroid function in dogs. *J Vet Intern Med* 2003; **17**: 463–472.
3 Parry N. Hypothyroidism in dogs: laboratory findings. *Companion Animal* 2013; **18**(3): 101–105.

HYPERADRENOCORTICISM IN DOGS AND CATS
(Cushing's disease)

Definition

Hyperadrenocorticism (HAC or Cushing's disease) is a constellation of symptoms that result from prolonged exposure to elevated serum cortisol concentrations, which may be spontaneous or iatrogenic.

Aetiology and pathogenesis

Most cases (80–85%) of spontaneous HAC in dogs are pituitary dependent (PDH): functional adenomas of the anterior pituitary secrete adrenocorticotrophic hormone (ACTH), resulting in adrenocortical hyperplasia. Of cases 15–20% are due to adrenal neoplasia, although this figure may be slightly higher in larger breed dogs. HAC is rare in cats, although iatrogenic and spontaneous cases with a similar proportion of PDH and adrenal tumours to dogs are seen.

Most cases of iatrogenic HAC result from long-term administration of glucocorticoid either orally or by depot injection. The risk of inducing iatrogenic HAC is dose and duration related, and may be minimised by administering oral prednisone (or prednisolone or methylprednisolone) on an alternate-day basis, although there is wide individual variation in steroid tolerance. Rarely, cases have been seen following topical administration (**Fig. 4.15**).

Clinical features

Animals of any age may be affected, but there is a steadily increasing risk with age up to 7–9 years old. There appears to be no sex predisposition to HAC, but females are predisposed to adrenal neoplasia. Any breed may be affected, but Terriers in particular are predisposed to HAC, Dachshunds to adrenal tumours and Boxers to pituitary neoplasia.

Dogs with HAC may exhibit a number of clinical signs. Common clinical signs are polyuria/polydipsia (PU/PD), a pendulous abdomen, hepatomegaly, polyphagia, weight gain, muscular weakness and atrophy, lordosis (ventral bowing of the spine) (**Fig. 4.16**), anoestrus, pendulous prepuce and testicular atrophy, panting, neurological or visual deficits (which can be associated with pressure from a pituitary macroadenoma) and insulin-resistant diabetes mellitus. Dermatological signs include the following:

- Dull, dry, faded coat that is easily epilated.
- Postclipping alopecia.
- Symmetrical-to-generalised, complete-to-diffuse non-inflammatory alopecia, particularly of the trunk, but sparing the head and distal limbs (**Fig. 4.16**).

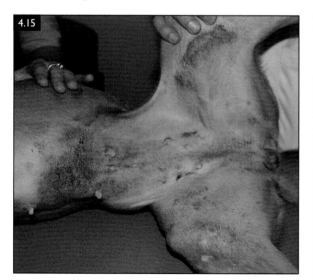

Fig. 4.15 Localised changes to the skin after long-term topical administration of betamethasone to an atopic Boxer.

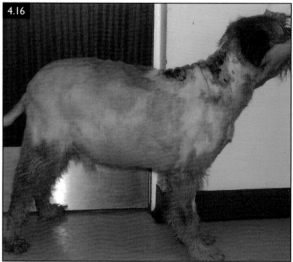

Fig. 4.16 Canine hyperadrenocorticism with truncal alopecia, pot-belly, lordosis and calcinosis cutis.

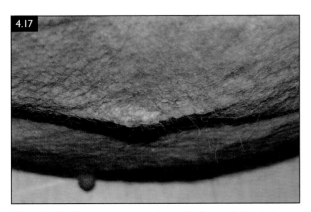

Fig. 4.17 Cutaneous atrophy with loss of elasticity, tenting and wrinkles.

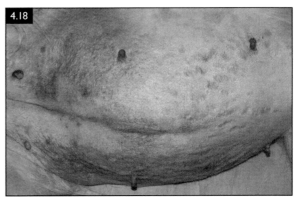

Fig. 4.18 Pot-belly, alopecia and cutaneous atrophy, with comedones, prominent blood vessels, haemorrhage, bruising and 'stretch marks'.

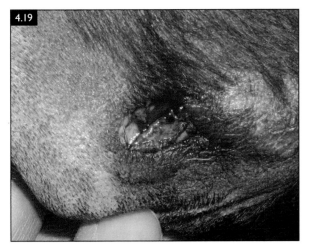

Fig. 4.19 Fragile skin and non-healing over the elbow.

- Mild-to-moderate scaling.
- Cutaneous atrophy, prominent blood vessels, loss of elasticity and wrinkling, especially on the abdomen (**Figs. 4.17, 4.18**).
- Comedones (**Fig. 4.18**).
- Easily bruised skin and poor wound healing (**Fig. 4.19**).
- Calcinosis cutis (**Figs. 4.20, 4.21**).
- Increased susceptibility to bacterial pyoderma, malassezia dermatitis, dermatophytosis and demodicosis.

Fig. 4.21 Close up of the lesions with well-demarcated pink to white papules and plaques. The lesions are firm and gritty.

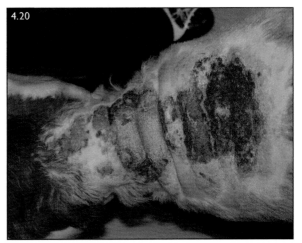

Fig. 4.20 Extensive inflamed plaques, ulceration and crusting associated with calcinosis cutis in a dog with iatrogenic hyperadrenocorticism. The dorsal neck is a frequently affected site.

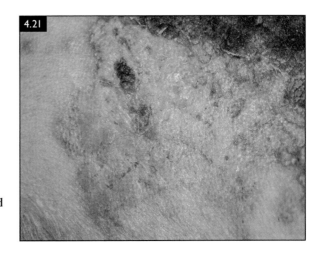

Dogs may present with any combination of clinical signs that can develop in any order. This can make the diagnosis difficult. Dogs with secondary infections and calcinosis cutis may be pruritic. Conversely, animals with pre-existing inflammatory disorders such as atopic dermatitis or osteoarthritis can improve as HAC develops.

Cats present with less well-defined clinical signs than dogs. These may be similar to the range seen in dogs, but affected cats often present with cutaneous atrophy and skin fragility. Such cats must be handled with extreme care to prevent further damage to the skin. Other skin changes include colour change, dullness, seborrhoea, scaling, matting, *Demodex* spp. and secondary infections. Polydipsia/polyuria is less likely unless there is concurrent diabetes mellitus, although many cats with HAC present as cases of insulin-resistant diabetes mellitus. Other clinical signs include neurological abnormalities, plantigrade stance, hepatomegaly and muscle atrophy.

Differential diagnoses

- Hypothyroidism.
- Sertoli cell neoplasia and other sex hormone dermatoses.
- Adrenal sex hormone dermatoses or alopecia of follicular arrest ('alopecia X').
- Follicular dysplasias.
- Telogen effluvium and anagen defluxion.
- Diabetes mellitus.

Diagnosis in dogs

Routine haematology, biochemistry and urinalysis are necessary in the diagnostic work-up of any dog with systemic illness. Dogs with HAC often have the following abnormalities:

- Stress leukogram: neutrophilia, lymphopenia, eosinopenia and monocytosis (rare).
- Hypercholesterolaemia.
- Mild-to-moderate hyperglycaemia.
- Increased serum ALT and ALP; the latter is very common in dogs (which have a steroid-induced isoenzyme) and usually out of proportion with the increase in ALT.
- Decreased total T_4 due to cortisol inhibition.
- Urine specific gravity generally <1.015 (i.e. hyposthenuric).

- Presence of urinary white blood cells, blood and protein due to urinary tract infections; these are common, but clinical signs can be masked by the anti-inflammatory action of cortisol.

None of the clinical signs and these findings is specific for HAC, and specific endocrine tests are required to confirm the diagnosis before starting treatment.

Low-dose dexamethasone suppression test

Low-dose dexamethasone suppression tests (LDDSTs) are the current diagnostic test of choice unless iatrogenic HAC is suspected.[1] The LDDST assesses the ability of the hypothalamic–pituitary–adrenal axis to respond to negative feedback, resulting in decreased ACTH release and adrenal cortisol production[1] (**Fig. 4.22**). LDDSTs are 85–100% sensitive and 44–73% specific (i.e. false negatives are uncommon but there may be false positives).[1] Dexamethasone is used because it does not cross-react with cortisol assays. The exact protocol varies with the laboratory, so it is advisable to check with the individual laboratory first. LDDSTs generally involve taking blood samples to measure blood cortisol levels immediately before, and then at 4 and 8 hours after giving 0.01–0.015 mg/kg of dexamethasone intravenously.

In about 30% of dogs there is adequate suppression at 4 h, but 'escape' at 8 h with cortisol concentrations rising again, which is diagnostic for PDH. In most cases of adrenal neoplasia, and some 25% of all spontaneous HAC cases (including PDH), there is no suppression at 4 or 8 h. In other cases, there may be some suppression but cortisol levels do not fall below 50% of the baseline measurement.

ACTH stimulation tests

In ACTH stimulations tests synthetic ACTH is used to stimulate cortisol production from the adrenal cortex (**Fig. 4.23**), and therefore assess adrenocortical reserve. ACTH stimulation tests are the current gold standard for diagnosis of iatrogenic HAC[1] and are used to monitor adrenal function during therapy. They are of less use for the diagnosis of spontaneous HAC,[1] because, although they are more specific than LDDSTs (i.e. false positives are uncommon), they are less sensitive (i.e. there may be false negatives).

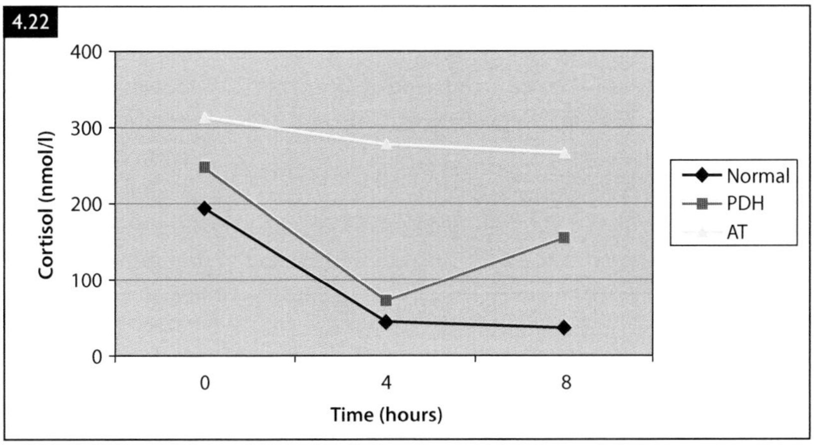

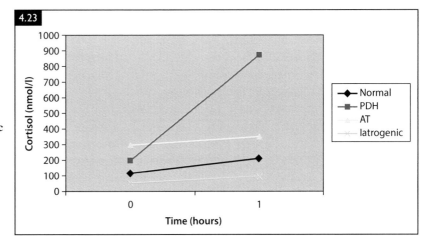

Fig. 4.22 Low-dose dexamethasone suppression test: typical results from cases of pituitary-dependent hyperadrenocorticism (PDH) and adrenal tumours (AT) after a low-dose dexamethasone suppression test.

Fig. 4.23 Adrenocorticotrophic hormone stimulation tests: typical results for various forms of hyperadrenocorticism. (AT, adrenal tumours; PDH, pituitary-dependent hyperadrenocorticism.)

Measurement of 17-hydroxyprogesterone (17OHP) can be useful in cases of 'atypical' HAC, where a strong clinical suspicion of HAC is not confirmed with adrenal tests based on the production of cortisol. This may be because some adrenocortical tumours release steroid precursors rather than cortisol.

Each laboratory has a normal range based on its protocol. Most tests involve taking blood samples before and 30–90 minutes after 250 µg ACTH given intravenously or intramuscularly.

Progestogens, glucocorticoids and ketoconazole decrease responses to ACTH.

Urinary cortisol:creatinine ratio

Urinary cortisol:creatinine ratio (UCCR) measurement is highly sensitive but poorly specific for HAC. A normal UCCR makes HAC very unlikely, but raised UCCRs are commonly seen in many other diseases associated with inflammation, systemic illness and PU/PD. Stress can also result in a raised UCCR, so samples should be collected at home by the owner before visiting the veterinary clinic. Pooled 3-day samples are most commonly used.

Endogenous ACTH assay

The test measures the circulating endogenous ACTH concentration to differentiate PDH from an adrenal tumour.[1] PDH cases have normal or high (>25 pg/ml) levels due to ACTH secretion from a functional pituitary tumour, independent of negative feedback from elevated cortisol. Adrenal tumours have low ACTH levels (<5 pg/ml) due to negative feedback from ACTH-independent cortisol production. ACTH is, however, very labile. Blood samples must be taken into chilled ethylenediaminetetraacetic acid (EDTA) tubes and centrifuged in a chilled centrifuge (placing a minicentrifuge in a refrigerator at 4°C for an hour is usually sufficient). The plasma should be immediately frozen and sent by overnight or same-day courier in a freezer pack. This test can also be used in cats.

High-dose dexamethasone suppression test

This should be performed as a differentiating test only if abdominal ultrasound (see below) or endogenous ACTH testing is unavailable.[1] This tests the resistance of the pituitary–adrenal axis to high doses of dexamethasone, because it has been shown that pituitary tumours in dogs with PDH may respond to high doses of dexamethasone, resulting in suppression of ACTH production and cortisol levels. Blood samples are taken before and then 4 and 8 hours after 1 mg/kg of iv dexamethasone. Any significant suppression of cortisol (>50% from the baseline) is diagnostic for PDH. There is no response to this test in about 15% cases of PDH and most dogs with adrenal neoplasia. However, given the relative frequencies of PDH and adrenal tumours, this results in only 50% specificity. High-dose dexamethasone suppression tests (HDDSTs) are therefore now used less often.

Diagnosis in cats

HAC occurs most frequently in cats as a cause of insulin-resistant diabetes mellitus.[2] Routine complete blood counts, serum biochemistries and urinalysis typically reflect changes secondary to diabetes. Cats lack steroid-induced ALP and dilute urine is an uncommon finding.

LDDSTs are the test of choice for diagnosis of feline HAC.[2] Dexamethasone is administered at 0.1 mg/kg iv (a higher dose than in dogs) and serum cortisol levels are measured at 4 and 8 h. The sensitivity is high, but the specificity is only moderate for the diagnosis of HAC in cats.[2]

ACTH stimulation testing is poorly sensitive in naturally occurring HAC in cats. However, it is sensitive for iatrogenic hyperadrenocorticism.[2] ACTH 125 μg is administered iv or im, and serum cortisol levels are measured generally 60 minutes later. Variation may occur among laboratories.

A combined ACTH stimulation/LDDST has been used in cats. A basal blood sample is followed by injection of 0.1 mg/kg of iv dexamethasone. Two hours later a second sample is obtained and followed by intravenous injection of 0.125 μg synthetic ACTH. The third blood sample is collected 1 hour later. Normal cats show 50% suppression of cortisol in the postdexamethasone sample and up to 400 nmol/l after ACTH. Cats with HAC exhibit little suppression after dexamethasone and exaggerated stimulation after ACTH.

The UCCR is a useful screening test for feline HAC. Collection of a morning sample at home will minimise the influence of stress on the test results (using non-absorbent litter, such as plastic or glass beads).[2] A negative result makes HAC unlikely, although a positive result can occur as the result of any illness.[2]

Imaging

Imaging is supportive of, but not diagnostic for, HAC.[1] Abdominal radiographs may reveal increased contrast due to additional intra-abdominal fat, distended bladder (PU/PD), hepatomegaly and/or dystrophic calcification of skin (calcinosis cutis), airways, blood vessels, kidneys, etc. Thoracic metastasis of an adrenal carcinoma can also be detected.

Ultrasonography can be very useful in both dogs and cats[2] to detect and assess adrenal tumours and will also detect bilateral hypertrophy in PDH.[1] Magnetic resonance imaging (MRI) and computed tomography (CT) will detect pituitary tumours, adrenal tumours and invasion of the vena cava.

Biopsy

Histopathological examination of skin biopsy samples may be helpful, but in many instances the cutaneous changes are non-diagnostic for both dogs and cats unless calcinosis cutis is present. The presence of calcinosis cutis is highly specific for HAC.

Treatment in dogs

If the cause of symptoms is due to exogenous steroid administration, the dose of steroids needs to be tapered to the minimum alternate-day dose that is needed. Other therapies should be used to spare the use of steroids when at all possible. The following treatments are for spontaneous HAC.

Trilostane is highly effective in canine HAC. It inhibits 3β-hydroxysteroid dehydrogenase, an enzyme essential for steroidogenesis.[3] It is effective in 67–100% of dogs. Trilostane is initially administered at 2–5 mg/kg po q24 h. Doses of 1.25–2.75 mg/kg po q12 h may also be used, and may control HAC symptoms more effectively than q24 h dosing.[4] Symptoms should improve steadily each month, and maximum improvement may take up to 1 year. Doses may need to be increased to up to 12 mg/kg per day depending on the response to therapy.[4] ACTH stimulation tests are required to monitor adrenocortical reserve during treatment. ACTH and serum chemistry (including renal and hepatic values and electrolytes) testing are performed 4–6 hours post-trilostane dosing, and should be performed 2, 4 and 12 weeks after initiation of treatment. If signs compatible with hypoadrenocorticism are detected, then the trilostane therapy should be discontinued until serum cortisol levels return to normal. Trilostane can then be restarted at a lower dose. Prednisone should be administered if the patient is experiencing an addisonian crisis.

Mitotane (*o,p'*-DDD) was once the treatment of choice, but is used much less now that trilostane is available. Mitotane exerts its effect by causing lysis of the adrenal gland. An induction dose (25–50 mg/kg q24 h) is usually given with food until effect (PU/PD [water intake <60 ml/kg per day], polyphagia resolves or if signs of hypoadrenocorticism occur) and an ACTH test performed to assess the adrenal reserve. Both basal and post-ACTH cortisol concentrations should be in the normal resting range. About 15% of dogs with PDH will still have elevated post-ACTH cortisol concentrations, and the induction course should be continued until the ACTH response is suppressed adequately. About 30% of dogs will have subnormal pre- and post-ACTH cortisol concentrations, and in these cases mitotane is withheld until normal cortisol concentrations recover. At this point, maintenance doses of mitotane (25–50 mg/kg per week) are given in two to three divided doses.[4]

The prognosis for dogs treated with mitotane is fair, but an appreciable number of dogs prove very hard to stabilise with frequent relapses and/or hypoadrenocortical (addisonian) crises. An alternative protocol is to continue the induction course at doses of 50–75 mg/kg until there is no adrenal reserve left, and then manage the dogs for hypoadrenocorticism. This protocol is now uncommon, because there are frequent crises during induction and many dogs eventually relapse.[4]

Very-high-dose mitotane therapy (50–75 mg/kg per day) for up to 11 weeks (with regular ACTH tests to assess response) may be necessary to reduce serum cortisol to normal levels in cases of adrenal tumours. These dogs may also need higher doses to maintain remission.

Other treatment options

Adrenal neoplasia may be managed by surgical resection. Surgery is difficult, has a significant complication rate, including perioperative death, and hypoadrenocortical crises are common. Histopathological features, tumour size and age do not appear to affect the outcome. Medical therapy with trilostane or mitotane can effectively control clinical signs in inoperable or partially resected adrenal tumours, although metastatic disease can still occur.

Ketoconazole inhibits adrenal steroid synthesis and has been used at 5–10 mg/kg po once daily to manage HAC. Its activity is, however, less specific and efficacious than trilostane.

Early reports suggested that selegiline (l-deprenyl) (2 mg/kg po q24 h) could be useful in the treatment of PDH, but later clinical trials demonstrated poor efficacy, and it is rarely used.

Surgical excision and radiation therapy may be used in cases of pituitary macroadenoma, if there are issues due to the mass effect or disease cannot be controlled medically.

Treatment in cats

Trilostane is effective in up to 86% of cats, and it is the most effective medical option.[2,3] The dose is 10 mg per cat po q24 h. ACTH stimulation testing is as for dogs.

Metyrapone may be considered if trilostane is unavailable. The dose is 30 mg/kg po q12 h. ACTH stimulation testing is as for trilostane. The maximum dose should not exceed 70 mg/kg q12 h.[2]

Surgical (hypophysectomy or adrenalectomy) and radiation therapies are also available for cats.[4]

Mitotane and ketoconazole are not recommended for cats.[2]

Hypoadrenocortical (addisonian) crisis

Most adverse effects from therapy are associated with decreased serum cortisol and an addisonian crisis, with signs such as lethargy, weakness, inappetence, vomiting, diarrhoea, bradycardia and collapse. Owners should be aware of these signs and instructed to withdraw therapy temporarily and administer prednisolone (0.2–0.25 mg/kg po) as necessary. Severe cases that present with circulatory collapse will need intravenous fluid support. Prednisolone treatment should cease for a minimum of 24 h before an ACTH stimulation test, because it will interfere with the cortisol assay.

Calcinosis cutis

Exacerbation of or the appearance of calcinosis cutis after medical or surgical treatment is reasonably common. This usually resolves over the course of therapy. Severe cases of calcinosis cutis may not fully resolve even with good control of HAC. Simple monitoring is appropriate if the lesions are quiescent with no ulceration or secondary infection. Daily topical application of dimethyl sulphoxide (DMSO) has been effective, but treated animals should be monitored for signs of hypercalcaemia.

Key points

- Daily, low-dose glucocorticoid administration is more likely to cause iatrogenic HAC than alternate-day glucocorticoid administration. This is true even if the alternate-day dose is higher than the daily dose.
- Any screening test for HAC may be negative. If a test is negative, but suspicion for HAC remains, then another test should be performed.

References

1 Behrend EN, Kooistra HS, Nelson R, Reusch CE, Scott-Moncrieff JC. Diagnosis of spontaneous canine hyperadrenocorticism: 2012 ACVIM consensus statement (small animal). *J Vet Intern Med* 2013; **27**: 1292–1304.
2 Niessen SJ, Church DB, Forcada Y. Hypersomatotropism, acromegaly, and hyperadrenocorticism and feline diabetes mellitus. *Vet Clin North Am Small Anim Pract* 2013; **43**: 319–350.
3 Scudder C, Kenny MP, Niessen S. Treatment of canine and feline hyperadrenocorticism: trilostane and the alternatives. *Companion Animal* 2015; **20**: 230–238.
4 Arenas C, Melian C, Pérez-Alenza MD. Evaluation of 2 trilostane protocols for the treatment of canine pituitary-dependent hyperadrenocorticism: twice daily versus once daily. *J Vet Intern Med* 2013; **27**: 1478–1485.

FELINE PARANEOPLASTIC ALOPECIA

Definition

Feline paraneoplastic alopecia is a non-pruritic syndrome of hair loss that is a marker for underlying internal malignancy.

Aetiology and pathogenesis

This condition is generally associated with a pancreatic adenocarcinoma, but in a small number of cases it has been reported in association with bile duct carcinoma.[1-4] The mechanism by which the tumour causes this dramatic hair loss is not known.

Clinical features

The syndrome occurs in older cats. Alopecia first appears on the ventral abdomen, thorax and limbs, and then may generalise.[1-4] Occasionally, the pinnae and periorbital regions may also be affected.

Hair adjacent to the advancing alopecia epilates easily. The alopecic skin has a characteristic smooth, shiny appearance (**Fig. 4.24**). It is thin and inelastic, but not fragile.[3] The footpads may be affected with translucent scale often arranged in rings.[3] Excessive grooming and secondary malassezia dermatitis may also develop.[2,3] Concurrent signs of underlying neoplasia include anorexia, weight loss and lethargy.

Differential diagnoses

- Psychogenic alopecia.
- Lymphocytic mural folliculitis.
- Thymoma-associated exfoliative dermatitis.
- Demodicosis.
- Hyperadrenocorticism.
- Telogen defluxion.

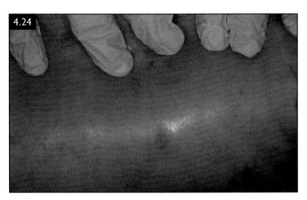

Fig. 4.24 Smooth, shiny, glistening skin and alopecia in a cat with feline paraneoplastic alopecia.

Diagnosis

The history and clinical findings are distinctive. Dermatohistopathology is supportive. Ultrasonography or exploratory laparotomy will confirm neoplasia.

Treatment

Complete surgical excision of the internal malignancy is curative. However, in most cases, tumour metastasis has occurred by the time a diagnosis is made and the prognosis is therefore poor.[1-3] Recurrence of the alopecia indicates metastatic disease and relapse.

Key points

- A condition with distinctive alopecic, smooth, shiny skin that is due to internal malignancy and has a poor prognosis.
- Pruritus is not a feature of this disease unless secondary malassezia dermatitis is present.

References

1 Brooks DG, Campbell KL, Dennis JS *et al.* Pancreatic paraneoplastic alopecia in three cats. *J Am Anim Hosp Assoc* 1994; **30**: 557–563.
2 Godfrey DR. A case of feline paraneoplastic alopecia with secondary *Malassezia*-associated dermatitis. *J Small Anim Pract* 1998; **39**: 394–396.
3 Pascal A, Olivry T, Gross TL *et al.* Paraneoplastic alopecia associated with internal malignancies in the cat. *Vet Dermatol* 1997; **8**: 47–52.
4 Tasker S, Griffon DJ, Nuttall TJ *et al.* Resolution of paraneoplastic alopecia following surgical removal of a pancreatic carcinoma in a cat. *J Small Anim Pract* 1999; **40**: 16–19.

ACQUIRED PATTERN ALOPECIA
(Pattern baldness, follicular miniaturisation)

Definition

Acquired pattern alopecia is a condition that results in thinning of hair or alopecia in specific symmetrical locations over the body.

Aetiology and pathogenesis

The pathogenesis of acquired pattern alopecia is unknown, although some form of genetic predisposition is suspected.

Clinical features

The syndrome is frequently seen in Dachshunds, but it can occur in other short-coated breeds such as the Boston Terrier, Chihuahua, Greyhound, Whippet and Miniature Pinscher. Common features of pattern alopecia include an insidious onset and slowly progressive, symmetrical and focal hair loss, which may result in well-demarcated patches of complete alopecia (**Fig. 4.25**). The underlying skin is usually normal. Very short and very fine hairs may be evident, especially in the earlier stages. Affected dogs show no systemic clinical signs, and the rest of the hair coat is normal. One pattern involves gradual alopecia and hyperpigmentation of the pinnae in male and, less commonly, female Dachshunds. This usually starts at age 6–12 months and is complete by 6–9 years. Another pattern is seen in young to adult Greyhounds that develop gradual hair loss of the caudal thighs. The most frequently seen pattern consists of bilateral thinning of hair that can progress to total hair loss in one or more of the following areas: pinna and areas just caudal to the pinna, areas between ear and eye, ventral neck, chest, ventral

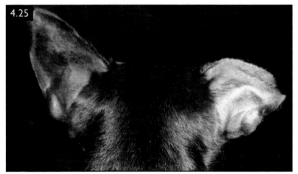

Fig. 4.25 Pattern baldness affecting the dorsal pinnae in a Patterdale Terrier.

abdomen and perianal and caudal thighs. Of these the pinna is most frequently affected. This pattern occurs in Dachshunds, but it is also recognised in other breeds (see also page 237).

Differential diagnoses
- Cushing's syndrome.
- Hypothyroidism.
- Sertoli cell tumour.
- Exposure to human topical hormone replacement therapy.
- Demodicosis.
- Dermatophytosis.
- Follicular dysplasia.
- Telogen effluvium and telogen defluxion.
- Alopecia areata.
- Vasculopathy.
- Dermatomyositis.

Diagnosis
Diagnosis is based on history, clinical findings and ruling out other differentials. Histopathology reveals normal skin with miniaturisation of hair follicles and very fine hair shafts.

Treatment
Acquired pattern alopecia is a benign cosmetic condition and does not need treatment. Melatonin (3–12 mg/dog po q12 h) may occasionally result in hair regrowth.

Key point
- Pattern baldness is a cosmetic, genetically predisposed condition. Regrowth of hair is only rarely achieved.

BLACK HAIR FOLLICULAR DYSPLASIA

Definition
Black hair follicular dysplasia is a rare disorder affecting growth of black hairs, with sparing of white hairs.[1]

Aetiology and pathogenesis
The underlying aetiology of the disorder is not understood. Abnormally large granules of melanin are present within the pigmented hair shafts, which may exhibit microscopic defects, and there are areas of epidermal pigment clumping, suggesting defects in pigment handling.[1] The dermatosis has been shown to be autosomally transmitted in one study on an affected crossbred litter,[2] although the mode of inheritance was not determined.[1] Breeds reportedly affected include the Bearded Collie, Border Collie, Beagle, Basset Hound, Papillon, Saluki, Jack Russell Terrier, American Cocker Spaniel, Cavalier King Charles Spaniel, Dachshund, Gordon Setter and Munsterlander.[1,3,4] As black hair follicular dysplasia and colour-dilution alopecia share clinical and histopathological features, it is possible that black hair follicular dysplasia is a localised form of colour-dilution alopecia.[5]

Clinical features
Only black-pigmented hair is affected. There is a patchy hypotrichosis associated with pigmented regions of skin (**Fig. 4.26**). Affected areas produce short, dry, lustreless hair, although the severity varies both within and between individuals. Affected animals are normal at birth. Abnormalities may be detected both microscopically and grossly from as early as 3 weeks of age[2] and, rarely, they are delayed later than 6 weeks[1] (see also page 236).

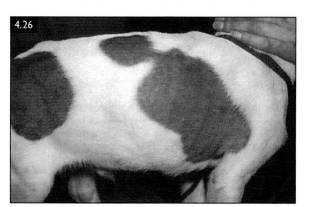

Fig. 4.26 Black hair follicle alopecia in a Jack Russell Terrier (photo courtesy of CM Knottenbelt).

Differential diagnoses

- Demodicosis.
- Dermatophytosis.
- Superficial pyoderma.
- Colour-dilution alopecia.
- Endocrinopathy.
- Alopecia areata.

Diagnosis

A history of normal pups developing lesions that are confined to the pigmented areas only is highly suggestive of black hair follicular dysplasia. Hair plucks, tape-strips and skin scrapes should be taken to rule out demodicosis. Hair plucks will often demonstrate abnormal hairs with macromelanosomes (see Colour-dilution alopecia, page 237). Histopathological examination of biopsy samples is diagnostic.

Treatment

The dermatosis is not responsive to treatment. Only the pigmented areas of the skin are affected and there are no systemic signs. Management should be symptomatic; mild shampoos and systemic antibacterial therapy may be indicated if secondary superficial pyoderma develops.

Key point

- Pathognomonic presentation where only black-coloured areas are affected.

References

1 Hargis AM, Brignac MM, Al-Bagdadi FAK *et al*. Black hair follicular dysplasia in black and white Saluki dogs: differentiation from color mutant alopecia in the Doberman Pinscher by microscopic examination of hairs. *Vet Dermatol* 1991; **2**: 69–83.
2 Selmanowitz VJ, Markofsky F, Orentreich N. Black hair follicular dysplasia in dogs. *J Am Vet Med Assoc* 1977; **171**: 1079–1081.
3 Harper RC. Congenital black hair follicle dysplasia in Bearded Collie pups. *Vet Rec* 1978; **102**: 87.
4 Scott DW, Miller WH, Griffin CE. Black hair follicular dysplasia. In: *Muller and Kirk's Small Animal Dermatology*, 6th edn. Philadelphia, PA: WB Saunders, 2001: pp. 959–970.
5 Gross TH, Ihrke PJ, Walder EJ, Affolter VK. Color-dilution alopecia and black hair follicular dysplasia. In: *Skin Diseases of the Dog and Cat: Clinical and Histopathologic Diagnosis*, 2nd edn. Oxford: Blackwell Publishing, 2005: pp. 518–522.

COLOUR-DILUTION ALOPECIA
(Colour-mutant alopecia, blue Doberman or blue dog syndrome)

Definition

Colour-dilution alopecia is an inherited disorder of colour-diluted (i.e. grey or 'blue', or red/fawn) dogs characterised by alopecia developing in the areas of the dilute-coloured hair.

Aetiology and pathogenesis

Colour-dilution alopecia is the result of an autosomal genetic mutation.[1,2] Affected animals have many large, irregularly shaped melanin granules in the basal keratinocytes, the hair matrix cells and the hair shafts.[1,3] The extensive melanin clumping in the hair and associated distortion of the cuticular–cortical structure of the hair are thought to lead to fragility and breaking of hair shafts.[3] Similar findings can be seen in non-alopecic animals with dilute-coloured coats as well, although the macromelanosomes appear to be smaller and do not affect hair follicle and shaft integrity. Cats with diluted coats are only very rarely affected by colour-dilution alopecia.

Clinical features

Colour-dilution alopecia was initially diagnosed in blue Doberman Pinschers, leading to the early name of blue Doberman syndrome. However, the syndrome has also been diagnosed in other breeds with blue colour dilution. The syndrome appears in approximately 93% of blue and 83% of fawn Doberman Pinschers.[1] Onset generally occurs in animals aged 4 months to 3 years. However, it has developed in some animals as late as 6 years of age.[4] Affected animals gradually develop a dull, dry, brittle, poor-quality coat with fractured hair (**Figs. 4.27, 4.28**). As the condition progresses, a moth-eaten partial alopecia develops, which may continue to worsen until there is total alopecia of dilute-coloured hair. Follicular papules often develop and may advance to comedo formation or secondary bacterial folliculitis and/or malassezia dermatitis. As the condition becomes chronic, the affected skin can become hyperpigmented and seborrhoeic. The severity of the syndrome varies. Lesions will be limited to the

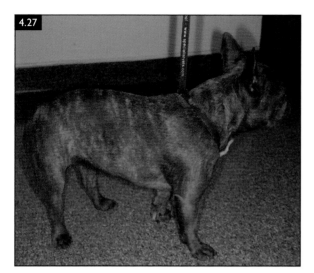

Fig. 4.27 Colour-dilute coat in a brindle Staffordshire Bull Terrier. The usual coat is black and brown. This dog was asymptomatic apart from mild thinning of the coat.

dilute-coloured parts of the coat in multi-coloured animals (see also page 236).

Differential diagnoses
- Hyperadrenocorticism.
- Hypothyroidism.
- Sex hormone dermatoses.
- Cyclical flank alopecia.
- Acquired pattern alopecia.
- Demodicosis.
- Dermatophytosis.
- Staphylococcal pyoderma.
- Malassezia dermatitis.

Diagnosis
Clinical examination will raise suspicion of the disorder. Microscopic examination of affected hair may demonstrate uneven distribution and clumping of melanin (**Fig. 4.29**) that may cause distortion of the hair shaft. Histopathological examination of biopsy samples will confirm the diagnosis.

Treatment
There is no specific treatment that will alter the course of the syndrome. Harsh, drying shampoos can accelerate coat damage. Gentle bathing with antimicrobial, keratolytic and moisturising

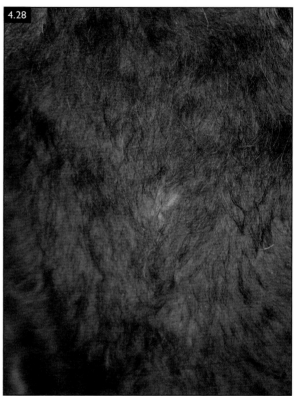

Fig. 4.28 Colour dilution in a blue German Shepherd dog. The dilute-coloured areas in this dog were severely affected with alopecia, follicular dysplasia and staphylococcal pyoderma.

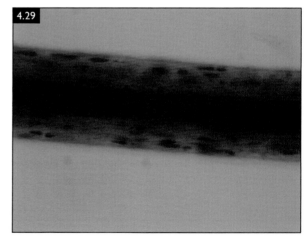

Fig. 4.29 Macromelanosomes in a hair pluck from the blue German Shepherd dog.

products should be tailored to the needs of each individual case. Systemic antibiotics would be appropriate if a secondary bacterial folliculitis is present. High-quality diets and essential fatty acids may also be helpful.

Key points
- Diagnosis depends on histopathological examination.
- There is no treatment that will alter the coat changes.

References
1 Miller WH. Color-dilution alopecia in Doberman Pinschers with blue or fawn coat colors: a study of the incidence and histopathology of this disorder. *Vet Dermatol* 1990; **1**: 113–121.

2 Miller WH. Alopecia associated with coat color dilution in two Yorkshire Terriers, one Saluki, and one mix-breed. *J Am Anim Hosp Assoc* 1991; **27**: 39–43.

3 Brignac MM, Foil CS, Al-Bagdadi FAK *et al.* Microscopy of color-mutant alopecia. In: von Tscharner, C Halliwell, REW (eds), *Advances in Veterinary Dermatology*, Vol. 1. London: Baillière Tindall, 1990: p. 448.

4 Gross TH, Ihrke PJ, Walder EJ, Affolter VK. Color-dilution alopecia and black hair follicular dysplasia. In: *Skin Diseases of the Dog and Cat: Clinical and Histopathologic Diagnosis*, 2nd edn. Oxford: Blackwell Publishing, 2005: pp. 518–522.

DERMATOPHYTOSIS

Definition
Dermatophytosis is an infection of the skin, hair or nails with fungi of the genera *Microsporum*, *Trichophyton* and *Epidermophyton*. This is a zoonotic condition (see also *Trichophyton*, page 85). Pathogenic fungi are being reclassified according to recent molecular findings and their nomenclature could change in the future, e.g. dermatophytes are being classified in the genus *Arthoderma*, and the *Arthoderma otae* complex includes *M. canis*, *M. furrugineum*, *M. equimum* and *M. audouinii*.

Aetiology and pathogenesis
The most common cause of dermatophytosis in cats is *M. canis*; in dogs the most common causes are *M. canis* and *M. gypseum*. Other less frequent species include *Trichophyton mentagrophytes*, *M. persicolor*, *T. erinacei*, *M. verrucosum*, *M. equinum* and *T. equinum*.

Infection occurs by contact with infected animals, fomites or environments. Dermatophytosis commonly affects cats; they can be asymptomatic carriers and unwitting sources of infection for other mammals. Infected hairs can contaminate collars, brushes, toys, etc. Dermatophyte-infected hair can remain viable in the environment for years; carpeting and upholstery are especially good environments for harbouring infected hairs but soil is also a source of exposure.

Predisposing factors for infection include: young age, immunosuppression, malnutrition, concurrent disease, high temperature and humidity and skin trauma.[1] The incubation period varies from 1–3 weeks. Dermatophytes infect growing hairs and living skin.

Dermatophytosis is often self-limiting in immunocompetent animals; these animals are more resistant to subsequent dermatophyte infections in the future.[1]

Clinical features
Classic signs include multi-focal alopecia and scaling, typically on the face, head and feet (**Figs. 4.30–4.33**). Other clinical signs include folliculitis and furunculosis, feline acne, onychomycosis, granulomas and kerions.[1] Pruritus and inflammation are usually minimal, but occasionally severely pruritic, pustular or crusting forms occur, especially in older or immunosuppressed individuals. These signs may mimic allergies, ectoparasites, miliary dermatitis, pyoderma or pemphigus foliaceus.

Dermatophyte mycetomas or pseudomycetomas are subcutaneous nodular and ulcerating forms with draining sinus tracts seen in Persian cats and occasionally other long-haired breeds (**Fig. 4.34**). This is often associated with a generalised greasy seborrhoea (**Fig. 4.35**).

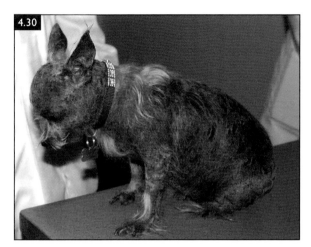

Fig. 4.30 Generalised dermatophytosis with *Microsporum canis* in a Yorkshire Terrier; despite the extensive alopecia and scaling there is only mild inflammation.

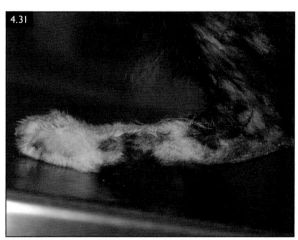

Fig. 4.31 Dermatophytosis: *M. canis* dermatophytosis usually results in focal alopecia.

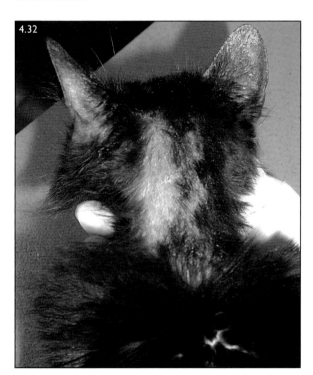

Fig. 4.32 Localised alopecia, erythema and scaling in cat with a *Microsporum canis* infection.

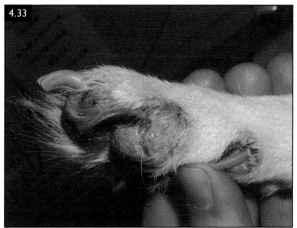

Fig. 4.33 Paronychia in a Jack Russell Terrier with a *Trichophyton mentagrophytes* infection.

Differential diagnoses

As the clinical presentation can be so variable, dermatophytosis should be considered in almost any animal, but especially a cat, that presents with: focal-to-multi-focal alopecia, scaling and crusting; diffuse alopecia, seborrhoea and scaling; nodules and draining sinus tracts; inflammation, erythema, erosions and ulcers; or folliculitis and furunculosis.

Diagnosis

The diagnosis of dermatophytosis and species identification relies on fungal culture of hair and scale.

T. mentagrophytes typically causes more severe inflammation, alopecia, furunculosis, crusting and granulomas of the face and feet, especially in small Terrier breeds (**Figs. 4.36, 4.37**).

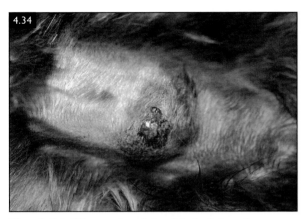

Fig. 4.34 Ulcerated nodule with draining sinus tracts.

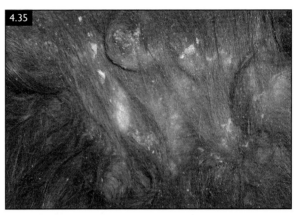

Fig. 4.35 Generalised greasy scaling and poor hair coat in a Persian cat with dermatophytosis.

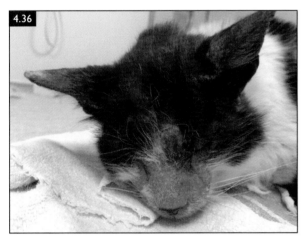

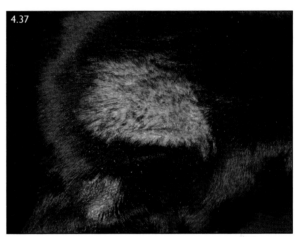

Figs. 4.36, 4.37 Dermatophytosis: *Trychophyton mentagrophytes* infection usually results in well-demarcated inflammatory lesions in both cats (Fig. 4.36; photo courtesy of Katarina Varjonen) and dogs (Fig. 4.37).

Hairs can initially be examined by microscopy for the identification of hyphae, destruction of the hair shaft, and ectothrix arthroconidia spores (**Figs. 4.38, 4.39**). It is sometimes possible to identify fungal elements on tape-strip or impression smear cytology (**Fig. 4.40**). Up to 50% of *M. canis* strains fluoresce green under a Wood's lamp (**Fig. 4.41**). Skin biopsies may be submitted, but histology is not as sensitive as culture and often requires special stains (e.g. periodic–acid Schiff [PAS] or Grocott–Gomori silver stains).

Dermatophytes readily produce whitish fluffy colonies on dermatophyte test medium (DTM), inducing a red colour change that coincides with early fungal growth, usually within 7–10 days (faster if incubated above 25°C) (**Figs. 4.42, 4.43**).

Pigmented or slimy colonies and/or colour changes that coincide with late fungal growth all indicate a saprophyte. *Trichophyton* spp. occasionally fail to induce a colour change.

Fungal elements should be examined under the microscope. A tape mount can be prepared and stained with new methylene blue. *M. canis* macroconidia spores are characterised by a spindle shape, thick wall, terminal knob and six or more cells. *Trichophyton* spp. typically have spiral hyphae, flask-shaped microconidia and smooth thin-walled macroconidia.

Dermatophytes develop characteristic colony morphology and more readily produce macroconidia on Saboraud's agar. However, this takes at least 3 weeks and specialised mycology skills to interpret.

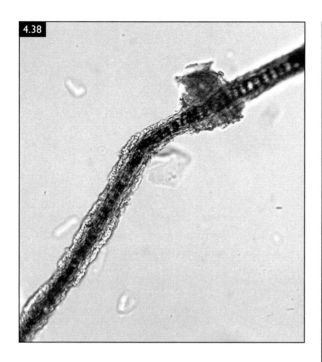

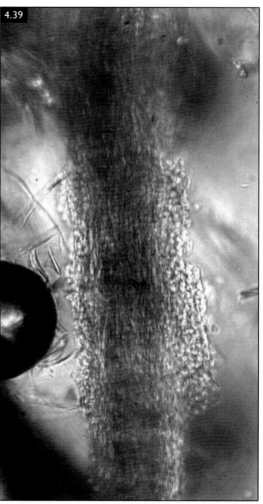

Figs. 4.38, 4.39 Dermatophytosis: photomicrograph of a hair shaft exhibiting spores and hyphae. Note that these impart a 'dirty', thickened appearance to the hair (Fig. 4.38, magnification ×40; Fig. 4.39, magnification ×100).

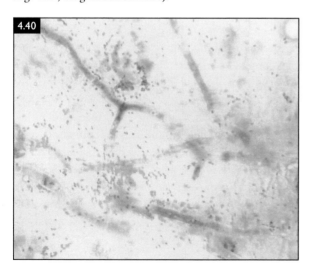

Fig. 4.40 Hyphae seen on tape-strip cytology from a dog with dermatophytosis (DiffQuik stain, magnification ×1000).

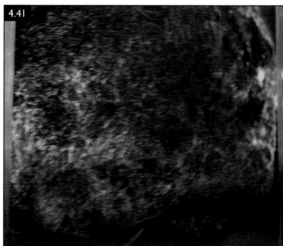

Fig. 4.41 Fluorescing hairs and scale in a Yorkshire Terrier with dermatophytosis caused by *M. canis*.

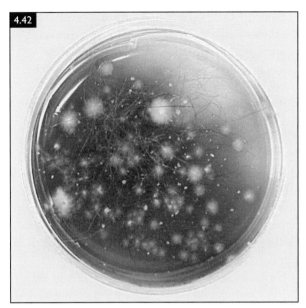

Fig. 4.42 Positive culture on dermatophyte test medium. The critical observation is the appearance of colour change at the same time as colony growth becomes apparent.

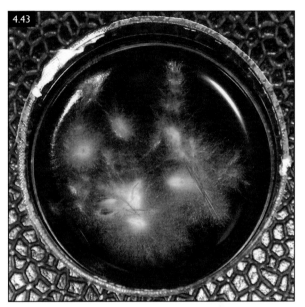

Fig. 4.43 This is a similar plate as in Fig. 4.42, but a week later. The uniform red colour now makes it impossible to tell if the fungal growth appeared after the colour change or before.

Polymerase chain reaction tests are highly sensitive but false positives can occur with transient nonpathogenic contamination of the skin or coat with dermatophyte elements. The results should therefore be interpreted in light of the clinical signs and other findings.

Treatment

Clipping is not necessary in all most cases, but it can facilitate topical therapy and remove infected hairs, reducing the pathogenic load and environmental contamination. This should be done with care to avoid skin trauma (which can spread and worsen the infection). Bear in mind that clipped hair and spores can easily be spread throughout the hospital environment on air currents, clothing and staff, creating a contamination nightmare.

Clinical cure occurs before mycological cure, and animals should not be regarded as cured until they have had two negative cultures at least 7 days apart. Duration of therapy may range from 2 months to 6 months; some cases need perpetual therapy.

Topical therapy

Topical therapy reduces environmental contamination and the time to clinical and fungal cure. Lime sulphur solutions are highly effective and well tolerated, although staining and pungent. Enilconazole dip is also highly effective and well tolerated by dogs, but idiosyncratic reactions including raised liver enzymes, muscle weakness and death are occasionally seen in cats. Chlorhexidine is less effective, but chlorhexidine/miconazole shampoo is an effective adjunct therapy. Many other antifungal shampoos are available and have variable efficacy. Topical therapy should be applied to the entire body once or twice a week until the patient has been cured. The topical antifungal creams and solutions for humans can be used on focal lesions, but are less effective in animals as the hair coat impedes application and hides the extent of lesions.

Systemic therapy

Severely affected or multiple pet households necessitate oral and topical therapy simultaneously.

Itraconazole (5 mg/kg q24 h) is highly effective and well tolerated in cats and dogs. It can be administered daily. It can also be administered daily on alternating weeks[1] or every other day.[2] Itraconazole persists in the hair for 3–4 weeks after dosing. Therapeutic concentrations are maintained in the skin and hair for at least 2 weeks after the final dose.

Ketoconazole (5–10 mg/kg q24 h) is effective and usually well tolerated, but it can cause anorexia and vomiting, and is potentially teratogenic and hepatotoxic. It should be administered with food. Cats are particularly susceptible to side effects, and itraconazole or terbinafine is a better treatment option.

Terbinafine (30 mg/kg q24 h) has been used successfully for dermatophytosis[3] and dermatophyte mycetomas. There is a long duration of activity and this may allow relatively short courses of therapy, followed by careful observation. Terbinafine appears to be well tolerated in cats and dogs.

Griseofulvin dosing depends on the formulation: micronised formulation 50–100 mg/kg q24 h and ultramicronised/PEG formulation 10–30 mg/kg q24 h. Doses can be divided and given twice daily with a (fatty) meal until the infection has resolved. It is well tolerated, but should not be used in animals aged under 6 weeks. Side effects include pruritus, anorexia, vomiting, diarrhoea, liver damage, ataxia and bone marrow suppression. Griseofulvin is teratogenic and may affect sperm quality. Griseofulvin should be used only if other treatment options are not available, and itraconazole, ketoconazole and terbinafine should be considered first.

Environmental decontamination[4]

The major source of environmental contamination of dermatophyte spores is infected hairs. These may be removed with a combination of disposal, physical cleaning (including daily vacuuming) and wiping surfaces with 1:10 bleach:water solution or enilconazole. Removal of infected hairs in the environment is particularly important for resolution of dermatophytosis.

Control of dermatophytosis in catteries and multi-cat households[4]

The principles for controlling dermatophytosis in catteries and multi-cat households are as follows:

- Isolate the cattery and suspend breeding until the outbreak is controlled.

- Separate infected and non-infected cats based on culture and use barrier precautions to prevent spread of the infection. If it is impossible to isolate culture-negative cats, they should all be treated as culture positive.
- Treat infected cats.
- Eliminate environmental contamination.
- Prevent reinfection.

Pregnant queens and kittens can be isolated and treated with topical lime sulphur, miconazole/chlorhexidine or enilconazole. Negative cats should be recultured and any that become positive, moved. Ideally, infected cats should not be moved until all of them are cured.

New cats and animals that have been to shows and/or stud should be isolated for 3–4 weeks and cultured using toothbrush technique if no lesions are seen within that time; many owners and shelter workers can be taught to use DTM in-house. Wood's lamp examination is also useful for identifying dermatophyte-positive cats. Prevention is better, less expensive and less time-consuming than treatment.

Key point
- Dermatophytosis is zoonotic.

References

1   Frymus T, Gruffydd-Jones T, Pennisi MG *et al*. Dermatophytosis in Cats: ABCD guidelines on prevention and management. *J Feline Med Surg* 2013; **15**: 598–604.

2   Middleton SM, Kubier A, Dirikolu L, Papich MG, Mitchell MA, Rubin SI. Alternate-day dosing of itraconazole in healthy adult cats. *J Vet Pharmacol Therapeut* 2016; **39**: 27–31.

3   Moriello K, Coyner K, Trimmer A, Newbury S, Kunder D. Treatment of shelter cats with oral terbinafine and concurrent lime sulphur rinses. *Vet Dermatol* 2013; **24**: 618–e150.

4   Newbury S, Moriello K, Coyner K, Trimmer A, Kunder D. Management of endemic *Microsporum canis* dermatophytosis in an open admission shelter: a field study. *J Feline Med Surg* 2015; **17**: 342–347.

FELINE DEMODICOSIS

Definition

Feline demodicosis is the proliferation of demodex mites within the hair follicles (*Demodex cati*) or on the epidermis (*D. gatoi*; see page 48). A putative third species, *D. felis*, may also be found in cats. Recently, *D. canis* has been isolated from the chin in cats.

Aetiology and pathogenesis

D. cati mites are normal inhabitants of the hair follicle. They proliferate when the immune system is compromised, similar to *D. canis* in dogs. Causes of immune compromise include: hyperadrenocorticism, diabetes mellitus, retroviral infection, squamous cell carcinoma, internal cancers and immunosuppressive drug therapy. Inhalant glucocorticoids can lead to localised demodicosis on the muzzle.[1] However, an underlying cause cannot be found in many cases.

D. gatoi mites are transmitted by contact between cats. These mites inhabit the epidermis, and are not considered commensal organisms of the skin.

Clinical features

Demodicosis in cats can be localised, generalised or otic. There may be variable, focal to multi-focal or generalised alopecia and scaling, with occasional erythema, papules, erosions, crusting, comedones and hyperpigmentation, especially of the eyelids, periocular area, chin, head and neck (**Fig. 4.44**). Infestation of the chin may result in the lesions of feline acne. The otic form may be associated with ears of normal appearance, where the mites are an incidental finding, or the ears may have a dark-brown ceruminous exudate. *Demodex* spp. have also been associated with facial or focal to generalised greasy seborrhoea, especially in Persian cats. Pruritus is variable, but typically absent with *D. cati*. *D. gatoi*, in contrast, may cause moderate-to-severe generalised or localised pruritus (see page 48).

Differential diagnoses

- Dermatophytosis.
- Bacterial folliculitis.
- Allergic dermatitis.
- Contact dermatitis.

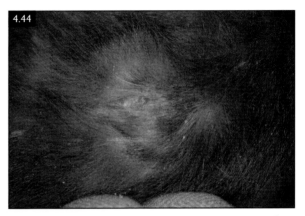

Fig. 4.44 Patchy alopecia, scaling and crusts on the rump of a cat with *Demodex gatoi*.

- Drug reaction (topical flea and tick preventives or oral medications such as methimazole).
- Flea-bite hypersensitivity or other ectoparasites.
- Other forms of chin acne, facial dermatitis, seborrhoea and otitis in cats.

Diagnosis

D. cati is easily diagnosed with multiple hair plucks, tape-strips and/or deep skin scrapings. Scrapings should be deep enough to induce capillary bleeding. *D. cati* can also be found in otic debris mounted in oil.

D. gatoi can be difficult to diagnose. It is sometimes found on tape-strips and skin scrapings, but many skin scrapings are required to collect the mite. The mite may also be identified on a faecal flotation. Response to treatment is often the only way to obtain a diagnosis, and unfortunately this mite is difficult to treat.

Treatment

For *D. cati*, any underlying disease should be treated and immunosuppressive therapy should be decreased or modified if possible. Treatment options include: milbemycin oxime 1 mg/kg po q24 h,[1] 2% lime sulphur dips, doramectin 0.6 mg/kg sc weekly[2] and ivermectin 0.2–0.3 mg/kg po q24–48 h. The lime sulphur dip should be sponged over the cat weekly for six treatments. This treatment is malodorous, staining and difficult to use on the face. Neurological side effects such as ataxia are possible with ivermectin. Topical administration of fluralaner every 8 weeks shows promise. Treatment should be continued until clinical cure and negative skin scrapings are obtained.

For *D. gatoi*, 2% lime sulphur dips have historically been the most reliable treatment. Dips are applied to the entire skin weekly for a total of six treatments. If no change in the skin condition is observed after three dips, then demodicosis is unlikely. Treatment should be continued for 2 weeks beyond a clinical cure (see page 48 for additional treatment options).

Key points
- *D. cati* is an important differential for feline chin acne.
- *D. gatoi* is transmissible to other cats.

References
1   Bizikova P. Localized demodicosis due to *Demodex cati* on the muzzle of two cats treated with inhalant glucocorticoids. *Vet Dermatol* 2014; **25**: 222–e58.
2   Beale K. Feline demodicosis A consideration in the itchy or over grooming cat. *J Feline Med Surg* 2012; **14**: 209–213.

CANINE DEMODICOSIS

Definition
Demodicosis is an abnormal proliferation of a commensal hair follicle mite, *Demodex canis*, resulting in alopecia and other clinical signs. Pruritus may be intense or non-existent. The longer-bodied mite (*D. injai*) has been associated with sebaceous hyperplasia and seborrhoeic dermatitis that mainly affects the dorsal trunk. A more superficial short-bodied mite can also be found alongside the long-bodied forms.

Aetiology and pathogenesis
D. canis mites are a part of the normal microfauna of canine skin. The mites are transmitted from the dam to the puppy through skin contact in the immediate postnatal period.[1] *D. canis* mites are not typically contagious between adult dogs except with very susceptible individuals and close contact.[2]

The demodex life cycle requires 20–35 days and consists of five stages: spindle-shaped eggs; small larvae with six short legs; six-legged protonymphs; nymphs with eight short legs; and adults with an obvious head, thorax and four pairs of jointed legs (**Fig. 4.45**).

D. canis mites proliferate when the immune system is suppressed[3] or compromised. Examples of underlying conditions include: endoparasiticism, malnutrition, neoplasia, hypothyroidism (although euthyroid sick syndrome is a common finding in severe demodicosis), hyperadrenocorticism or other systemic disease.[1] Drugs such as chemotherapeutics, glucocorticoids and oclacitinib may also induce demodicosis. Many times, an underlying cause cannot be found,[1] and demodicosis develops in an otherwise apparently healthy dog. There may be a genetic predisposition to idiopathic generalised demodicosis.

Clinical features
Demodicosis can occur as mild, localised disease or moderate-to-severe generalised disease.

Localised demodicosis is generally defined as four or fewer skin lesions with each lesion 2.5 cm in diameter or smaller.[1] Lesions are multi-focal, asymmetrical and well circumscribed with scaling, thinning of the hair, alopecia and/or erythema (**Fig. 4.46**). The skin can have a blue–grey colour, comedones and follicular casts. Commonly affected sites are the face, head, neck, forelimbs and trunk. Demodicosis is a rare cause of otitis externa. Secondary bacterial or (rarely) *Malassezia* infection can cause papules,

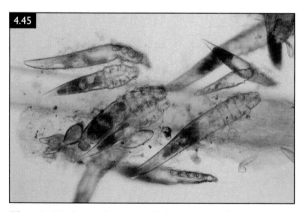

Fig. 4.45 *Demodex canis* **adults, eggs and larvae.**

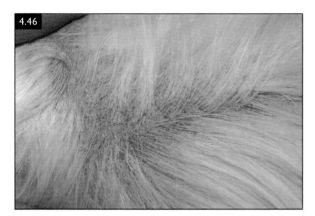

Fig. 4.46 Localised demodicosis with alopecia and prominent follicular casts in a West Highland White Terrier.

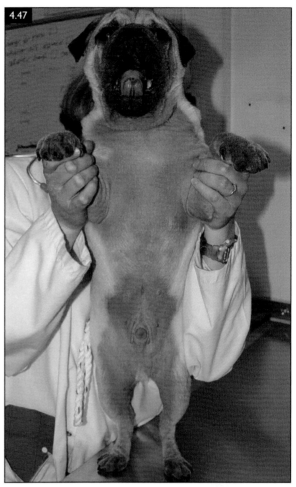

Fig. 4.47 Generalised demodicosis in a Pug; large numbers of tightly apposed comedones give the skin a characteristic grey colour.

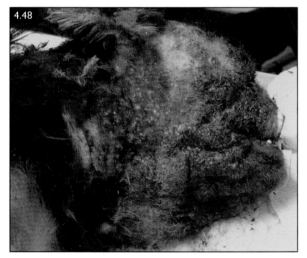

Fig. 4.48 Severe generalised demodicosis with a secondary bacterial furunculosis affecting a Cavalier King Charles Spaniel; the extent and severity of the infections in these cases can be life threatening.

pustules, scaling, crusts, seborrhoea, pruritus and pain.

Generalised demodicosis is generally defined as more than four lesions, or lesions that affect an entire body region or one or more paws. The clinical signs include multi-focal-to-generalised alopecia with scaling, hyperpigmentation, comedones and follicular casts (**Fig. 4.47**). Secondary bacterial infections are common, and lesions include papules, pustules, furunculosis, draining sinus tracts, crusts, pruritus and pain (**Fig. 4.48**). Severe secondary infections can be associated with enlarged lymph nodes, pyrexia,

depression, septicaemia and death. Pododemodicosis is characterised by swelling of the feet, interdigital furunculosis ('cysts'), draining sinus tracts, pain and lameness (**Fig. 4.49**). Erythema and pruritus can be intense and easily confused with atopic dermatitis (**Fig. 4.50**).

Demodicosis is also characterised by age of onset. Juvenile-onset disease occurs between 1 and 10 months of age, but is most common between 3 and 6 months. Localised juvenile-onset disease typically self-resolves. Generalised disease is, however, less likely to resolve spontaneously and can persist into adulthood. Adult-onset demodicosis can be secondary to immunosuppressive conditions, but often an underlying cause is not found.

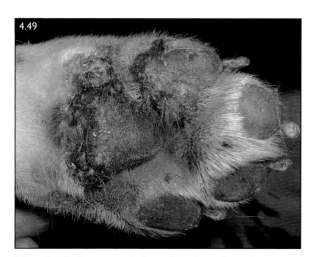

Fig. 4.49 Severe pododemodicosis and pyoderma.

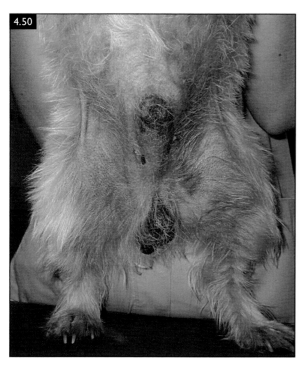

Fig. 4.50 Pruritic demodicosis in a West Highland White Terrier. This can be very similar to atopic dermatitis, but note the follicular papules, erythema and casts compared with the more diffuse erythema seen in atopic dermatitis.

Differential diagnoses

Demodicosis may present in a variety of ways and can mimic nearly every other skin condition – both pruritic and non-pruritic. Demodicosis may also occur concurrently with other skin diseases.

As a result, many skin conditions require deep skin scrapings and/or a hair plucks to rule demodicosis in or out. Many skin conditions (i.e. atopic dermatitis) wax and wane, and it should always be considered as a possible cause of worsening or non-responsive skin disease.

Diagnosis

Deep skin scrapings are the preferred method of diagnosis.[1] The clinician should use a scalpel blade to scrape the epidermis until capillary bleeding occurs. Squeezing the skin before or while scraping helps to force mites out of the hair follicle. Hair plucks are not as sensitive as skin scrapings, but are good for sampling areas that are difficult to scrape (eyelids, chin and paws) or for sampling fractious animals. The sensitivity of the hair pluck increases with the number of hairs that are plucked. Adhesive tape-strip can be used to collect material expressed on to the skin surface by very firmly squeezing the skin. *Demodex* spp. can also be found in material expressed from draining sinus tracts in cases with furunculosis. Skin biopsies may be necessary in dogs with severely scarred and/or thickened skin (e.g. chronic pododermatitis or Shar Peis).

Treatment

Localised demodicosis

Simple monitoring is appropriate for localised demodicosis without secondary infection in young, healthy dogs. Disease in these cases usually resolves spontaneously. Dogs should be examined every 2–3 weeks to check for generalised disease and/or infection.

Generalised demodicosis

Isoxazolines[5] (i.e. sarolaner, fluralaner, lotilaner and afoxolaner) are a new class of parasiticides that have great efficacy against demodicosis at label doses. Isoxazolines are safe for ivermectin-sensitive dogs. Side effects are uncommon and mainly gastrointestinal, but some should be avoided in dogs with a history of seizures.

Amitraz[1] is applied in the USA as a 250 ppm (0.025%) dip every 14 days and in Europe as a 500 ppm (0.05%) dip once weekly. In each case the dip is allowed to dry on the animal (wetting reduces efficacy).

Long-haired animals should be clipped and bathed with benzoyl peroxide or other keratolytic shampoo to enhance contact. Reported efficacy ranges from 0% to 90%. Off-licence uses include applying 1000–1250 ppm solutions once or twice weekly to alternate halves of the body and using 0.15–0.5% solutions in mineral oil daily for pododemodicosis and otitis externa. Amitraz-containing collars and spot-ons are not effective. Adverse effects include vomiting, sedation, hypothermia, hypotension, bradycardia, pruritus, exfoliative erythroderma, hyperglycaemia and death, especially in Chihuahuas. Some of the effects can be reversed with atipamezol or yohimbine. Amitraz is not pleasant to use and compliance can be poor. It should be applied in a well-ventilated area and the owners should wear impervious aprons and gloves. Potential adverse effects in humans include sedation, migraines, hyperglycaemia, dyspnoea and contact reactions. Amitraz is a monoamine oxidase inhibitor (MAOI) and it can have potential adverse effects in individuals taking other MAOIs (e.g. some antihistamines, antidepressants and antihypertensives) and can dysregulate blood sugar in diabetic dogs or cats.

Imidacloprid 10%/moxidectin 2.5% spot-on applied weekly to twice weekly has been reported to be effective in 5 of 26 dogs with severe, generalised demodicosis.[4,5] It is likely to be more effective in dogs with only mild-to-moderate demodicosis. Adverse effects are uncommon, but can include seborrhoea, erythema and vomiting. Ingestion can result in ataxia, tremors, dilated pupils and poor papillary light reflex, nystagmus, dyspnoea, salivation and vomiting, especially in Collies, Old English Sheepdogs and related breeds.

Milbemycin oxime[1] (0.5–2 mg/kg po q24 h) is effective in many cases. Higher doses have a greater success rate than lower doses. However, MDR1 mutant individuals, such as Collies, may experience adverse neurological events with higher doses. Generally, adverse events are rare and are generally limited to mild, transient ataxia and tremors, inappetence and vomiting. These can be managed by reducing the dose and administering with food.

Ivermectin[1] (0.3–0.6 mg/kg po q24 h) is effective in many cases. Higher doses have a greater success rate than lower doses. MDR1 mutant individuals

may experience severe adverse neurological events ranging from mild ataxia to coma and death. Ivermectin is very well tolerated in breeds without this mutation. The clinician should consider starting the patient with a low dose (0.1 mg/kg po q24 h) and gradually increase to full dose over the course of approximately 1 week.[1] Genetic testing should be considered in dogs where the probability of an MDR1 mutation is unknown. Chronic neurotoxicity can be seen in any dog. It is usually mild and can be managed by reducing the dose and/or frequency of treatment.

Other treatment considerations

Pyoderma should be treated with an appropriate bactericidal systemic antibiotic (see Superficial folliculitis, page 66 and Deep pyoderma, page 195). Topical antibacterials may also be beneficial, and will help remove surface scale and crust. Secondary malassezia dermatitis can be managed with an antifungal shampoo, or systemically with ketoconazole (see Malassezia dermatitis, page 31). Ketoconazole must not be administered concurrently with ivermectin because this will interfere with cytochrome metabolism and increase the risk of neurological side effects. This is less likely to occur with itraconazole.

Managing an underlying condition can result in remission of adult-onset demodicosis. A poor response to treatment, in contrast, is often associated with failure to control underlying conditions. Topical therapy, Cytopoint (lokivetmab) or antihistamines can be used to manage pruritus if necessary. Glucocorticoid use without concurrent acaricidal therapy will lead to worsening of demodicosis. Relapses can be associated with oestrus and affected bitches should be neutered. Affected dogs and their relatives should not be bred from.

Monitoring treatment

Skin scrapes and/or hair plucks should be repeated every 4–6 weeks and should reveal decreasing numbers of mites with an increasing ratio of dead and adult mites to live and immature mites. If not, the treatment should be re-evaluated and an underlying cause looked for. Treatment should be continued for

1 month beyond two to three negative skin scrapes. Some dogs with demodicosis can achieve clinical but not parasitological cure. These individuals will need to receive one of the above-described treatments indefinitely. Treatment can often be administered less frequently when the goal is to maintain clinical remission of demodicosis.

Key points
- Demodicosis can be intensely pruritic in some cases.
- Breeding from individuals that have had idiopathic generalised demodicosis is not recommended.

References

1 Mueller RS, Bensignor E, Ferrer L *et al*. Treatment of demodicosis in dogs: 2011 clinical practice guidelines. *Vet Dermatol* 2012; **23**: 86–e21.

2 Nayak DC, Tripathy SB, Dey PC, Biswal S, Parida GS. Therapeutic efficacy of some homeopathic preparations against experimentally produced demodicosis in canids. *Indian Vet J* 1998; **75**: 342–344.

3 Ferrer L, Ravera I, Silbermayr K. Immunology and pathogenesis of canine demodicosis. *Vet Dermatol* 2014; **25**: 427–e65.

4 Paterson TE, Halliwell RE, Fields PJ *et al*. Canine generalized demodicosis treated with varying doses of a 2.5% moxidectin + 10% imidacloprid spot-on and oral ivermectin: Parasiticidal effects and long-term treatment outcomes. *Vet Parasitol* 2014; **205**: 687–696.

5 Fourie JJ, Liebenberg JE, Horak IG, Taenzler J, Heckeroth AR, Frénais R. Efficacy of orally administered fluralaner (Bravecto) or topically applied imidacloprid/moxidectin (Advocate) against generalized demodicosis in dogs. *Parasites Vectors* 2015; **8**: 187.

ALOPECIA AREATA

Definition
Alopecia areata is an uncommon autoimmune disease that results in non-pruritic alopecia in dogs and other mammals.

Aetiology and pathogenesis
Alopecia areata is a T-cell-mediated, autoimmune disease.[1] The hair follicle bulb becomes inflamed, leading to distortion and eventual loss of the hair.

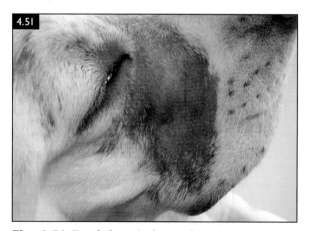

Fig. 4.51 Focal alopecia due to alopecia areata. Note the complete absence of primary and secondary lesions apart from alopecia.

Clinical features
Alopecia areata is characterised by focal-to-multi-focal areas of well-circumscribed alopecia (**Fig. 4.51**). These are usually irregular and asymmetrical, but can appear symmetrical in some cases. The head, neck and distal limbs are most commonly affected. In some animals the disease may restrict itself to one hair colour. The underlying skin appears normal, although hyperpigmentation may be present in chronic cases. Rarely, it can be associated with nail disorders.[2] Alopecia areata is not reported to be pruritic and the skin does not appear outwardly inflamed.

Differential diagnoses
- Postinjection alopecia.
- Pseudopelade.
- Dermatomyositis.
- Vasculitis and vasculopathy.
- Demodicosis.
- Dermatophytosis.
- Follicular dysplasia.
- Acquired pattern alopecia.
- Leishmaniasis.
- Bacterial pyoderma.

Diagnosis

The history and clinical signs are highly suggestive. Hair plucks can reveal characteristic 'exclamation-mark' hairs – these are short and stubby with dystrophic, proximally tapered portions and frayed, damaged distal portions. Skin scraping, fungal culture and skin cytology should be performed to rule out infectious causes, which are much more common causes of alopecia. Histopathology will usually confirm the presence of lymphocyte infiltrates targeting the hair bulb.

Treatment

Oral ciclosporin has been used successfully in many cases[1] (see Immunosuppressive Drug Therapy Table, page 289, for dosing). Treatment should be administered daily for as long as new hair growth is evident. In cases where ciclosporin is effective, the coat may continue to develop over the course of 12 months or more.[1] If no new hair is observed after 3 months of treatment, then ciclosporin should be discontinued for lack of efficacy. New hair growth may be unpigmented. More than half the dogs affected with alopecia areata may spontaneously regrow hair.[1] Other dogs will not respond to any type of treatment. Some dogs may respond to oral glucocorticoids[2] or topical tacrolimus ointment.

Key point

- Definitive diagnosis is important, because some of the differentials are more serious conditions that require specific treatment.

References

1 Ginel PJ, Blanco B, Pérez-Aranda M, Zafra R, Mozos E. Alopecia areata universalis in a dog. *Vet Dermatol* 2015; **26**: 379–e87.
2 Jonghe D. Trachyonychia associated with alopecia areata in a Rhodesian Ridgeback. *Vet Dermatol* 1999; **10**: 123–126.

TAIL GLAND HYPERPLASIA
(Stud tail)

Definition

Tail gland hyperplasia is characterised by hypersecretion of sebum with resulting folliculitis and pyoderma.

Aetiology and pathogenesis

The tail gland is an oil gland (also called the supracaudal organ) located a third of the way distal to the base of the tail on the dorsal side. It secretes sebaceous material that is periodically expressed when the arrector pili muscles contract.[1] The gland can become hyperplastic in intact male cats and dogs. Neutered animals can also be affected, although typically to a lesser degree. The hyperplastic gland becomes impacted with sebum with resulting folliculitis, furunculosis and pyoderma (**Fig. 4.52**). Other skin conditions, such as allergy and endocrine abnormalities, can exacerbate tail gland hyperplasia and folliculitis.

Clinical signs

This condition is seen in dogs and cats. Waxy, sebaceous debris accumulates on the dorsal surface of the tail. Variable erythema, crusting, folliculitis, furunculosis, pain, pruritus and alopecia result.

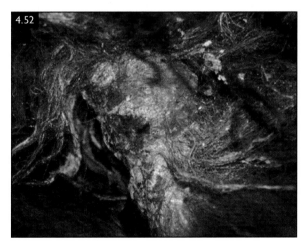

Fig. 4.52 Swelling, alopecia, seborrhoea and secondary infection of the caudal (tail) gland in in an intact male dog with hyperandrogenism.

Differential diagnosis
- Demodicosis.
- Trauma.
- Dermatophytosis.
- Allergic dermatitis.
- Ectoparasites.

Diagnosis
The diagnosis is made based on history, physical exam and ruling out the other differentials. Surface cytology is necessary to identify the presence of pyoderma; skin scrapings and cultures should be performed if needed.

Treatment
Diffuse tail pyoderma can be treated systemically with appropriate topical or systemic antibacterials. Ear ointments that contain gentamicin and betamethasone are effective for treating focal bacterial pyoderma. The tail may need to be shaved to facilitate topical treatments. If the skin is very inflamed, a systemic steroid can be used to reduce inflammation and pain. Once pain, inflammation and infection have been controlled, the hypersecretion of sebum can be addressed. Castration is helpful in some cases. Topical 1% phytosphingosine preparations applied weekly or topical steroid-containing products may also help. Topical retinoic acid is effective if applied two to four times a day until resolution of lesions (approximately 1 month), then less frequently to maintain the skin.[2] There are many owner precautions to consider with retinoid therapy.

Key point
- Life-long topical therapy may be necessary in cases that are not completely responsive to castration.

References
1   Shabadash SA, Zelikina TI. The tail gland of canids. *Biol Bull Russian Acad Sci* 2004; **31**: 367–376.
2   Ural K, Acar A, Guzel M, Karakurum MC, Cingi CC. Topical retinoic acid in the treatment of feline tail gland hyperplasia (stud tail): a prospective clinical trial. *Bull Vet Instit Pulawy* 2008; **52**: 457–459.

INJECTION SITE ALOPECIA

Definition
Injection site alopecia occurs at the site of subcutaneously administered drugs, including vaccines.

Aetiology and pathogenesis
Vaccine-associated alopecia is caused by ischaemia to the skin as a result of a localised vasculitis; the most commonly reported vaccine to cause this reaction is rabies. Steroid-associated alopecia is caused by cutaneous atrophy.

Clinical features
In vaccine-associated disease the focal alopecia occurs 2–6 months after the rabies vaccine injection.[1] Areas overlying the injection site become hyperpigmented and alopecic, and may measure 2–10 cm in diameter. In rare instances animals may become depressed, lethargic and febrile, and develop alopecia over the face, limbs, margins of the pinnae and tip of the tail. Erosions and ulcers have also been noted on the tongue, footpads, elbows and lateral canthi. Focal decreased muscle mass has also been noticed in severe cases.[2,3] Lesions may be exacerbated on revaccination.[2] Poodles and Bichon Frise are at increased risk, but the condition has been reported in many dog breeds.[2]

Subcutaneous injections with glucocorticoids or progestogen suspensions result in focal alopecia at the site of injection (**Fig. 4.53**). Corticosteroid injections can cause alopecia and sometimes severe, slowly healing severe cutaneous atrophy at the injection site.

Differential diagnoses
- Demodicosis.
- Dermatophytosis.
- Bacterial dermatitis.
- Alopecia areata.
- Other causes of vasculitis or cutaneous atrophy.
- Systemic lupus erythematosus.

Diagnosis
Clinical history and examination are normally sufficient to suggest the diagnosis, especially if records indicate clearly the location of injections given.

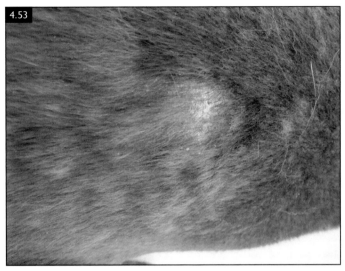

Fig. 4.53 Focal alopecia and cutaneous atrophy after depot glucocorticoid injections.

Examination of skin scrapings and fungal culture will rule out infectious causes, and histopathological examination of biopsy samples will confirm the diagnosis.

Treatment

In vaccine-associated simple monitoring is an option because hair regrowth without treatment can occur, although this may take up to a year. Pentoxifylline (15–25 mg/kg po q8–12 h) is reported to be beneficial for lesions resulting from vasculitis.[3] Other potential treatments include 0.1% tacrolimus ointment (applied q12 h), and tetracycline and niacinamide (250 mg each po q8 h if the animal is <15 kg and 500 mg each po q8 h if the animal is >15 kg; doxycycline 10 mg/kg po q24 h can be used instead of tetracycline).[4] In some animals, the atrophic changes are permanent. Surgical removal, prednisolone and/or other immunosuppressive drugs may be necessary to manage the vasculitis in severe, recalcitrant cases. Repeating the same vaccine can cause previously resolved areas to flare up (see Vasculitis, page 221). It may be best to avoid prominent locations when injecting show animals of predisposed breeds.

For steroid-associated lesions, therapy is supportive until the lesion resolves on its own, but there may be a permanent scar. Surgical removal may have delayed wound healing.

Key point

• This condition is usually cosmetic but is disturbing to owners.

References

1 Wilcock BP, Yager JA. Focal cutaneous vasculitis and alopecia at sites of rabies vaccination in dogs. *J Am Vet Med Assoc* 1986; **188**: 1174–1177.

2 Gross TH, Ihrke PJ, Walder EJ, Affolter VK. Post rabies vaccination panniculitis. In: *Skin Diseases of the Dog and Cat: Clinical and Histopathologic Diagnosis*, 2nd edn. Oxford: Blackwell, 2005: pp. 538-541.

3 Vitale CB, Gross TL, Margro CM. Case report: vaccine-induced ischemic dermatopathy in the dog. *Vet Dermatol* 1999; **10**: 131–142.

4 Medleau L, Hnilica KA. Injection reaction and post-rabies vaccination alopecias. In: *Small Animal Dermatology: A Color Atlas and Therapeutic Guide*. St Louis, MO: Elsevier, 2006: p. 267.

POSTCLIPPING ALOPECIA

Definition
Postclipping alopecia (PCA) results from failure of hair growth after clipping.

Aetiology and pathogenesis
PCA is relatively common in dogs, but rare in cats. The exact mechanism of hair cycle arrest varies between individuals, but some dogs normally have a very long hair cycle with prolonged telogen (resting phases). In Labrador Retrievers, normal postclipping regrowth takes 2.5–5 (mean 3.7) months and there is no relationship to the season in which the dogs are clipped.[1] PCA can also be a sign of any condition that causes hair cycle arrest, including underlying endocrine and metabolic diseases.

Clinical features
Although PCA may occur in any breed, it occurs primarily in long-coated breeds such as Siberian Huskies, Alaskan Malamutes, Samoyeds, Chow Chows and Keeshonds.[2] Clinically, the hair does not regrow after clipping (**Fig. 4.54**). In some cases, there appears to be an association with lumbar epidural anaesthesia. Occasionally, a few guard hairs will regrow in the affected area. Pyoderma is rare, but may be related to the trauma of clipping or underlying immunosuppressive conditions (**Fig. 4.55**). Rarely, PCA can be associated with dermatophytosis triggered by the trauma of clipping and preparing the skin in a contaminated clinic environment. With no underlying cause, hair growth generally resumes within 6–12 months, but full regrowth can take 18–24 months.

Differential diagnoses
- Hyperadrenocorticism.
- Hypothyroidism.
- Sex hormone endocrinopathies (Sertoli cell tumour, exogenous steroids).
- Many underlying systemic diseases can cause hair cycle arrest.
- Alopecia X, flank alopecia, pattern alopecia.

Diagnosis
Diagnosis is based on history and clinical findings as well as ruling out conditions in the differential diagnosis. Affected dogs should be screened for hypothyroidism and other underlying conditions. Cytology should be used to check for pyoderma.

Treatment
Although the clipping did not cause the hair cycle arrest, the clipping did cause the alopecia, and so it is typical for owners to blame this condition on the act of clipping. Education is important, as is keeping this dog's prolonged hair cycle in mind next time clipping is considered. Underlying causes of hair cycle arrest should be investigated. Melatonin (3–12 mg/dog po q12 h) may result in hair regrowth in rare cases. Other potential treatments

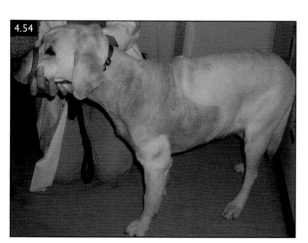

Fig. 4.54 Postclipping alopecia in a Labrador Retriever.

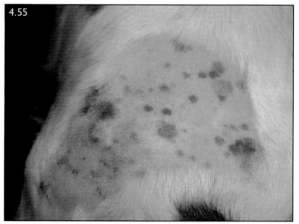

Fig. 4.55 Postclipping alopecia and pyoderma in an English Springer Spaniel.

include low-level laser therapy (LLLT) and micro-needling (see page 96), but there is little evidence of efficacy.

Key point
- With time, and no underlying disease conditions, hair will regrow in most animals.

References
1 Diaz SF, Torres SMF, Dunstan RW *et al.* An analysis of canine hair re-growth after clipping for a surgical procedure. *Vet Dermatol* 2004; **15**: 25–30.
2 Gross TL, Irhke PJ, Walder EJ. Post-clipping alopecia. In: *Veterinary Dermatopathology*. St Louis, MO: Mosby Year Book, 1992: pp. 285–286.

TOPICAL CORTICOSTEROID REACTION

Definition
Topical corticosteroid reaction is a thinning of the skin (cutaneous atrophy) with prominent comedones, associated with topical application of potent corticosteroid medications.

Aetiology and pathogenesis
Corticosteroids are catabolic to the skin. A wide variety of corticosteroid-containing sprays, creams, ointments and gels may cause cutaneous atrophy, but many cases are associated with products containing triamcinolone or betamethasone.

Clinical features
Due to the difficulty of applying topical preparations to densely haired areas of the body, lesions are generally found in the glabrous skin of the ventral abdomen, pinnae or axilla. Lesions appear as focal areas of alopecic, thin, almost translucent skin, often with prominent comedones (**Fig. 4.56**) and/or milia. Varying degrees of erythema and hyperpigmentation may be present. Long-standing lesions may become eroded, ulcerated or torn, or show evidence of scarring. Other lesions include localised demodicosis and/or bacterial folliculitis, telangiectasia and poor wound healing.

Differential diagnosis
- Exposure to topical oestrogen.[1]

Diagnosis
Diagnosis is based on history of topical corticosteroid use and the observation of dermal atrophy.

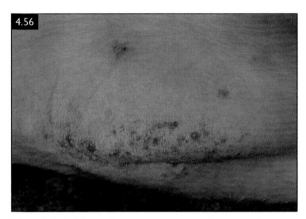

Fig. 4.56 Alopecia, cutaneous atrophy, comedones, milia and telangiectasia at the site of topical corticosteroid application in a dog.

Treatment
Discontinue application of topical corticosteroids. Return of the skin to normal appearance may take several months or years. The skin should be monitored for secondary pyoderma and protected from trauma.

Key point
- Topical steroids such as hydrocortisone aceponate or mometasone may be less likely to cause dermal atrophy.

Reference
1 Berger DJ, Lewis TP, Schick AE, Miller RI, Loeffler DG. Canine alopecia secondary to human topical hormone replacement therapy in six dogs. *J Am Animal Hosp Assoc* 2015; **51**: 136–142.

CHAPTER 5

DERMATOSES OF ABNORMAL KERATINISATION

TOPICAL THERAPIES FOR SEBORRHOEA (TABLE 5.1)

Table 5.1 **Topical therapies for seborrhoea**
ANTIBACTERIAL
Benzoyl peroxide (keratolytic*, drying)
Chlorhexidine
Ethyl lactate
Salicylic acid (keratolytic)
Selenium sulphide (keratolytic)
Sulphur (keratolytic)
Tar (keratolytic, drying)
MOISTURISING
Aloe vera
Colloidal oatmeal
Fatty acids
Lanolin
Phytosphingosine
50:50 propylene glycol and water (keratolytic)
Urea (keratolytic)
Sodium lactate

* Keratolytic: removes excess skin cells.

GENERAL APPROACH TO KERATINISATION DISORDERS (FIG. 5.1)

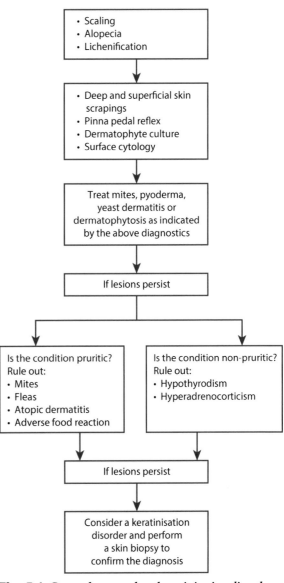

Fig. 5.1 General approach to keratinisation disorders.

ICHTHYOSIS

Definition

Ichthyosis is a congenital disease characterised by non-pruritic, excessive flaking or scaling of the skin. Golden Retrievers, American Bulldogs, Jack Russell Terriers (JRTs) and Norfolk Terriers are predisposed, although other breeds can be affected. The disease has a juvenile age of onset and persists throughout adulthood.

Aetiology and pathogenesis

Ichthyosis is an autosomal recessive genetic disease. The specific genetic mutation varies depending on the breed of dog. In every case, however, the gene mutation results in a cornification abnormality.[1–5]

Clinical features

This condition is non-pruritic unless secondary infections or atopic dermatitis is present. Ichthyosis predisposes to skin infections. Variable amounts of large, loosely adhered flakes of skin become apparent when the dog is only a few weeks old (**Fig. 5.2**). More severely affected individuals, particularly JRTs, may have tightly adherent flakes of skin that accumulate into thick sheets. The groin is usually most severely affected, but flakes also occur on the trunk. The skin may become hyperpigmented and also develop a roughened texture (**Fig. 5.3**). The hair coat quality may be poorer than normal, but alopecia is not a feature of this disease in Golden Retrievers. The clinical signs may become more pronounced with age. The footpads, nose and teeth are not affected in the Golden Retriever.[4] American Bulldogs and JRTs with ichthyosis have striking *Malassezia* overgrowth. Severely affected dogs may be alopecic and have a peripheral lymphadenopathy.

Differential diagnoses

- Pyoderma.
- Malassezia dermatitis.
- Dermatophytosis.
- *Demodex* spp.
- *Cheyletiella* spp. (generally pruritic).
- Atopic dermatitis (generally pruritic).
- Sebaceous adenitis (adult age of onset).
- Hypothyroidism (adult age of onset).
- Exfoliative cutaneous lupus erythematosus.

Diagnosis

The history, signalment and clinical signs are highly suggestive. Other conditions such as pyoderma should be ruled out with surface cytology (i.e. tape preparations). Ectoparasites should be ruled out with flea combing, adhesive tape-strips, skin scrapings and a treatment trial of appropriate parasiticides. Histopathology reveals hyperkeratosis with variable amounts of hyperplasia and absent dermal inflammation unless there is secondary infection. Histopathology alone is not likely to yield a definitive diagnosis. Genetic testing is available to determine the carrier status of the genetic mutation (*PNPLA1*) in Golden Retriever dogs,[3] American Bulldogs (deficiency of *NIPAL4*)[5] and JRTs (*TGM1* deficiency).

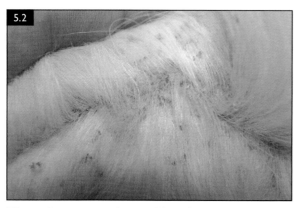

Fig. 5.2 Large, profuse and loosely adherent scales in the coat of a Golden Retriever with ichthyosis.

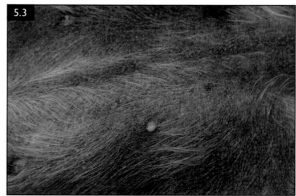

Fig. 5.3 Scaling, lichenification and hyperpigmentation on the ventral abdomen of a West Highland White Terrier with more severe ichthyosis.

Treatment

Secondary infections should be treated and prevented. Concurrent conditions, such as atopic dermatitis should be controlled. Administering daily omega₃-fatty acids (180 mg/5 kg of body weight) may help reduce flaking. Some fish-based diets contain therapeutic levels of omega-fatty acids. Bathing the patient every few days with products containing phytosphingosine may also help reduce flaking. Dogs with thick accumulations of scale should also be bathed with shampoos that contain benzoyl peroxide, salicylic acid or other keratolytic ingredients, although moisturisers may be required after or between baths.

It is not uncommon for dogs to have both ichthyosis and atopic dermatitis. This results in an individual with multiple aetiologies causing excessive dander. All conditions need to be addressed for therapy to be successful.

Key points

- This is a condition that is controlled but not cured.
- Some individuals have both ichthyosis and atopic dermatitis. Secondary infections are common.

References

1 Credille KM, Minor JS, Barnhart KF *et al.* Transglutaminase 1-deficient recessive lamellar ichthyosis associated with a LINE-1 insertion in Jack Russell terrier dogs. *Br J Dermatol* 2009; **161**: 265–272.

2 Credille KM, Barnhart KF, Minor JS *et al.* Mild recessive epidermolytic hyperkeratosis associated with a novel keratin 10 donors splice-site mutation in a family of Norfolk terrier dogs. *Br J Dermatol* 2005; **153**: 51–58.

3 Grall A, Guaguère E, Planchais S *et al.* PNPLA1 mutations cause autosomal recessive congenital ichthyosis in golden retriever dogs and humans. *Nature Genet* 2012; **44**: 140–147.

4 Guaguere E, Bensignor E, Kury S *et al.* Clinical, histopathological and genetic data of ichthyosis in the golden retriever: a prospective study. *J Small Anim Pract* 2009; **50**: 227–235.

5 Mauldin EA, Wang P, Evans E *et al.* Autosomal recessive congenital ichthyosis in American bulldogs is associated with *NIPAL4* (ICHTHYIN) deficiency. *Vet Pathol* 2015; **52**: 654–662.

SEBACEOUS ADENITIS

Definition

Sebaceous adenitis is an immune-mediated disease characterised by destruction of the sebaceous glands with subsequent scaling, alopecia and variable pruritus.

Aetiology and pathogenesis

The aetiology is immune mediated and is heritable in many, if not all, cases. A specific gene mutation is yet to be found. Standard Poodles,[1] Akitas, Havanese,[2] Vizslas and Samoyed dogs are predisposed.

Clinical features[3]

Sebaceous adenitis occurs in young adult to middle-aged dogs, with no sex predilection.

In general, sebaceous adenitis is characterised by focal, progressing to generalised, scaling and alopecia. The scaling tends to form casts that encompass hairs (**Figs. 5.4, 5.5**). Affected individuals may have pruritus that ranges from non-existent to severe and refractory.

Certain breeds may manifest signs of sebaceous adenitis in different ways. For example, Standard Poodles develop discoloration and straightening of the hair in addition to scaling and alopecia. Samoyeds tend to develop plaques of scale. Akitas may have more extensive alopecia, seborrhoea and even deep bacterial folliculitis and furunculosis

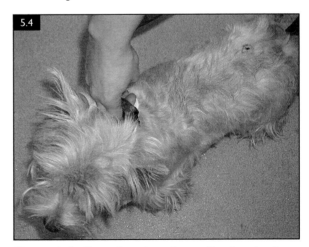

Fig. 5.4 Scaling, alopecia and coat discoloration in a West Highland White Terrier with sebaceous adenitis and secondary pyoderma.

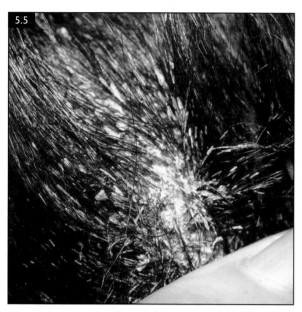

Fig. 5.5 Severe scaling and numerous follicular casts in a Bernese Mountain dog with sebaceous adenitis.

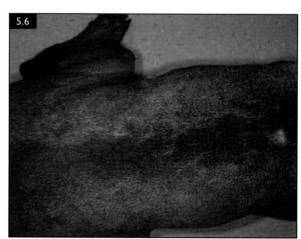

Fig. 5.6 Sebaceous adenitis in a short-coated Hungarian Vizla. There is a patchy and serpiginous alopecia, but the scaling typical in longer-coated dogs is mild to absent.

compared with other breeds. They may also manifest systemic signs of malaise, fever and weight loss, especially if there is a severe secondary infection. Vizslas and other short-coated breeds have clinical signs that are characterised by multi-focal, annular and serpiginous areas of alopecia and fine white scaling that occur progressively over the head, ears and trunk (**Fig. 5.6**). Scaling may be the most prominent sign in Springer Spaniels. Havanese dogs often have scaling that is initially evident in their ear canals.

Sebaceous adenitis is also seen in cats and rabbits, although there are clinical and histopathological differences from the canine condition.

Differential diagnoses
- Atopic dermatitis.
- *Cheyletiella* spp. or other parasites.
- Pyoderma.
- Epitheliotrophic lymphoma.
- Dermatophytosis.
- Pemphigus foliaceus.
- Leishmaniasis.
- Endocrinopathy
- Zinc-responsive dermatosis.
- Vitamin A-responsive dermatitis.
- Primary keratinisation defects.
- Exfoliative cutaneous lupus erythematosus.

Diagnosis
The presence or absence of pruritus helps narrow the list of differentials. Adhesive tape-strips, superficial and deep skin scrapings and surface cytology will help rule in mites and secondary infections. A treatment trial with a parasiticide may be needed to rule out ectoparasites. A hair pluck will reveal the typical profuse follicular casts. These are often macroscopically visible and mat the hairs together. Skin biopsy is diagnostic, revealing inflammation targeting sebaceous glands and the absence of sebaceous glands in chronic cases. Multiple biopsies are frequently necessary to observe the diagnostic pathology.

Treatment
The prognosis is fair to guarded because response to therapy varies among individuals. Mild cases may require only topical therapy. Moderate-to-severe cases often need a combination of systemic and topical therapy. Topical therapy should be directed at removing scale and then infusing moisture into the skin and coat to replace the sebum. Shampoos and spot-on products containing phytosphingosine or ceramides may be particularly helpful. Topical olive oil and/or a solution of 50:50 propylene glycol and water are effective, albeit messy. Shampoos containing phytosphingosine or ceramide should

be used weekly, or sometimes as frequently as daily, for 1 month to reduce scaling and replace moisture. Olive oil, 50:50 propylene glycol:water solution and spot-on products are typically needed one to three times a week for the first month, then weekly to every other week thereafter. Bathing followed by a body soak in 50:50 propylene glycol and coconut oil weekly to remission, and then as required, can be very effective but it is messy and time-consuming. Olive oil or spot-on treatments can be used to treat focal areas that are not particularly responsive to shampooing.

Essential fatty acid supplementation (180 mg/5 kg po q24 h) and vitamin A[4] (10 000 IU po q24 h given with food, maximum 800–1000 IU/kg/day) may be helpful as adjunct therapies.

Systemic glucocorticoids administered at anti-inflammatory doses (see Immunosuppressive Drug Therapy Table, page 289) may be of value in early cases. However, glucocorticoids are of less value in chronic and minimally inflamed cases.

Combined doxycycline or tetracycline with niacinamide (see Immunosuppressive Drug Therapy Table, page 289) is an effective treatment for many dogs with sebaceous adenitis. This treatment may take 2–3 months to reach maximum effect.

Ciclosporin[5] (see Immunosuppressive Drug Therapy Table, page 289) is effective in many cases of sebaceous adenitis. This treatment may take 6–8 weeks to reach maximum effects. This is the only treatment that has been demonstrated to lead to regeneration of sebaceous glands.

A combination of systemic therapies may be necessary in dogs with severe disease.

Key points
- Prominent follicular casts are highly suggestive of sebaceous adenitis.
- Diagnosis is only made by histopathological examination of multiple biopsy samples.
- A combination of systemic and topical treatments is often required except in the mildest of cases.

References
1 Pedersen NC, Liu H, McLaughlin B, Sacks BN. Genetic characterization of healthy and sebaceous adenitis affected Standard Poodles from the United States and the United Kingdom. *Tissue Antigens* 2012; **80**(1): 46–57.
2 Frazer MM, Schick AE, Lewis TP, Jazic E. Sebaceous adenitis in Havanese dogs: a retrospective study of the clinical presentation and incidence. *Vet Dermatol* 2011; **22**: 267–274.
3 Simpson A, McKay L. Applied dermatology: sebaceous adenitis in dogs. *Compend Contin Educ Vet* 2012; **34**(10): E1–7.
4 Lam AT, Affolter VK, Outerbridge CA, Gericota B, White SD. Oral vitamin A as an adjunct treatment for canine sebaceous adenitis. *Vet Dermatol* 2011; **22**: 305–311.
5 Palmeiro BS. Cyclosporine in veterinary dermatology. *Vet Clin North Am Small Anim Pract* 2013; **43**(1): 153–171.

ZINC-RESPONSIVE DERMATOSIS

Definition
Zinc-responsive dermatosis in dogs occurs due to an impaired ability to absorb zinc from the gut (type 1) or a relative or absolute deficiency of zinc in the diet (type 2).[1–3] Naturally occurring zinc deficiency has not been reported in cats.

Aetiology and pathogenesis
Zinc is found in high levels in the epidermis and is important in keratinocyte differentiation. Zinc deficiency causes hyperkeratosis, especially at pressure points, and predisposes to infections. There are two types of zinc-responsive dermatosis.

Type 1 disease is most frequently seen in Siberian Huskies, Samoyeds and Alaskan Malamutes (possibly due to autosomal recessive inheritance), although it has been recognised in other breeds.[1] These animals appear unable to absorb adequate zinc, even when fed a nutritionally balanced diet.

Type 2 disease, due to an absolute dietary zinc deficiency, is rare in animals fed high-quality, commercially prepared diets.[1,2] More commonly, there is a relative deficiency due to interaction with other dietary components or an inability to utilise dietary zinc. Absorption of zinc from the gut is inhibited by iron, copper and calcium.[1,2] Phytates and inorganic

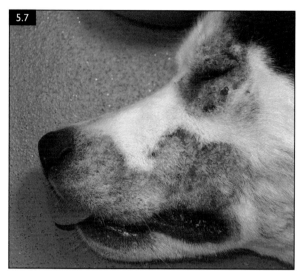

Fig. 5.7 Zinc-responsive dermatosis in a Siberian Husky.

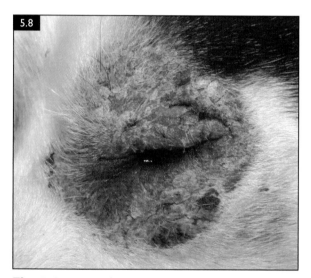

Fig. 5.8 Severe alopecia, inflammation and crusting around the eye.

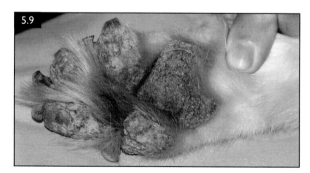

Fig. 5.9 Hyperkeratosis of the footpads.

phosphate bind zinc and hinder absorption in the intestine. This is most likely to be seen in rapidly growing animals, particularly giant breeds, fed inadequate diets or diets in which nutritional antagonism occurs, particularly due to high phytate content or over-supplementation with calcium.

Clinical features

There is no sex predisposition, although clinical lesions may be associated with or exacerbated by oestrus, pregnancy and lactation in intact females. Most cases of type 1 disease are seen between age 1 and 3 years, although there is a wide age range of up to 11 years at first presentation.[1] Type 2 is normally seen in young, growing dogs fed inappropriate diets, although it can be seen in older animals depending on the dietary history.

Cutaneous lesions include well-demarcated, symmetrical areas of scaling, crusting, lichenification, hyperkeratosis and erythema, predominantly around the mouth, eyes, pressure points,[4] footpads and scrotum (**Figs. 5.7–5.9**). Pruritus is variable, but it may be severe. Affected skin may fissure and ulcerate, which is often painful.[1] Secondary bacterial and yeast dermatitis may occur. The coat is generally dull and harsh and may exhibit multi-focal hypopigmentation. Other clinical signs include lymphadenopathy (especially if there is fissuring, inflammation and/or pyoderma), poor wound healing, anoestrus, infertility, inappetence (possibly due to altered taste and/or smell), failure to thrive and weight loss.

Differential diagnoses

- Atopic dermatitis.
- Demodicosis.
- Staphylococcal pyoderma.
- Malassezia dermatitis.
- Dermatophytosis.
- Pemphigus foliaceus.
- Superficial necrolytic dermatitis.
- Leishmaniasis.

Diagnosis

The history (particularly the breed and diet) and clinical signs are highly suggestive.[1] Cytology reveals numerous nucleated keratinocytes in confluent sheets consistent with widespread parakeratosis, with or without yeast, bacteria and/or neutrophils. Histopathology will confirm hyperkeratosis with diffuse parakeratosis. Parakeratosis may, however, be focal or minimal in some cases.[2] Plasma and hair zinc levels are generally the least useful information in the diagnosis of this disease.[3] Final confirmation of the diagnosis relies on response to treatment.[1,2]

Treatment

The prognosis is generally good. Therapy involves correction of any dietary factors and zinc supplementation with starting doses of 1–3 mg/kg per day of elemental zinc.[1,2] Zinc compounds have different doses (e.g. zinc sulphate 10 mg/kg per day, zinc gluconate 5 mg/kg per day[3] or zinc methionine 4 mg/kg per day) and it is important to check the level of elemental zinc in the supplement. Higher doses may be necessary in some dogs.[2] Zinc sulphate is more likely to cause vomiting and diarrhoea, so zinc gluconate or methionine is generally preferred. Higher doses produce a better response, especially initially, but these doses may be less well tolerated. Anecdotal evidence indicates that treatment with essential fatty acids (EFAs) and a low dose of oral glucocorticoids may dramatically enhance response to therapy. It is unclear whether this is associated with enhanced uptake or utilisation of zinc or reduction of cutaneous inflammation. Retinoids may also be of help in severe cases.[2] Animals that do not respond to oral medication may benefit from zinc sulphate given intramuscularly or slowly intravenously (weekly doses to a maximum of 600 mg/month),[2] although this can be painful and irritating to surrounding tissues. The most common cause of treatment failure is improper dosing of zinc. There is some rationale to feeding zinc- and EFA-supplemented diets. Antibiotics may be necessary to control secondary infections. Zinc supplementation may be required for life in type 1 disease, whereas it should be possible to maintain affected animals on a nutritionally balanced diet once the clinical signs have resolved in type 2 disease.

Key points

- May occur in dogs on a commercially prepared diet given calcium and/or cereal supplements.
- Common in northern breed dogs.
- This condition is variably pruritic.

References

1 Colombini S. Canine zinc-responsive dermatosis. *Vet Clin North Am Small Anim Pract* 1999; **29**: 1373–1383.
2 White SD, Bourdeau P, Rosychuk R *et al*. Zinc-responsive dermatosis in dogs: 41 cases and literature review. *Vet Dermatol* 2001; **12**: 101–109.
3 Hensel P. Nutrition and skin diseases in veterinary medicine. *Clinics Dermatol* 2010; **28**: 686–693.
4 Outerbridge CA. Cutaneous manifestations of internal diseases. *Vet Clin North Am Small Anim Pract* 2013; **43**: 135–152.

LEISHMANIASIS

Definition

Canine leishmaniasis is a serious systemic disease with a variable clinical presentation resulting from an infection by diphasic leishmania protozoa. Leishmaniasis is endemic in the Mediterranean basin[1] and in Central and South America. The disease has been reported in other countries including: southern Russia, India, China, eastern Africa and the USA.

Aetiology and pathogenesis

Leishmania spp. are transmitted by blood-feeding sandflies (*Phlebotomus* spp. in Europe and Asia; *Lutzomyia* spp. in the Americas). Dogs are the main vertebrate hosts, although rats and foxes are minor hosts. Female flies feeding on infected hosts ingest amastigotes. These multiply and become flagellated promastigotes in the gut of the sandfly. These are transferred when a fly feeds on another vertebrate host. The promastigotes are phagocytosed by macrophages and dendritic cells in the new host. They become non-flagellated amastigotes within 2–5 days and start to multiply. Infected cells eventually burst, releasing free amastigotes to infect adjacent cells. The organisms can disseminate to bone marrow, skin, liver, pancreas, kidneys, adrenal glands, digestive tract, eyes, testes, bone and joints. The onset of clinical signs can vary from 1 month to 7 years. Vertical transmission has been seen in areas without sandflies. Transmission by direct contact, blood transfusions and placenta has been reported in humans. There are rare reports of leishmaniasis developing in dogs from non-endemic areas that have been in close contact with infected dogs.

Dogs that mount a cell-mediated immune response are resistant to infection. Dogs that mount a humoral (antibody) immune response develop clinical signs of leishmaniasis. Chronic dermal inflammation and cutaneous parasite loads are directly related to the severity of clinical disease in New World canine visceral leishmaniasis. The parasite causes tissue damage through two pathogenic mechanisms:

- Non-suppurative granulomas, seen in skin, hepatic, enteric and bone lesions.
- Circulating immune complexes that lodge in the blood vessels, renal glomeruli and joints, resulting in vasculitis, glomerulonephritis, ocular lesions and lameness.

Clinical features

Canine leishmaniasis is an insidious, slowly progressive, multi-systemic condition. The clinical signs can vary widely among individuals. The time course of infection is variable; exposure to infected bites may result in no infection, a rapid establishment of a patent infection within 2 months, a prolonged sub-patent infection (4–22 months), before progression to overt clinical signs, or a transient subpatent period followed by 10–21 months of apparent *Leishmania*-negative status before progression. Leishmaniasis is rare in cats, but isolated cases with localised papular-to-nodular, erosive and crusting lesions have been reported. Cats can act as reservoir hosts for Old World leishmaniasis, transmitting viable organisms to sandflies.[2]

Cutaneous lesions (**Figs. 5.10–5.13**) affect up to 80%[3] of infected dogs. These include:

- Localised or generalised exfoliative dermatitis with characteristic small, adherent silvery-white scales.
- Nasodigital hyperkeratosis.
- Nodules and papules of the skin and mucocutaneous junctions.
- Ulcerations, especially pressure points, extremities and mucocutaneous junctions.
- Onychogryphosis, onychorrhexis and paronychia.
- Focal alopecia, predominately on the head and pinnae and/or periocular.
- Dry and dull hair coat.
- Sterile pustular dermatitis, especially ventral.
- Diffuse erythema and erythematous plaques.
- Nasal depigmentation, erosion and crusting.
- Secondary pyoderma and demodicosis.

Systemic signs are variable and include:

- Generalised lymphadenopathy.
- Anaemia and pale mucous membranes.
- Polydipsia, polyuria, glomerulonephritis and renal failure.
- Hepatic and splenic enlargement; possibly with hepatitis, jaundice and ascites.
- Exercise intolerance, weight loss, muscle wasting and pyrexia.
- Uveitis, keratitis, conjunctivitis and other ocular disease.
- Epistaxis, melena and other coagulopathies.
- Vasculitis and vasculopathy.
- Lameness, polyarthritis, polymyositis or osteomyelitis.

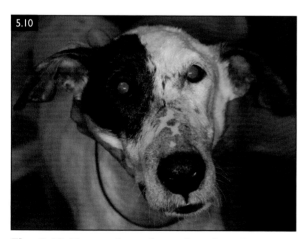

Fig. 5.10 Temporal muscle wasting, alopecia and scaling of the face in a dog with leishmaniasis. This UK-based dog had been imported from Cyprus 2 years earlier.

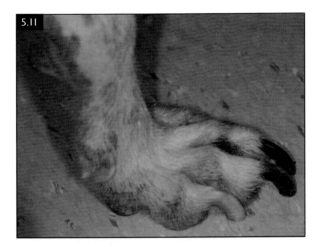

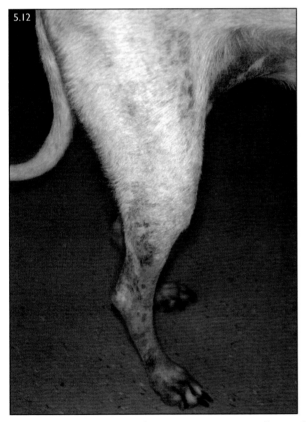

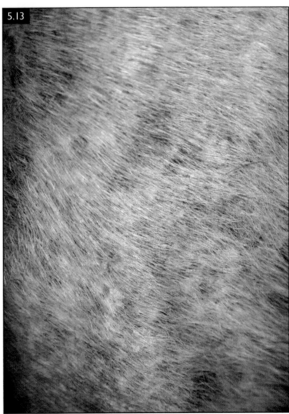

Figs. 5.11–5.13 Same dog as in Fig. 5.10: onychogryphosis (hypertrophy and curling of the claws) (Fig. 5.11); alopecia and scaling of the lower limb and bony points (Fig. 5.12); profuse, fine, silver–white scaling of the trunk (Fig. 5.13).

- Meningitis and neurological disorders.
- Anorexia, vomiting and diarrhoea.
- Sneezing and coughing.
- Atrophic masticatory myositis.

Differential diagnoses
- Pemphigus foliaceus.
- Cutaneous or systemic lupus erythematosus.
- Exfoliative cutaneous lupus erythematous.

- Vasculitis.
- Sebaceous adenitis.
- Zinc-responsive dermatitis.
- Bacterial folliculitis.
- Dermatophytosis.
- Demodicosis.
- Superficial necrolytic dermatitis.
- Epitheliotrophic lymphoma.

Due to the variable clinical presentation, *Leishmania* spp. should also be considered in many other cases, especially in, or if there has been travel to, endemic areas.

Diagnosis

Clinical examination and the knowledge that the affected animal lives in or has come from an area where leishmaniasis is prevalent will raise clinical suspicion. Most cases have a non-regenerative, normochromic/normocytic anaemia, hypergamma-globulinaemia, hypoalbuminaemia, a low albumin: globulin ratio and proteinuria with a protein: creatinine ratio of >1. Antinuclear antibody (ANA) tests are positive in roughly 50% of cases.

Organisms can be detected on cytology (**Fig. 5.14**) of scrapes from superficial lesions or aspirates from lymph nodes (30%), bone marrow (50%) or spleen. Cytology may be more sensitive than serology in early cases.

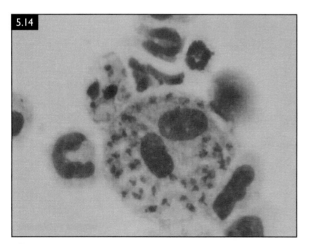

Fig. 5.14 *Leishmania* organisms in a macrophage from a lymph node aspirate (courtesy of Genevieve Marignac).

Histopathological inflammatory patterns are variable and often non-specific. Most cases have orthokeratotic hyperkeratosis with mononuclear inflammatory infiltrates, which may be perifollicular, perivascular, interstitial to diffuse, nodular, interface, pustular or mixed. Vasculitis, ischaemia and necrosis may also be present. Organisms can be seen in about 50% of cases with Giemsa stains.

Polymerase chain reaction (PCR) is highly sensitive and widely used, although contamination and false-positive results can be seen. False-negative PCR is also seen, because organisms may not be present in all tissues. PCR on bone marrow and tissue samples is almost 100% sensitive; PCR on blood, lymph node and cerebrospinal fluid (CSF) is less sensitive.

Leishmania-specific IgG serology is usually highly sensitive, but positive serology is associated with exposure and not necessarily disease. It is therefore less useful in endemic areas, where most dogs will be infected but only a minority will develop clinical signs. Titres remain high for prolonged periods after infection and successful treatment, although the response to individual antigens is variable. An indirect immunofluorescent antibody test (IFAT) to detect whole organisms is 98–99% sensitive and high titres are associated with clinically affected dogs or infected dogs that will develop clinical signs. Enzyme-linked immunosorbent assay (ELISA) tests detect a variety of antigens and are approximately 90% sensitive.

Definitive diagnosis relies on demonstrating organisms in affected tissues, although this is not possible in all cases. Therefore, diagnosis is often based on compatible clinical signs together with supportive evidence from a range of other tests. In one study of 160 dogs diagnosed with leishmaniasis, approximately 42% were positive by PCR, 46% by IFAT and 19% by lymph node aspirate cytology.

Treatment[1,4]

Dogs should be treated only if the health legislation of the country concerned permits therapy, because euthanasia is necessary in some countries. It is also important to determine if the patient's condition will allow a reasonable chance of successful treatment, as renal failure is a poor prognostic indicator. It is important to remember that parasite burdens may

Table 5.2 Treatment regimens for leishmaniasis and adverse effects

DRUG	DOSE	ROUTE	DURATION	POTENTIAL ADVERSE EFFECTS
Meglumine antimonite	75–100 mg/kg q24 h or 40–75 mg/kg q12 h	Subcutaneous injection	4 weeks	Nephrotoxicity, cutaneous abscess
Miltefosine	2 mg/kg q24 h	By mouth	4 weeks	Vomiting, diarrhoea
Allopurinol	10 mg/kg q12 h	By mouth	6–12 months	Xanthine urolithiasis

remain after treatment, permitting possible relapse or transmission. Treatment recommendations (*Table 5.2*) vary depending on the stage of disease.

Therapy for mild disease. Allopurinol or meglumine antimonite; or miltefosine/allopurinol combined with meglumine antimonite; or allopurinol combined with miltefosine. The prognosis is good.

Therapy for moderate disease. Allopurinol combined with meglumine antimonite or allopurinol combined with miltefosine. The prognosis is guarded to good.

Therapy for severe disease. Allopurinol combined with meglumine antimonite or allopurinol combined with miltefosine. An internal medicine text should be consulted for simultaneous treatment of renal disease. The prognosis is guarded to poor.

Therapy for severe disease accompanied by end-stage renal disease. Allopurinol alone. The prognosis is poor.[1]

Treatment can stop if the animal is in clinical remission and if haematology, biochemistry, urinalysis and the protein:creatinine ratio, serum protein electrophoresis (SPE), serology (IFAT) and PCR are all normal. Two negative PCRs 6 months apart are needed to demonstrate a parasitological cure.

Protection against sandfly bites is very important in endemic areas. The products must have repellent activity to prevent bites. Useful products include deltamethrin-impregnated collars and washes, imidacloprid and flumethrin collars, and permethrin/imidacloprid or dinotefuran/pyriproxyfen/permethrin spot-on products.[1,5] Avoiding times and places

that sandflies are most active may reduce the risk of bites.

Vaccines are available to prevent and block transmission of canine visceral leishmaniasis; however, the efficacy is not complete and they must be used together with antisandfly measures.[5,6]

Key points

- A disease with many clinical presentations that should always be considered as a differential or concomitant diagnosis in regions where *Leishmania* spp. are endemic.
- Always ask about an animal's travel history.
- Potentially zoonotic.

References

1 Solano-Gallego L, Miró G, Koutinas A *et al*. LeishVet guidelines for the practical management of canine leishmaniosis. *Parasit Vectors* 2011; **4**(1): 86.

2 Pennisi MG, Hartmann K, Lloret A *et al*. Leishmaniosis in cats ABCD guidelines on prevention and management. *J Feline Med Surg* 2013; **15**: 638–642.

3 Saridomichelakis MN, Koutinas AF. Cutaneous involvement in canine leishmaniosis due to *Leishmania infantum* (syn. *L. chagasi*). *Vet Dermatol* 2014; **25**: 61–e22.

4 Oliva G, Roura X, Crotti A *et al*. Guidelines for treatment of leishmaniasis in dogs. *J Am Vet Med Assoc* 2010; **236**: 1192–1198.

5 Maroli M, Gradoni L, Olivia G *et al*. Guidelines for prevention of leishmaniasis in dogs. *J Am Vet Med Assoc* 2010; **236**: 1200–1205.

6 Foroughi-Parvar F, Gholamreza H. Vaccines for canine leishmaniasis. *Adv Prevent Med* 2014; **8**: e3172.

EXFOLIATIVE CUTANEOUS LUPUS ERYTHEMATOSUS OF THE GERMAN SHORT-HAIRED POINTER

Definition

Exfoliative cutaneous lupus erythematosus (ECLE) is a familial form of lupus that affects German Short-haired Pointers. Spontaneous cases of ECLE have also been seen in other breeds. ECLE is one of the forms of cutaneous lupus that have been associated with systemic lupus erythematosus (SLE), especially in German Short-haired Pointers.

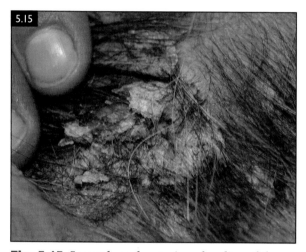

Fig. 5.15 Severe hyperkeratosis and scaling of the ventral abdomen in a Bearded Collie with ECLE.

Aetiology and pathogenesis

There is a strong genetic predisposition to the development of this disease, although the exact gene mutation is unknown. The inflammation of the skin is lupus like and autoantibodies have not been found.

Clinical features

The disease usually occurs in puppies and young adults, although it may be seen in older dogs in other breeds. Sex predilection has not been noted. ECLE is characterised by widespread scaling, depigmentation, alopecia, and ulceration and crusting on the muzzle, pinnae, trunk and limbs (**Figs. 5.15–5.17**). Dogs may be pruritic.[1] Systemic abnormalities such as lymphadenopathy, intermittent pyrexia, joint pain, infertility, hyperglobulinaemia and thrombocytopenia may also be present in dogs that develop SLE. Dogs often assume a 'hunched stance'.[2,3] Complications may include secondary pyoderma, yeast dermatitis and otitis.

Differential diagnoses

- Sebaceous adenitis.
- Primary idiopathic keratinisation defect (seborrhoea).
- Ichthyosis.
- Demodicosis.
- Dermatophytosis.

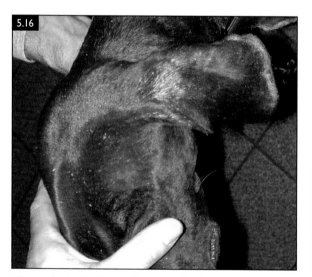

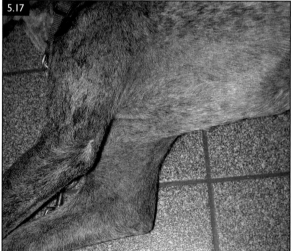

Figs. 5.16, 5.17 Scaling over the head and ear (Fig. 5.16), and forelimb and trunk (Fig. 5.17) of a German Short-haired Pointer with exfoliative cutaneous lupus erythematosus (photos courtesy of Pat McKeever).

- Follicular dysplasia.
- Leishmaniasis.
- Systemic lupus erythematosus.

Diagnosis

The diagnosis is based on the history, physical exam, skin cytology and skin biopsies. The skin should not be clipped or cleaned before punch biopsies. Multiple specimens should be selected from lesions of varying stages. Histopathology reveals lymphocytic interface dermatitis with marked hyperkeratosis and apoptotic keratinocytes. Destruction of sebaceous glands may also be observed.

Treatment

Glucocorticoids, ciclosporin and hydroxychloroquine can temporarily relieve clinical signs.[2] Leflunomide shows some promise[1] (see Immunosuppressive Drug Therapy Table, page 289). The prognosis in German Short-haired Pointers is generally guarded, but it can be better in other breeds without systemic involvement.

Key point

- This disease may wax and wane. German Short-haired Pointers eventually succumb to the disease, but treatment can improve quality of life in some dogs for several months to years.

References

1 Bryden SL, White SD, Dunston SM *et al*. Clinical, histopathological and immunological characteristics of exfoliative cutaneous lupus erythematosus in 25 German short-haired pointers. *Vet Dermatol* 2005; **16**: 239–252.

2 Werner A. All in the family: chronic dermatitis and German shorthaired pointers. Available from: http://www.cliniciansbrief.com/sites/default/files/attachments/MYD_Chronic%20Dermatitis%20in%20German%20Shorthaired.pdf (accessed: 2 April 2018).

3 Mauldin EA, Morris DO, Brown DC *et al*. Exfoliative cutaneous lupus erythematosus in German shorthaired pointer dogs: disease development, progression and evaluation of three immunomodulatory drugs (ciclosporin, hydroxychloroquine, and adalimumab) in a controlled environment. *Vet Dermatol* 2010; **27**: 373–382.

VITAMIN A-RESPONSIVE DERMATOSIS

Definition

Vitamin A-responsive dermatosis is a rare dermatosis characterised by epidermal hyperkeratosis with markedly disproportionate follicular hyperkeratosis.

Aetiology and pathogenesis

The aetiology is not known. Retinoic acid (a derivative of vitamin A) is essential for a wide range of cell and tissue functions. It is particularly important in keratinocyte proliferation and differentiation by regulating the expression of keratins. Even though the clinical signs resolve with vitamin A supplementation, there is no evidence that affected animals are deficient in vitamin A.

Clinical features

The dermatosis is almost entirely confined to Cocker Spaniels. The clinical signs usually begin between age 2 and 5 years, and clinical signs get more severe with time. Dogs develop prominent, frond-like follicular casts and multi-focal, frond-like, erythematous, crusted plaques, particularly on the lateral thorax and ventrum (**Fig. 5.18**). Affected animals are often pruritic and have malodorous skin, especially with concomitant bacterial or *Malassezia* infections.

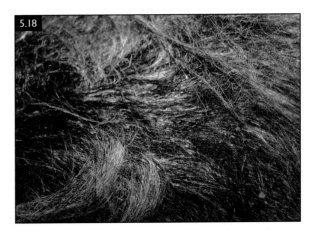

Fig. 5.18 Alopecia, seborrhoea and scaling with prominent follicular casts in a Cocker Spaniel with vitamin A-responsive dermatosis.

Differential diagnoses

- Sarcoptic mange.
- Demodicosis.
- Flea allergic dermatosis.
- Atopic dermatitis.
- Cutaneous adverse food reaction.
- Primary idiopathic keratinisation defect (seborrhoea).
- Sebaceous adenitis.
- Ichthyosis.

Diagnosis

The clinical signs and history are highly suggestive. Histopathology will help confirm the presence of a follicle-oriented keratinisation defect, but the final diagnosis relies on the response to vitamin A therapy. Cytology should be performed to identify secondary bacterial and/or yeast infections, which will need appropriate management.

Treatment

The prognosis is generally good. Treatment with 10 000 IU (maximum 800–1000 IU/kg per day) vitamin A in food once daily usually resolves the clinical signs within 4–8 weeks.[1] Appropriate keratolytic and/or antimicrobial treatment will speed clinical resolution. Once in remission, affected dogs can be maintained with daily (or less frequently if possible) vitamin A supplementation. At these doses vitamin A is very well tolerated, but potential adverse effects include hepatopathy, hyperostosis and keratoconjunctivitis sicca. Affected individuals generally require lifelong supplementation with vitamin A.[1]

Key point

- An uncommon dermatosis that is ultimately diagnosed by response to vitamin A.

Reference

1   Hensel P. Nutrition and skin diseases in veterinary medicine. *Clinics Dermatol* 2010; **28**: 686–693.

IDIOPATHIC KERATINISATION DEFECTS (Primary seborrhoea)

Aetiology and pathogenesis

Primary keratinisation defects (seborrhoea) in Cocker Spaniels is an uncommon, possibly familial, dermatosis associated with abnormal basal epidermal cell kinetics. Compared with normal dogs, basal epidermal cells in affected dogs undergo accelerated cellular proliferation and turnover.[1-3] There is an increase in the number of actively dividing basal cells, a shortened cell cycle and a decreased transit time to the stratum corneum (7–8 days compared with 21–23 days). Hair follicles and sebaceous glands are similarly affected. This results in marked scaling, greasiness and alopecia. The disrupted epidermal barrier and altered cutaneous microenvironment predispose to secondary pyoderma and malassezia dermatitis. Similar conditions are recognised in other Spaniels, especially English Springers **(Fig. 5.19)** and, less commonly, in other breeds.[4] The condition may be associated with less greasiness in other breeds.

Clinical features

Most animals display abnormal keratinisation from an early age. The clinical signs vary in severity and extent, but tend to worsen with time. Mildly affected dogs exhibit adherent, greasy scales around the nipples, lip folds and external ear canals **(Fig. 5.20)**. More severely affected animals have more severe and generalised lesions in skin folds, ventral neck, ventral body, medial limbs, trunk and feet. Severely affected dogs are malodorous, greasy, alopecic and pruritic, with a papular scaling and, occasionally, crusting dermatosis **(Figs. 5.21, 5.22)**. Chronic or recurrent and, often severe, otitis externa is common.

Differential diagnoses

- Sebaceous gland hyperplasia or dysplasia.
- Ectoparasite infestation, particularly *Cheyletiella* and *Demodex* spp.
- Atopic dermatitis.
- Cutaneous adverse food reaction.
- Endocrinopathies, especially hypothyroidism.
- Sebaceous adenitis.

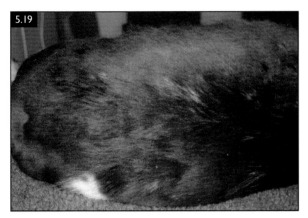

Fig. 5.19 Primary keratinisation defect in an English Springer Spaniel.

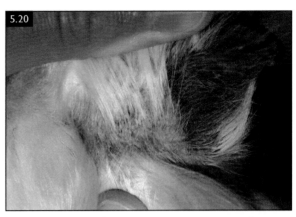

Fig. 5.20 Same dog as in Fig. 5.19: severe scaling.

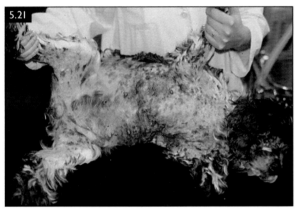

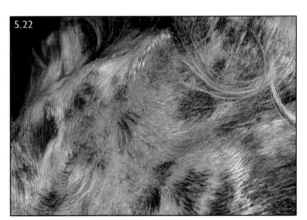

Figs. 5.21, 5.22 Primary keratinisation defect in a Cocker Spaniel with severe erythema, alopecia, scaling and superficial spreading pyoderma.

- Dietary deficiency (especially EFAs).
- Vitamin A-responsive dermatosis.
- Dermatophytosis.
- Leishmaniasis.
- Pemphigus foliaceus.
- Epitheliotrophic lymphoma.
- Allergic or irritant contact dermatitis.

Some of these conditions may be concurrent (especially parasites and hypersensitivities) and/or triggers for secondary scaling and seborrhoea. These conditions can result in secondary pyoderma and malassezia dermatitis. The seborrhoea may resolve once secondary infections have been treated and controlled.

Diagnosis

The diagnosis of a primary keratinisation defect relies heavily on ruling out other diseases. Pruritic dogs should be evaluated for atopic dermatitis, cutaneous adverse food reactions, ectoparasites, and secondary pyoderma and/or malassezia dermatitis. Clinicians should ensure that affected dogs are receiving an easily digestible, balanced diet that is rich in EFAs. Affected dogs should also be evaluated for endocrine disease, particularly hypothyroidism and hyperadrenocorticism.

If the dog continues to have seborrhoea after other conditions have been identified and managed properly, then a skin biopsy should be performed. Primary keratinisation defects are characterised histologically by non-inflammatory orthokeratotic (i.e. non-nucleated) hyperkeratosis and keratin plugs in the hair follicles. Histopathology can be non-specific, but it is particularly useful for ruling out other skin diseases. Histological interpretation will be hindered by inflammation from pyoderma and yeast dermatitis, so it is important to ensure that secondary infections have been properly treated before procuring a skin biopsy.

Treatment

If a primary cause cannot be identified and controlled, then lifelong therapy is necessary. It is very important to maintain rigorous flea control and to treat secondary skin and ear infections promptly.[4–6]

Topical therapy

Topical therapy can be very effective, is generally safe and is traditionally the mainstay of treatment.[7] It does, however, require an amenable patient, adequate facilities and a committed owner, and is not suitable in every case. Topical therapy should be keratolytic (to soften and remove existing scale), keratoplastic (suppress basal cell turnover and excessive keratinistion) and degreasing or moisturising to help restore the epidermal barrier and reduce transepidermal water loss (*Table 5.3*). The relative importance of these factors varies with each case. Treatment may require a combination of products, which are best selected by trial and error.

Topical therapy should be instituted two to three times weekly with a 10- to 15-minute contact time. Once in remission the frequency can be reduced. It may also be possible to switch to less aggressive products and/or reduce the number of different products employed.

Systemic therapy

Systemic therapy can be used in cases where topical therapy is ineffective or inappropriate. EFA supplementation can help restore normal epidermal barrier function.[4] Synthetic retinoids (e.g. isotretinoin or acitretinoin [1–2 mg/kg q24 h, reducing to 1 mg/kg q48 h for maintenance]) can be effective in

Table 5.3 Topical therapies for idiopathic keratinisation defects

INGREDIENT	ANTIBACTERIAL	MOISTURISING	DRYING	KERATOLYTIC	KERATOPLASTIC[1]
Benzoyl peroxide	X		X	X	
Chlorhexidine	X				
Ethyl lactate	X			X	X
Salicylic acid	X			X	X
Selenium sulphide	X				X
Sulphur	X		X	X	X
Tar	X		X	X	X
Aloe vera		X			
Colloidal oatmeal		X			
Fatty acids		X			
Lanolin		X			
Phytosphingosine[2]	X	X			
Propylene glycol		X		X	
Mineral oil		X		X	
Urea		X		X	
Sodium or ammonium lactate		X			X

[1] Keratoplastic = modifies and normalises keratinocyte turnover.

[2] Phytosphingosine = modifies sebaceous gland activity and normalises sebaceous secretion.

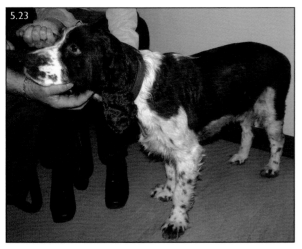
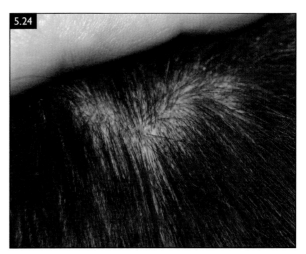

Figs. 5.23, 5.24 Same dog as in Fig. 5.19: good response to treatment with essential fatty acids, keratolytic and emollient shampoos and vitamin A.

suppressing the accelerated cellular kinetics and associated keratinisation defects.[5,6] Vitamin A (10 000 IU q24 h, maximum 800–1000 IU/kg q24 h (see Vitamin A-responsive dermatosis, page 146) can also be effective, and is less expensive and better tolerated than synthetic retinoids (**Figs. 5.23, 5.24**). This blurs the distinction between what is vitamin A-responsive dermatosis and primary keratinisation defect in Cocker Spaniels.

Key points

- Primary seborrhoea is rare, but secondary seborrhoea is common. Secondary seborrhoea responds best when the underlying condition is treated.
- Primary seborrhoea is a disease that is not cured, and treatment is required for the life of the pet.

References

1   Kwochka KW, Rademakers AM. Cell proliferation of epidermis, hair follicles and sebaceous glands of Beagles and Cocker Spaniels with healthy skin. *Am J Vet Res* 1989; **50**: 587–591.

2   Kwochka KW, Rademakers AM. Cell proliferation kinetics of epidermis, hair follicles and sebaceous glands of Cocker Spaniels with idiopathic seborrhea. *Am J Vet Res* 1989; **50**: 1918–1922.

3   Kwochka KW. Cell proliferation kinetics in the hair root matrix of dogs with healthy skin and dogs with idiopathic seborrhea. *Am J Vet Res* 1990; **51**: 1570–1573.

4   Scott DW, Miller WH. Primary seborrhea in English springer spaniels: a retrospective study of 14 cases. *J Small Anim Pract* 1996; **37**: 173–178.

5   Fadok VA. Treatment of canine idiopathic seborrhea with isotretinoin. *Am J Vet Res* 1986; **47**: 1730–1733.

6   Power HT, Ihrke PJ, Stannard AA *et al*. Use of etretinate for treatment of primary keratinization disorders (idiopathic seborrhea) in Cocker Spaniels, West Highland White Terriers, and Bassett Hounds. *J Am Vet Med Assoc* 1992; **201**: 419–429.

7   Rosenkrantz W. Practical applications of topical therapy for allergic, infectious, and seborrheic disorders. *Clin Tech Small Anim Pract* 2006; **21**: 106–116.

CANINE EAR MARGIN SEBORRHOEA

Definition
Canine ear margin seborrhoea is a cornification abnormality that results in scaling and alopecia on the margins of the pinnae.

Aetiology and pathogenesis
Canine ear margin seborrhoea can be a primary idiopathic condition or secondary to other diseases such as atopy, vasculitis or hypothyroidism.

Clinical features
Primary idiopathic ear margin seborrhoea tends to affect dogs with pendulous pinnae, especially Dachshunds, Springer Spaniels and Cocker Spaniels. Initially, excessive adherent keratin accumulation is noted on the pinnal margins. In some cases, the accumulations may be waxy or greasy and follicular casts may be present. Focal areas of alopecia may develop along the ear margins (**Fig. 5.25**). If a thick layer of keratin debris accumulates, it may fissure and bleed. The lesions are only occasionally pruritic and may be secondarily infected. Associated fissures and ulcerations are painful.

Differential diagnoses
- Atopic dermatitis (especially German Shepherd dogs, Cocker Spaniels and Springer Spaniels).
- Early vasculitis (vasculitis will eventually have focal areas of tissue necrosis).
- Sarcoptic mange (usually very pruritic).

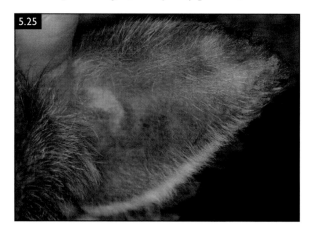

Fig. 5.25 Ear margin seborrhoea with scaling, alopecia, fissures and crusts of the pinna tip and margin.

- Frostbite.
- Sebaceous adenitis.
- Ichthyosis.
- Zinc-responsive dermatosis.
- Vitamin A-responsive dermatosis.

Diagnosis
The diagnosis is based on the clinical findings and ruling out other differentials. Surface cytology should be performed to investigate secondary bacterial or yeast dermatitis. Dermatohistopathology can provide supporting evidence. Biopsy of the ear margin can cause persistent haemorrhage and a lesion that is slow to heal due to head shaking. Taking narrow full-thickness wedges, closing the wound with a double-layer suture pattern and closing the dorsal and ventral skin separately avoids the cartilage and may encourage healing.

Treatment
Simple monitoring is an appropriate treatment option if the ear margins are not painful, pruritic or infected.

Excessive scale can be removed with keratolytic shampoos or ointments. Topical phytosphingosine products may be useful to decrease the accumulation of scale and production of sebum. These products should be used daily or every other day until the desired effect is achieved, and then approximately weekly to prevent recurrence. Topical emollient and moisturising creams and ointments can help prevent drying and fissuring.

Inflammation can be treated with a topical glucocorticoid, such as fluocinolone acetonide 0.1% in 60% dimethyl sulphoxide (DMSO), or 0.1% betamethasone valerate cream, applied twice daily until the desired effect is reached, and then periodically as needed to prevent recurrent inflammation. The pinnae should be monitored for dermal atrophy, which is a potential side effect of continuous topical glucocorticoid applications.

Bacterial or *Malassezia* infections can be treated with appropriate topical or systemic antimicrobials.

Key points
- This is usually an idiopathic condition that is generally controlled but not cured.
- This condition is generally non-pruritic.

NASAL AND DIGITAL HYPERKERATOSIS

Definition

Nasal hyperkeratosis is characterised by excessive amounts of keratin on the nasal planum. Digital hyperkeratosis presents similarly and affects the footpads.

Aetiology and pathogenesis

Hyperkeratosis occurs because of increased production or retention of keratinised tissue. It may be genetic, conformational or idiopathic. Familial nasal and/or footpad hyperkeratosis has been reported in Dogues de Bordeaux and Irish Terriers.[1] Nasal parakeratosis is a type of hereditary hyperkeratosis that has been reported in young adult Labrador Retrievers.[1] Poor conformation (particularly English Bulldogs), obesity and degenerative joint disease can also lead to fronding hyperkeratosis on the footpad margins, because dogs with these conditions (and declawed cats) tend to walk and bear weight abnormally. Spontaneous idiopathic disease, particularly of the older dog, is the most common cause of nasal and digital hyperkeratosis.

Clinical features

Nasal hyperkeratosis is confined to the nasal planum and presents as a variably thickened, fissured accumulation of dry, frond-like, keratinised tissue (**Figs. 5.26, 5.27**). Pedal hyperkeratosis is more variable in presentation (**Fig. 5.28**). Areas of hyperkeratosis may fissure, leading to secondary bacterial or *Malassezia* infection. Fissured and infected lesions can be very painful. Both nasal and digital hyperkeratosis may occur in the same individual. With conformational abnormalities and degenerative joint disease, focal, fronding hyperkeratosis typically occurs on the periphery of footpads.

Differential diagnoses

- Canine distemper virus infection.
- Canine papillomavirus infection.
- Pemphigus foliaceus.
- Superficial necrolytic dermatitis.
- Zinc-responsive dermatosis.
- Cutaneous lupus erythematosus.
- Epitheliotrophic lymphoma.

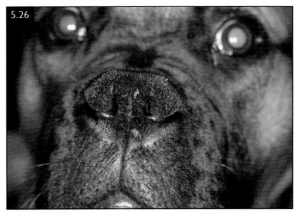

Fig. 5.26 Nasal hyperkeratosis in a Boxer dog.

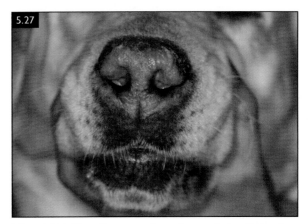

Fig. 5.27 Hereditary nasal parakeratosis in a Labrador.

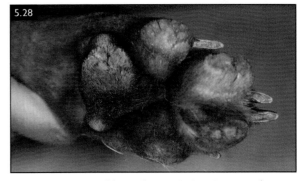

Fig. 5.28 Digital hyperkeratosis in a Dogues de Bordeaux.

Diagnosis

Consideration of the vaccine history and the risk of exposure to the virus are particularly important in establishing the likelihood of canine distemper or papillomavirus infection. Canine distemper virus is rare in areas where vaccination against distemper is standard practice. Canine papillomavirus only rarely causes focal, fronding hyperkeratosis of the footpads, and is more likely to be associated with endophytic footpad corns or exophytic interdigital lesions.

Dietary history and signalment will raise suspicions of absolute or relative zinc deficiency. Zinc-responsive dermatosis, pemphigus foliaceus and superficial necrolytic dermatitis may affect the nasal planum and footpads, although the lesions tend to be more crusted than hyperkeratotic. Cutaneous lupus erythematosus and epitheliotrophic lymphoma should be considered in cases with nasal ulceration.

Cytology should be performed to rule out secondary bacterial or yeast infections. If the diagnosis is uncertain based on history and physical exam, then a skin biopsy is recommended.

Treatment

Treatment is not needed for mild cases. For moderate to severe, painful hyperkeratosis, a mixture of 50% propylene glycol and warm water can be used to soak the footpads daily until the hyperkeratosis has receded to an acceptable level. The softened, hyperkeratotic fronds can be carefully trimmed with a scissors or filed with a pumice stone. The footpads will need to be periodically soaked in the propylene glycol and water mixture to prevent the hyperkeratosis from returning, drying and fissuring.[1] Additional topical treatment options include: petroleum jelly, tretinoin gel, fluocinolone acetonide in 60% DMSO or other keratolytic or keratoplastic agents.

The fissures in the hyperkeratotic tissue may become infected. Mild infections can be treated with topical ointments that contain betamethasone, gentamicin and clotrimazole. Deep and severely inflamed infections may require systemic glucocorticoid, antibacterial and/or antiyeast treatment.

Hyperkeratosis that is secondary to other diseases generally improves when the primary disease is treated.

Key points
- Idiopathic hyperkeratosis is usually a cosmetic condition. Treatment is medically indicated only if secondary infection or pain occurs.
- This is a condition that is not cured, but can be controlled with continuous treatment.

Reference
1 Peters J, Scott DW, Erb HN, Miller WH. Hereditary nasal parakeratosis in Labrador retrievers: 11 new cases and a retrospective study on the presence of accumulations of serum ('serum lakes') in the epidermis of parakeratotic dermatoses and inflamed nasal plana of dogs. *Vet Dermatol* 2003; **14**: 197–203.

CALLUS FORMATION

Aetiology and pathogenesis
A callus is a defined area of hyperkeratosis, which is sometimes lichenified and typically occurs over bony pressure points. The hyperkeratosis and thickening of the skin are due to irritation resulting from frictional contact with a hard surface on the exterior of the skin and pressure from an underlying bony prominence (see also Decubital ulcers, page 179).

Clinical features
Callus development occurs more frequently in large, short-haired dogs that sleep on hard surfaces. Lesions usually develop on the lateral aspect of the elbows or hocks (**Fig. 5.29**). They may also develop on the sternum of deep-chested dogs or dogs with short limbs in which the sternum may continually contact objects such as stairs. Calluses appear as focal areas of alopecia, hyperkeratosis and lichenification with a light grey surface. Milia and/or comedones can also be seen. Entrapment of hair and/or sebum in a callus may result in a foreign body reaction with furunculosis, draining tracts and secondary deep pyoderma (**Fig. 5.30**). Fissuring and secondary infection can be painful. Calluses may erode, ulcerate and form non-healing wounds in dogs with underlying disorders such as hyperadrenocorticism. Calluses with subcutaneous hygromas may present as fluctuant, mobile masses.

Differential diagnoses
- Demodicosis.
- Neoplasia.
- Dermatophytosis.
- Deep pyoderma.
- Zinc-responsive dermatosis.

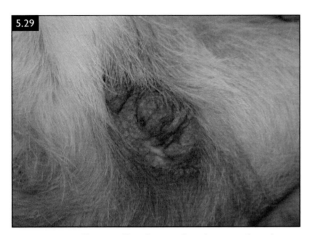

Fig. 5.29 Elbow callus: large, deeply convoluted lesions on the lateral aspect of elbows are typical of callus.

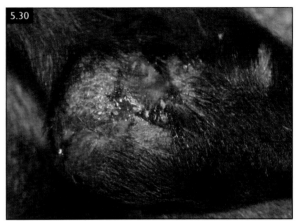

Fig. 5.30 Infected callus on a dog's hock.

Diagnosis

Diagnosis is generally based on the history and clinical features. Further investigation for underlying causes may be necessary in cases of non-antibiotic-responsive infections or non-healing wounds.

Treatment

The sleeping habits should be modified if possible, so that the patient rests on soft bedding material such as foam rubber padding. Custom or homemade pads over the affected pressure points are also useful. Feminine hygiene pads, small beanbags and DogLeggs® (custom-fit, wearable joint padding) can be used for elbow padding.

Degenerative joint disease may contribute to the development of pressure necrosis and pyoderma of calluses. Proper pain management of the underlying joint disease reduces the amount of time that a patient spends recumbent, and so reduces pressure necrosis in the callused area.

Inflamed calluses should be treated with twice-daily fluocinolone acetonide in DMSO; this topical product can be absorbed deep into affected tissue. Petroleum jelly-type products are useful if the callus needs to be softened. Care must be exercised to avoid excessive treatment that creates an erosion or ulcer.

Infected calluses should be treated with a systemic antibiotic. Culture and sensitivity testing are helpful for guiding antibiotic selection. Adjunctive treatment with mupirocin ointment should be

considered, because it can penetrate thickened tissue. Treatment should be continued for 2–4 weeks beyond resolution of lesions. This may require 4–8 weeks of treatment depending on the severity and depth of secondary infections.

Calluses and subcutaneous hygromas should not be surgically removed, as this frequently results in a non-healing wound (Fig. 5.31). Severely proliferative lesions may be carefully removed or ablated with a CO_2 laser.

Key points

- Management of pressure necrosis is key for resolution and prevention of infected calluses.
- Surgical resection of elbow calluses frequently result in a non-healing wound.

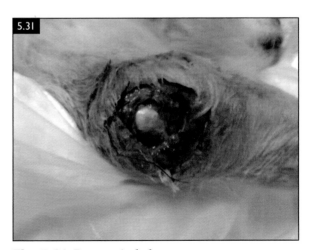

Fig. 5.31 Postsurgical ulcer.

SCHNAUZER COMEDO SYNDROME

Definition
Schnauzer comedo syndrome is a follicular keratinisation disorder of Miniature Schnauzers characterised by comedone formation along the dorsal midline.

Aetiology and pathogenesis
The syndrome is probably associated with an inherited developmental defect of the hair follicles, leading to abnormal keratinisation, comedone formation and in some cases a secondary bacterial folliculitis.[1]

Clinical features
Non-pruritic comedones develop in young to adult Miniature Schnauzers. They extend laterally from the dorsal midline and are located from the neck to the sacrum. In many cases, lesions are more prominent on the lumbosacral region. In early or mild cases the lesions may not be visualised, but small papules can be palpated over the dorsum; these may be crusted and firm or soft and waxy. With progression, there is thinning of the hair and the papular comedones become more obvious (**Fig. 5.32**). A secondary bacterial folliculitis may develop and cause crusts, pruritus and pain.

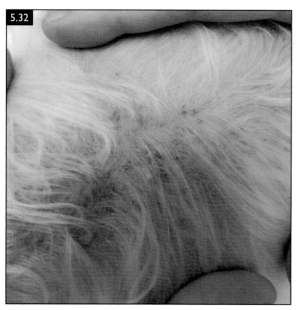

Fig. 5.32 Schnauzer comedo syndrome – alopecia, erythema, comedones and crust on the dorsal–lumbar sacral skin.

Differential diagnoses
- Demodicosis.
- Hypothyroidism.
- Bacterial folliculitis.
- Dermatophytosis.
- Fleabite hypersensitivity.
- Contact dermatitis.

Diagnosis
The history and clinical signs are highly suggestive, and the diagnosis can be confirmed with a skin biopsy. Skin scrapes, cytology, fungal culture, diet trial and flea control trials can be helpful to rule out the differential diagnoses. Hair plucks, adhesive tape-strips, deep skin scrapings and surface cytology are required to accurately evaluate comedones.

Treatment[1]
The prognosis is variable but generally good, although lifelong treatment will be necessary. Mild cases with few lesions may not require treatment. More severe cases can be managed with shampoos that contain phytosphingosine and/or benzoyl peroxide. Daily bathing for the initial 4 weeks of treatment is helpful to reduce the size of comedones. Weekly to twice-monthly baths are often necessary to prevent recurrence of large comedones. Weekly to twice-monthly topical 'spot-on' products containing phytosphingosine can also help to prevent development of large comedones. Spot-on products may be used in place of baths in some cases. Vitamin A (10 000 IU; maximum 800–1000 IU/kg per day) in food once daily may also help prevent comedone formation.

Topical steroids are helpful if inflammation, pruritus and pain are present from follicular rupture. Secondary bacterial folliculitis should be treated with appropriate antibacterial therapy (see Superficial pyoderma, page 70).

Key point
- This is a condition that is not cured, but it can be controlled with lifelong therapy.

Reference
1   Hannigan MM. A refractory case of schnauzer comedo syndrome. *Can Vet J* 1997; **38**: 238.

CUTANEOUS HORN

Definition
Cutaneous horns are localised, benign outgrowths of keratin or sometimes serocellular debris, with the appearance of small horns.

Aetiology and pathogenesis
Cutaneous horn is a descriptive term and the lesions may be associated with viral papillomas, actinic keratoses, bowenoid in-situ carcinoma, invasive squamous cell carcinoma and infundibular keratinising acanthoma.[1] Multiple cutaneous horns have been reported in cats associated with feline leukaemia virus (FeLV) infection.[2,3]

Clinical features
Cutaneous horns are localised and non-pruritic (**Fig. 5.33**). Multiple lesions may be seen in some individuals. In cats, cutaneous horns may affect the footpads.[2,3] There is no breed, age or sex predilection. The horn is firm to the touch, and not easily removed from the underlying skin. If pulled off, the base tends to haemorrhage and the horns typically recur.

Differential diagnoses
- Papillomavirus.
- Actinic keratoses.
- Bowenoid in-situ carcinoma or squamous cell carcinoma.
- Infundibular keratinising acanthoma.
- Cutaneous horn of feline footpad caused by FeLV infection.

Diagnosis
To determine the specific aetiology, the entire base of the horn should be surgically removed and submitted for histopathological evaluation. Cats should be screened for FeLV infection.

Treatment
Surgical excision is generally curative, although this depends on the specific aetiology of the lesion. Further treatment depends on the aetiology. Cutaneous horns of the footpads of FeLV-positive cats will often recur after surgery.[3]

Key point
- Cutaneous horn is a keratin outgrowth sometimes associated with cancerous conditions.

References
1 Gross TH, Ihrke PJ, Walder EJ, Affolter VK. Cutaneous horn of feline pawpad. In: *Skin Diseases of the Dog and Cat: Clinical and Histopathological Diagnosis*, 2nd edn. Oxford: Blackwell Publishing, 2005: p. 562.
2 Scott DW. Feline dermatology, 1979–1982: introspective retrospections. *J Am Anim Hosp Assoc* 1984; **20**: 537.
3 Center SA, Scott DW, Scott FW. Multiple cutaneous horns on the footpads of a cat. *Feline Pract* 1982; **12**: 26–30.

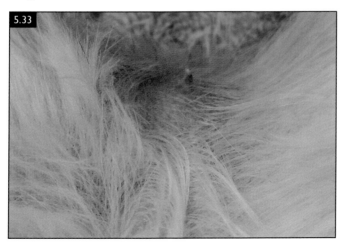

Fig. 5.33 A cutaneous horn emerging from an infundibular keratinising acanthoma.

SPICULOSIS

Definition
Spiculosis is a rare condition of Kerry Blue Terriers, characterised by pruritus and hard brittle spicules of keratin protruding from hair follicles.

Aetiology and pathogenesis
The pathogenesis of spiculosis is unknown. It is possible that the condition is congenital, with 6 months to 1 year needed for expression of the clinical disease.

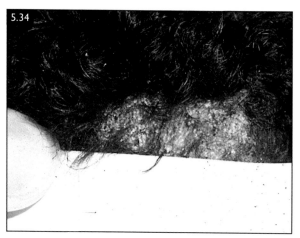

Fig. 5.34 Spicule protruding from a papule on a Kerry Blue Terrier with spiculosis (photo courtesy of Pat McKeever).

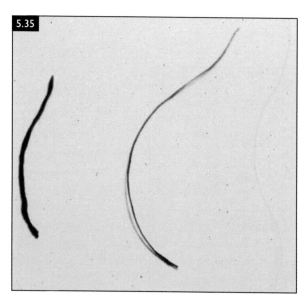

Fig. 5.35 Spicules of varying sizes (left and centre) and a normal hair (right) from a dog with spiculosis (photo courtesy of Pat McKeever).

Cells of the hair bulb show premature keratinisation that results in an amorphous keratinised mass, shaped by the outer root sheath and follicular wall into a spicule.[1] Multiple spicules occurring in the same location may result in secondary infection and furunculosis.

Clinical features
Spiculosis is a disease of Kerry Blue Terriers. It is characterised by hard brittle spicules that are 1.0–2.5 mm in diameter and 0.5–3.0 cm in length (**Figs. 5.34, 5.35**). In the reported cases of young intact males, onset of lesions occurred spontaneously at between age 6 months and 1 year.[1] Lesions may be found on any haired area of the body, but they are found most frequently over the lateral aspect of the hocks and other pressure points. Affected animals may be asymptomatic or may lick and chew excessively at the involved areas to the point that they develop acral lick granulomas.[1]

Differential diagnoses
Spiculosis is highly distinctive clinically. The only time confusion could arise is if secondary acral lick granulomas were present.

Diagnosis
Diagnosis is based on the history and clinical findings.

Treatment
Mild or asymptomatic cases do not need treatment. Isotretinoin (1 mg/kg po q24 h) resulted in complete remission in two reported cases and marked improvement in one.[1] As the commercial availability of this drug is limited, the alternative would be acitretin (0.5–2.0 mg/kg po q24 h). Secondary infections and inflammation need to be addressed, if present.

Key point
- A breed-specific condition characterised by hard spicules protruding from the skin.

Reference
1 McKeever PJ, Torres SMF, O'Brien TD. Spiculosis. *J Am Animal Hosp Assoc* 1992; **28**: 257.

GENERAL APPROACH TO ULCERATIVE DERMATOSES

Ulcerative lesions extend from the surface of the skin into the dermis. These lesions are generally a secondary lesion and are often the result of a bullous, necrotic or vasculitic process. Ulcers can also occur if crusts are removed from the skin. Ulcers that move with the skin are more superficial and are characteristic of diseases that target the basement membrane and basal epidermis (e.g. discoid lupus erythematosus [DLE], pemphigus vulgaris and autoimmune subepidermal blistering diseases). Movement of the skin over the ulcer suggests a deeper lesion with full-thickness necrosis into the deep dermis or subcutis, as seen with more destructive conditions (e.g. toxic epidermal necrolysis, vasculitis and German Shepherd dog pyoderma).

Ulcers often indicate more severe disease, and the prognosis tends to be guarded. Systemic disease is possible with several of the ulcerative dermatoses.

Ulcerative lesions should be checked for pyoderma with impression smears (see Superficial pyoderma, page 65, and Deep pyoderma, page 195). Ulcerative lesions are susceptible to bacterial infection, even if pyoderma is not present on initial presentation.

Ulcerative lesions almost always require a biopsy for diagnosis and additional tests may also be indicated if systemic disease is possible. Of particular importance is the biopsy technique for ulcerative dermatoses. The skin should not be shaved or cleansed before biopsy. Erythematous skin directly adjacent to an ulcer is more likely to give a diagnostic result than biopsy of the centre of an ulcer. Biopsies should always include abnormal epidermis, dermis and subcutis. It is not worthwhile to biopsy normal appearing epidermis when an ulcerative dermatosis is present.

FELINE IDIOPATHIC ULCERATIVE DERMATITIS

Definition

Feline idiopathic ulcerative dermatitis is a rare disease of cats characterised by focal ulceration of the dorsal neck and severe self-mutilation of the area.

Aetiology and pathogenesis

The aetiology and pathogenesis are unknown and probably multi-factorial. The underlying cause may vary among patients because individual cases respond to treatments differently. Factors in the development of this condition may include one or more of the following: application of topical spot-on flea control products, injection of vaccines and depot products, neuropathy and allergic dermatitis. Unfortunately, many cases prove to be idiopathic. (See page 63.)

Clinical features

The lesion is a 2- to 5-cm, well-demarcated, single ulcer located on the caudal dorsal neck or area between the scapulae (**Fig. 6.1**). Lesions are rarely found elsewhere. There is a firm elevated border

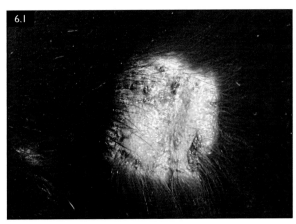

Fig. 6.1 Crusted ulcer on the dorsal neck of a cat with feline idiopathic ulcerative dermatitis.

with peripheral swelling and erythema. Cats often severely self-traumatise the lesion.[1] If self-trauma is minimal, a thick crust will form over the lesion.

Differential diagnoses

- Trauma.
- Burn.
- Injection reaction.
- Foreign body reaction.
- Localised trauma due to allergic dermatitis.
- Neoplasia.
- Ectoparasites.
- Eosinophilic plaque or granuloma.

Diagnosis

The location of the lesion and the intense scratching of the affected skin are highly suggestive. Cytology is predominantly neutrophilic with variable numbers of macrophages, lymphocytes, plasma cells and eosinophils. Secondary bacterial infection may be seen in ulcerated and traumatised lesions. Skin biopsy of the epithelialised margin of the lesion supports the diagnosis.

Treatment

Cases often present with severe pruritus that may persist despite administration of glucocorticoids. Multi-modal therapy is often necessary. This is a condition that is generally not cured, but controlled with continuous therapy. The first step (after the diagnosis has been confirmed) is to determine if there is an underlying cause for the lesion such as recent application of a topical product, recent injection or allergy. Topical spot-on preparations and injections in this area should be avoided in these patients.

The next step is to diagnose and treat secondary infections. Surface cytology should be performed to determine if the lesion is infected. Topical treatments such as mupirocin 2% ointment or silver sulfadiazine cream are usually helpful to treat and prevent local bacterial infection. The topical antibiotic should be applied daily until the skin has healed. The area should be periodically cleansed with a chlorhexidine solution to remove accumulation of debris and medication. A bandage needs to be fashioned to cover the lesion. Feminine hygiene pads work well as a wrap around the neck. These can be changed daily to maintain cleanliness of the skin, and they do not fall apart easily even if the cat scratches it.

While the infection is being treated and the lesion is being covered, the next step is to determine if there is an underlying hypersensitivity. Some cats will improve with glucocorticoids such as dexamethasone. Ideally, potent glucocorticoids such as dexamethasone should be used only as temporary therapy because of the risk of serious systemic side effects with long-term use. While the glucocorticoids are being administered, the pet should receive a novel protein or hydrolysed diet to determine whether a food allergy is an underlying cause. If scratching persists while the pet is receiving the glucocorticoid, then the clinician should start the cat on concurrent gabapentin 10 mg/kg po q12–24 h. If the lesions are not ultimately responsive to a 2-month diet trial, then ciclosporin treatment should be attempted. The ciclosporin dose is 5–7 mg/kg po q24 h for 6–8 weeks, then as needed to prevent the lesion from returning. Some cats require a combination of gabapentin and immunosuppressive drugs such as modified ciclosporin to prevent return of the lesion. Some cats also require lifelong application of a bandage to prevent recurrence of the lesion.

Surgical excision of the lesion may be curative, but also comes with the strong possibility of dehiscence or recurrence. Phenobarbital 12.5 mg per cat po q12–24 h may be effective in some cases. One cat responded to topiramate 5 mg/kg po q12 h.[1]

Key point

- Bandaging the lesion is an important part of therapy and may be a lifelong requirement.

Reference

1 Grant D, Rusbridge C. Topiramate in the management of feline idiopathic ulcerative dermatitis in a two-year-old cat. *Vet Dermatol* 2014; **25**: 226–e60.

FELINE CUTANEOUS HERPESVIRUS AND CALICIVIRUS INFECTIONS

Definition

Feline herpesvirus (feline viral rhinotracheitis virus/ FHV) and feline calicivirus (FCV) are viruses that are common among cats and can cause upper respiratory tract infections, conjunctivitis and skin and oral ulceration.[1,2]

Aetiology and pathogenesis

Calicivirus is spread through direct contact with infected cats, and herpesvirus is spread through direct or airborne transmission.[1] Immunosuppression associated with poor body condition, stress, feline immunodeficiency virus (FIV) or feline leukaemia virus (FeLV), steroids or other immunosuppressive treatments may predispose cats to more generalised viral infections with cutaneous involvement. Highly virulent systemic strains of calicivirus associated with oedema, cutaneous ulceration and high mortality, have been described.

Clinical features

Cats infected with either FHV or FCV may exhibit concurrent oral ulceration and/or upper respiratory tract infection. Lesions usually occur on the distal limbs (**Fig. 6.2**) or head (**Figs. 6.3, 6.4**) (particularly the periocular skin and nasal philtrum), although they may be more generalised. The most common cutaneous lesions are poorly-defined, moist ulcers, although more discrete crusted lesions are occasionally seen. Lesions may appear to be mildly pruritic, especially in the early stages. There may also be local lymphadenopathy.

Differential diagnoses

- Contact dermatitis.
- Feline poxvirus infection.
- Eosinophilic granuloma complex lesions.
- Atopic dermatitis.
- Adverse reaction to food.
- Mosquito bite hypersensitivity.
- Pemphigus foliaceus.

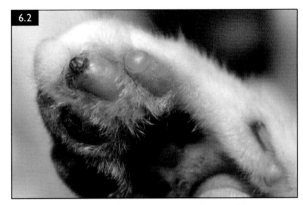

Fig. 6.2 Crusted, digital erosions due to feline calicivirus infection (courtesy of Jan DeClercq).

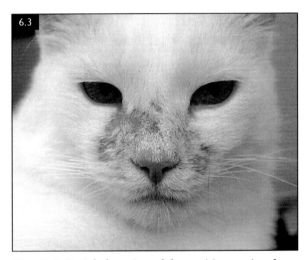

Fig. 6.3 Facial alopecia and dermatitis associated with feline herpes virus.

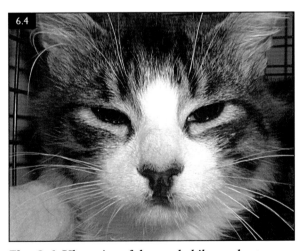

Fig. 6.4 Ulceration of the nasal philtrum due to feline calicivirus.

Diagnosis

The presence or prior history of an oral or upper respiratory tract viral infection with cutaneous ulceration, particularly if there has been treatment with glucocorticoids, ciclosporin and/or any form of stress, is highly suggestive. Affected cats should be checked for FeLV and FIV infection. Histopathological examination of affected tissue can identify cytopathic changes typical of viral infections. Viral isolation from affected tissue, particularly if it is disinfected before sampling, may help confirm active viral infection rather than simple contamination.[1,2] Immunohistochemistry, in-situ hybridisation and polymerase chain reaction (PCR) can be used to detect FHV-1 antigen and DNA in affected skin.[1,2]

Treatment

Affected cats should not be given systemic glucocorticoids or ciclosporin. If necessary, systemic broad-spectrum antibacterial drugs should be administered in severe cases to manage or prevent secondary bacterial infection. Cats should be fed a high-quality diet and kept as free from stress as possible. For mild disease, or recurrent symptoms, lysine (500 mg po q12–24 h) may help prevent replication of herpesvirus.[2] For more severe or ulcerated herpesvirus lesions, famciclovir (62.5–90 mg/kg po q12–24 h or 125 mg/cat po q8 h) can be effective and well tolerated.[2] Various treatments with interferon have also been described.[1] Topical antiviral eyedrops, including cidofovir, trifluridine and idoxuridine, may also be used for ulcerative keratitis.[1] Aciclovir should be avoided because it is minimally effective, and can cause bone marrow suppression and nephrotoxicity.

Affected cats may become persistent virus carriers.[1] Immunosuppression or stress can trigger recurrent infections. Calicivirus can persist in the environment for up to 1 month.[1]

Key points

- Do not give steroids or ciclosporin to cats with viral dermatitis.
- A positive PCR may be an incidental finding due to a cat's previous exposure to the virus.[1,2]
- Supportive care is very important, because specific antiviral treatments may be ineffective.

References

1   Nagata M. Applied dermatology: cutaneous viral dermatoses in dogs and cats. *Compend Contin Educ Vet* 2013; **35**(7): E1.
2   Quimby J, Lappin MR. Feline focus – update on feline upper respiratory diseases: condition-specific recommendations. *Intern Med* 2010; **32**: 548–557.

FELINE COWPOX INFECTION

Definition

Feline cowpox is due to infection with an orthopox virus.

Aetiology and pathogenesis

This virus exists within a reservoir population of small, wild mammals.[1,2] Cats are initially infected, presumably by bite wounds, and there is local multiplication at the site of inoculation. Viraemia then occurs, with multiple, generalised papulocrustous lesions appearing over the subsequent 7–10 days. These lesions gradually resolve and the cats usually make a complete recovery. A fatal variant with a fulminating generalised infection and vasculitis has recently been described.

Clinical features

There is no breed, age or sex predisposition, but hunting cats are most likely to be affected.[1] Most cases are seen in the late summer and autumn period. The primary lesion, a papulovesicle, is usually on the head or forelimb and may become secondarily infected. Multiple (usually >10) secondary lesions follow, most occurring on the head and trunk. These secondary lesions begin as small, firm papules, which enlarge to become flattened, crusted, alopecic areas between 0.5 and 2.0 cm in diameter (**Fig. 6.5**). Occasionally, secondary lesions are erythematous and exudative. In most cases the lesions heal within 4 weeks. The primary lesions may be mildly irritating, but pruritus is not a major feature of this condition. Systemic signs such as fever, anorexia, depression and diarrhoea may occur 1–3 weeks after infection.

Systemic complications are rare unless cats are treated with systemic glucocorticoids or other immunosuppressive agents and/or are systemically immunosuppressed (i.e. FIV), although fulminant and fatal cases have been described in the UK. Systemic involvement can include pulmonary lesions (**Fig. 6.6**), widespread vasculitis and secondary bacterial infection (**Fig. 6.7**).

Differential diagnoses
- Cat bite abscess.
- Flea bite hypersensitivity.
- Calicivirus or herpesvirus infection.
- Dermatophytosis.
- Superficial pyoderma.
- Mycobacterial infection (feline leprosy).
- Eosinophilic granuloma complex.
- Miliary dermatitis.
- Systemic fungal infection.

Diagnosis
The history, clinical signs and local knowledge are suggestive. It is particularly important to differentiate the numerous small crusted papules seen in miliary dermatitis from the less numerous, larger 'pocks' (papules with a depressed necrotic centre) seen in cowpox. The diagnosis can be confirmed by biopsy and histopathology, serology, electron microscopy and virus isolation.[1,2]

Treatment
Therapy is supportive and may include fluids, nutritional support and antibiotics.[1] Cowpox is zoonotic and barrier precautions should be instituted.

Key points
- Do not give steroids to these cats.
- Potentially zoonotic.

References
1   Nagata M. Applied dermatology: cutaneous viral dermatoses in dogs and cats. *Compend Contin Educ Vet* 2013; **35**(7): E1.
2   Wiener DJ, Welle MM, Origgi FC. Cutaneous lesions associated with dual infection caused by canine distemper virus and orthopoxvirus in a domestic cat. *Vet Dermatol* 2013; **24**: 543–e130.

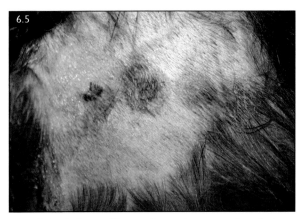

Fig. 6.5 Soft, eroding and crusting secondary lesion ('pox') in a cat with cowpox infection.

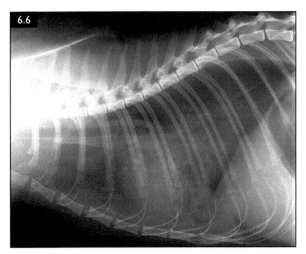

Fig. 6.6 Pulmonary lesions in the cat in Fig. 6.5.

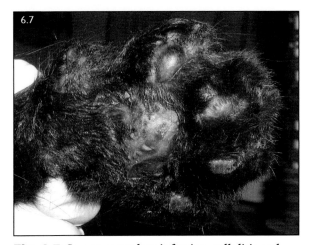

Fig. 6.7 Severe secondary infection, cellulitis and oedema in a cat with a highly virulent, fulminant form of cowpox.

PEMPHIGUS VULGARIS

Definition

Pemphigus vulgaris (PV) is a very rare, autoimmune, blistering disease of dogs and cats. There are no breed or age predispositions.

Aetiology and pathogenesis

Autoantibodies target desmoglein-3, a protein critical for appropriate adhesion of an epithelial cell, particularly in the basal epidermis, mucocutaneous junctions and epithelia. The cleavage of desmoglein-3 results in the separation of epithelial cells from each other and subsequent formation of vesicles.[1] The vesicles rapidly rupture leaving ulcers.

Clinical features

Characteristic lesions are dramatic and include flaccid vesicles, erosions and ulcers. Mucosal lesions are generally observed first, followed by lesions that may occur on the face, concave pinnae and nasal planum. Pressure points, footpads and intertriginous areas are also usually affected (**Fig. 6.8**). Lesions in cats are concentrated in the oral cavity and the head, and systemic signs are less common. Nikolskiy's sign may be present.

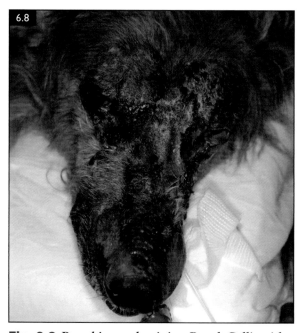

Fig. 6.8 **Pemphigus vulgaris in a Rough Collie with severe ulcers and crusts over the face.**

Differential diagnoses

- Bullous pemphigoid.
- Epidermolysis bullosa.
- Mucous membrane pemphigoid.
- Drug eruption.
- Erythema multiforme.
- Epitheliotrophic cutaneous lymphoma.
- Mucocutaneous candidiasis.

Diagnosis

The history, physical examination, impression smears and skin biopsy lead to the diagnosis of PV. PV results in acantholytic keratinocytes, but these are much less obvious than in pemphigus foliaceus because the cells often remain attached to the basement membrane. A direct impression smear from an intact vesicle, under a moist crust or from an ulcer pustule, may reveal non-degenerate neutrophils and acantholytic keratinocytes, but the findings are usually non-specific. Bacteria may be present in secondarily colonised or infected lesions.

The punch biopsy technique is appropriate for diseases in this category. The skin should not be shaved or cleaned before obtaining the biopsy, and crusts should not be removed. With rare exception, skin devoid of epithelium should not be biopsied because epithelium is required for a histological diagnosis. Moist, tightly adhered crusts, vesicles and the epithelialised edge of an erosion are the ideal lesions to biopsy. In cases where mucosal erosions predominate, a wedge biopsy may be preferred over a punch biopsy. It can be helpful to biopsy induced lesions in the surrounding skin (i.e. Nikolskiy's sign).

Treatment

Treatment involves immunosuppression with glucocorticoids combined with azathioprine and/or ciclosporin (modified), chlorambucil or tetracycline/niacinamide. Steroids should be administered at a high dose until lesions have improved (7–10 days), and then tapered eventually to the lowest alternate-day dose that maintains remission. Multi-drug therapy (i.e. azathioprine combined with steroids) increases the likelihood of successful outcome. (See Immunosuppressive Drug Therapy Table, page 289, for dosages. See also Pemphigus foliaceus, page 81.)

Complications include lethargy, anorexia, weight loss and secondary skin infections. Prognosis is guarded because PV can be refractory to therapy.

Key point
- A potentially devastating disease that requires aggressive treatment.

Reference
1   Olivry T, Linder KE. Dermatoses affecting desmosomes in animals: a mechanistic review of acantholytic blistering skin diseases. *Vet Dermatol* 2009; **20**: 313–326.

BULLOUS PEMPHIGOID

Definition
Bullous pemphigoid (BP) is an autoimmune vesiculobullous disease that affects middle-aged dogs and cats. It is one of a group of similar conditions known as autoimmune subepidermal blistering diseases (AISBDs), which can be hard to fully differentiate on histopathology alone.

Aetiology and pathogenesis
The aetiology is unknown, although genetic susceptibility to environmental triggers and adverse drug reactions may both be factors. The condition is characterised by autoantibodies directed against 180-kDa type XVII collagen (BP180, BPAG2) and/or the 230-kDa plakin epidermal isoform BPAGle (BP230) in the hemidesmosomes and, possibly, the basement membrane zone of the skin and mucosa.[1] This results in disruption of dermoepidermal cohesion, separation and subepidermal vesicle formation. The vesicles quickly rupture and most animals present with ulcers and crusting.

Clinical features
The condition has been reported in both dogs and cats.[2] Breed and sex predilections have not been identified. The initial lesions are erythematous macules and patches that progress to turgid vesicles (which may be haemorrhagic with an erythematous margin), and then ulcers with crusts (**Figs. 6.9, 6.10**). The lesions are not pruritic, but can be painful. The footpads and mucosa are generally (but not always) spared, which helps differentiate this condition from other AISBDs. BP and epidermolysis bullosa acquisita generally feature tense vesicles, whereas the vesicles of vesicular cutaneous lupus erythematosus and pemphigus vulgaris are more flaccid.

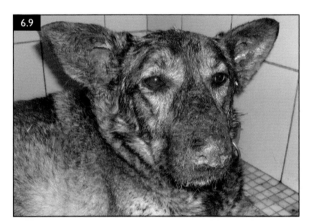

Fig. 6.9 Widespread ulcers and crusts on the nasal planum, face and ears of a dog with bullous pemphigoid (courtesy of Ekaterina Mendoza-Kuznetsova).

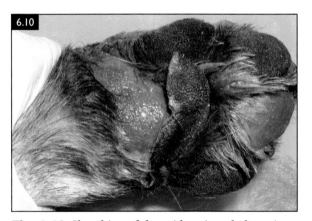

Fig. 6.10 Sloughing of the epidermis and ulceration of the footpads in the same dog (courtesy of Ekaterina Mendoza-Kuznetsova).

Differential diagnoses
- Pemphigus variants.
- Epidermolysis bullosa acquisita (typically involves footpads).

- Systemic lupus erythematosus.
- Vesicular cutaneous lupus erythematosus.
- Mucous membrane pemphigoid (typically involves mucosa).

Diagnosis[3]

The clinical signs are very suggestive of a subepidermal, ulcerating, immune-mediated disease. Diagnosis is via skin biopsy and immunofluorescence. Bullae or vesicles should be sampled via wedge biopsy. If only erosions and ulcers are present, then the clinician should obtain a wedge biopsy encompassing both margins of an erosive lesion. It is important to include epidermis in the sample. A biopsy that includes only dermis will yield minimal diagnostic information. The lack of mucosal involvement is the primary way to differentiate BP from mucous membrane pemphigoid.

Treatment

Treatment involves topical steroids for mild cases and oral steroids, tetracyclines with niacinamide and/or azathioprine for more severe cases. (See Immunosuppressive Drug Therapy Table, page 289, for dosages.)

Complications include secondary bacterial infections.

Spontaneous remission has been reported although it should be anticipated that life-long therapy could be necessary.

Key point
- Do not limit the biopsy sample to eroded skin.

References

1 Olivry T. Chan LS. Autoimmune blistering dermatoses in domestic animals. *Clinics Dermatol* 2001; **19**: 750–760.
2 Olivry T, Chan LS, Xu L *et al*. Novel feline autoimmune blistering disease resembling bullous pemphigoid in humans: IgG autoantibodies target the NC16A ectodomain of type XVII collagen (BP180/BPAG2). *Vet Pathol Online* 1999; **36**: 328–335.
3 Olivry T. An autoimmune subepidermal blistering skin disease in a dog? The odds are that it is not bullous pemphigoid. *Vet Dermatol* 2014; **25**: 316–318.

MUCOUS MEMBRANE PEMPHIGOID

Definition

Mucous membrane pemphigoid (MMP) is a rare autoimmune blistering disease of dogs and cats that affects the mucous membranes.[1] Dogs are affected in adulthood, with no recognised sex predilection. German Shepherd dogs may be predisposed.

Aetiology and pathogenesis

Circulating autoantibodies target basement membrane adhesion proteins (collagen 17). This results in dermoepidermal cleavage and subsequent vesicle formation.

Clinical features (Fig. 6.11)

Lesions are characterised by subepidermal vesicles that progress to form erosions, ulcers and crusts. The oral cavity, nasal planum, eyes, genitalia and concave pinnae can be affected.[2] Footpads are rarely affected. Hypopigmentation and atrophic scarring may occur in some cases. The lesions are non-pruritic, but may be painful. Lymphadenopathy may be present.[2]

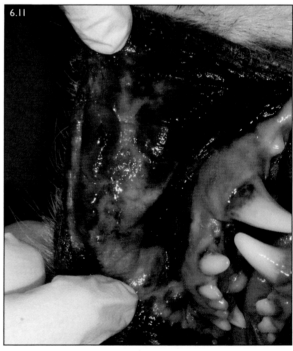

Fig. 6.11 Mucous membrane pemphigoid in a Labrador with severe turgid erythematous vesicles and ulcers of the oral cavity and lips.

Differential diagnoses

- Pemphigus vulgaris.
- Erythema multiforme.
- Bullous drug eruption.
- Bullous pemphigoid (typically does not affect mucosa).
- Epidermolysis bullosa acquisita (typically affects paw pads).
- Vesicular cutaneous lupus erythematosus.

Diagnosis[3]

The clinical signs are very suggestive of a subepidermal, mucosa-only, slowly progressive, ulcerating, immune-mediated disease. Diagnosis is via skin biopsy and immunofluorescence. Bullae or vesicles should be sampled via wedge biopsy.[3] If only erosions and ulcers are present, then the clinician should obtain a wedge biopsy encompassing both margins of an erosive lesion. It is important to include epidermis in the sample. A biopsy that includes only dermis will yield minimal diagnostic information.

Response to therapy and lesion appearance can also guide the diagnosis. Bullous pemphigoid and mucous membrane pemphigoid are fairly glucocorticoid responsive, whereas epidermolysis bullosa acquisita is more glucocorticoid resistant. The mucous membranes are predominantly affected in mucous membrane pemphigoid.

Treatment

Treatment involves immunosuppression, although mild cases may not need treatment. Lesions are generally not severe and tend to respond easily to therapy. Tetracycline and niacinamide should be considered as initial treatment. Steroids and other immunosuppressants may be considered if the lesions are severe or do not respond readily. (See Immunosuppressive Drug Therapy Table, page 289, for dosages.)

Prognosis is good to guarded. Complications include secondary infections of the lesions.

Key point

- Do not limit biopsy sample to eroded skin.

References

1 Olivry T. Chan LS. Autoimmune blistering dermatoses in domestic animals. *Clinics Dermatol* 2001; **19**: 750–760.
2 Olivry T, Dunston SM, Schachter M *et al.* A spontaneous canine model of mucous membrane (cicatricial) pemphigoid, an autoimmune blistering disease affecting mucosae and mucocutaneous junctions. *J Autoimmun* 2001; **16**: 411–421.
3 Olivry T, Jackson HA. Diagnosing new autoimmune blistering skin diseases of dogs and cats. *Clin Techniques Small Anim Pract* 2001; **16**: 225–229.

MUCOCUTANEOUS PYODERMA

Definition

Mucocutaneous pyoderma is a syndrome characterised by bacterial infection of the mucocutaneous junctions.

Aetiology and pathogenesis

Mucocutaneous pyoderma can be primary or secondary. Primary mucocutaneous pyoderma is an uncommon condition that is most commonly seen in German Shepherd dogs. It may be related to mucocutaneous lupus erythematosus (MCLE – see page 180).[1] Secondary mucocutaneous pyoderma is more common and often associated with atopic dermatitis, food allergies, contact reactions, lip-fold dermatitis and self-trauma. *Staphylococcus pseudintermedius* is the most common bacterium isolated, but a range of oral organisms can been seen in mixed infections.

Clinical features (Figs. 6.12, 6.13)

Primary mucocutaneous pyoderma is characterised by erythema, erosion, ulceration, crusting, alopecia and eventual depigmentation of the mucocutaneous junctions. The clinical appearance is similar to cutaneous lupus erythematosus and epitheliotrophic T-cell lymphoma. The clinical suspicion of primary mucocutaneous pyoderma is increased if multiple mucocutaneous junctions are affected. The lesions are variably pruritic, and severe lesions may be painful. Age or sex predilections have not been noted, but German Shepherd dogs and their

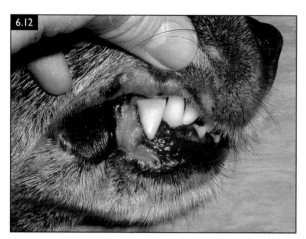

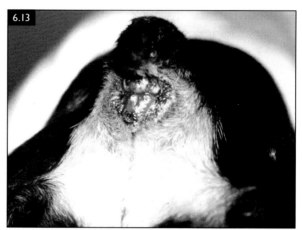

Fig. 6.12 Erythema and erosions along the lip margins in a German Shepherd dog with mucocutaneous pyoderma. The clinical signs can be very similar to epitheliotrophic T-cell lymphoma and cutaneous lupus erythematosus.

Fig. 6.13 Ulceration of the anus of a dog with mucocutaneous pyoderma (courtesy of Pat McKeever).

crosses are predisposed.[2] The lesions respond to appropriate antibiotic medication, which helps to differentiate the condition.

Secondary mucutaneous pyoderma has similar features, but fewer mucocutaneous junctions are involved and the lesions can be more purulent and crusted. Secondary mucocutaneous pyoderma is generally accompanied by additional clinical signs (such as pruritus) associated with an underlying cause (such as allergy). Lesions are present on other areas of the body besides mucocutaneous junctions. In addition, secondary mucocutaneous pyoderma is generally not completely antibiotic responsive until underlying causes have been controlled.

Differential diagnoses
- Mucous membrane pemphigoid.
- Erythema multiforme.
- Pemphigus foliaceus.
- Pemphigus vulgaris.
- Drug reactions.
- Discoid lupus erythematosus.
- Cutaneous lymphoma.
- Zinc-responsive dermatosis.

Diagnosis
The diagnosis is based on history, signalment, physical examination and response to antibiotic therapy.

Skin scrapings must be performed if haired skin is involved. Superficial cytology must be performed to identify bacteria. Culture may be required if antibiotic resistance is suspected. Biopsy should be performed to rule out other conditions, especially if the lesions persist despite antibiotic therapy.[1] Biopsies should be obtained ideally when infections are resolved.

Treatment
- Exudate and crust should be removed by soaking the lesion with warm water or a solution containing chlorhexidine or an appropriate antimicrobial.
- Topical antibiotics (e.g. mupirocin, polymyxin B, fusidic acid or gentamicin) should be applied every 12 h for 3 weeks (until healed). Concurrent use of topical steroids can improve response to therapy.
- If the lesions do not respond to topical treatment oral antibiotics can be administered as for superficial pyoderma (see page 70). Cephalosporins are a good first-choice antibiotic for this condition. The lesions should be cultured if bacteria persist despite antibiotic therapy.

Mucocutaneous pyoderma may be an earlier stage in MCLE. Biopsy and histopathology should be performed to rule out immune-mediated disease in cases that stop responding to antibacterial therapy.

Key points

- Mucocutaneous pyoderma is a condition that is controlled for but not cured.
- It is important to rule out causes of secondary mucocutaneous pyoderma.

EPIDERMOLYSIS BULLOSA ACQUISITA

Definition

Epidermolysis bullosa acquisita (EBA) is an autoimmune vesiculobullous disease targeting collagen VII. It is one of a group of diseases known as autoimmune subepidermal blistering diseases (AISBDs), which can be hard to differentiate on histopathology alone.

Aetiology and pathogenesis

In EBA, circulating autoantibodies target collagen VII in anchoring fibrils[1] that bind to the basement membrane zone. This results in dermoepidermal cleavage and subsequent vesicle formation. The condition is rare, but makes up 25% of the reported AISBDs. Great Danes are overrepresented as a breed, which indicates a genetic predisposition.

References

1. Olivry T, Rossi MA, Banovic E, Linder KE. Mucocutaneous lupus erythematosus in dogs (21 cases). *Vet Dermatol* 2015; **26**(4): 256-e55.
2. Wiemelt SP, Goldschmidt MH, Greek JS, Jeffers JG, Wiemelt AP, Mauldin EA. A retrospective study comparing the histopathological features and response to treatment in two canine nasal dermatoses, DLE and MCP. *Vet Dermatol* 2004; **15**: 341–348.

Clinical features

Young adult Great Danes and male dogs are overrepresented.[1,3] Initial lesions include patchy erythema and vesicles of the face, oral cavity, concave pinna, axilla and groin. Of cases 75% show footpad sloughing or ulceration. The vesicles are typically turgid and erythematous, and may be haemorrhagic. Areas of friction tend to have the most obvious lesions (**Figs. 6.14, 6.15**). The groin and axilla develop erosions quickly. The oral mucosa and footpads usually feature extensive sloughing. Affected individuals may show systemic signs of illness.[1,3]

A localised variant of EBA exists that does not have systemic signs.

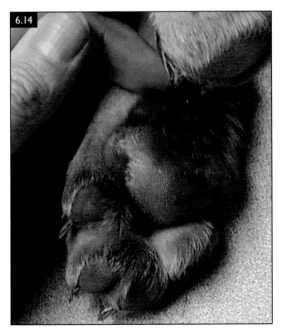

Fig. 6.14 Ulceration of the footpad in a dog with epidermolysis bullosa acquisita (courtesy of Pat McKeever).

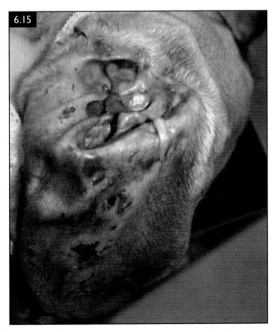

Fig. 6.15 Ulcers on the ventral pinna of a Great Dane with epidermolysis bullosa acquisita.

Differential diagnoses

- Bullous pemphigoid.
- Vesicular cutaneous lupus erythematosus.
- Systemic lupus erythematosus (in cases with systemic signs).
- Pemphigus vulgaris.
- Erythema multiforme/Stevens–Johnson syndrome.
- Bullous drug eruptions.
- Mucous membrane pemphigoid.

Diagnosis

The presence of vesicles and ulcers in a Great Dane is highly suggestive. The diagnosis is made via skin biopsy and immunofluorescence.

Bullae or vesicles should be sampled via wedge biopsy. If only erosions and ulcers are present, then the clinician should obtain a wedge biopsy encompassing both margins of an erosive lesion. It is important to include epidermis in the sample. A biopsy that includes only dermis will yield minimal diagnostic information.

Treatment[2,3]

Treatment involves immunosuppressive therapy, including intravenous immunoglobulin.[2] (See Immunosuppressive Drug Therapy Table, page 289, for drug dosages.) Remission of lesions may take several weeks. Combination therapy with oral steroids and ciclosporin, azathioprine, colchicine or dapsone is often helpful. The steroids can be slowly tapered as soon as lesions begin to resolve. Affected dogs may require life-long steroids combined with a steroid-sparing agent.

Complications include lethargy, fever and sepsis. Anaemia and thrombocytopenia were observed in one dog.

The prognosis is guarded because this disease does not always respond readily to treatment.[3]

Key point

- Areas of friction and trauma (i.e. footpads) are predominantly affected in EBA.

References

1　Olivry T, Chan LS. Autoimmune blistering dermatoses in domestic animals. *Clinics Dermatol* 2001; **19**: 750–760.
2　Hill PB, Boyer P, Lau P, Rybnicek J, Hargreaves J, Olivry T. Epidermolysis bullosa acquisita in a great Dane. *J Small Anim Pract* 2008; **49**: 89–94.
3　Bizikova P, Linder KE, Wofford JA, Mamo LB, Dunston SM, Olivry T. Canine epidermolysis bullosa acquisita: a retrospective study of 20 cases. *Vet Dermatol* 2015; **26**: 441–e103.

VASCULOPATHY OF GREYHOUNDS
(Cutaneous and renal glomerular vasculopathy, Alabama rot, Greenetrack's disease)

Definition

Vasculopathy of Greyhounds is a condition characterised by painful, ulcerative skin lesions and renal disease. More recent cases in the UK have affected a wider range of breeds.

Aetiology and pathogenesis

The pathogenesis is postulated to be due to a Shiga-like toxin produced by *Escherichia coli*.[1] This may be similar to the acute renal failure associated with *E. coli* O157 infections in humans. However, no such toxin has been identified in dogs and the cause remains unknown.

Clinical features (Figs. 6.16–6.18)

Vasculopathy of Greyhounds is observed predominantly in young adult racing Greyhounds that are often fed a raw meat diet. However, it has also been reported in Great Danes, English Springer Spaniels, mixed breeds, Retrievers, Whippets, Border Collies, Jack Russell Terriers and Doberman Pinschers.[2] In the UK, the condition is most common from November to March (particularly during cold wet weather) and there is no association with feeding raw meat. There is no age or sex predisposition.

Most lesions occur on the hindlimbs, but they can occasionally be seen on the forelimbs, trunk and inguinal region.[1] Lesions may also affect the face and oral cavity. In Greyhounds, there is initial oedema of the skin, which is followed by erythema.[1] The erythematous skin darkens and becomes black as it becomes necrotic. Sloughing of the skin results in deep ulcers.[1] In other breeds, the lower limbs or feet are usually first affected, with a patch of swelling and purple discoloration that may ooze serum or blood. The initial lesions can resemble rashes, stings, bites or wounds caused by trauma, and vary in size from 0.5 cm to 5 cm in diameter. Patches of oedema, haemorrhage and necrosis subsequently develop elsewhere. The necrotic, sloughed and ulcerated skin can be painful.

Acute kidney injury usually develops in 4–5 days, although some cases may not progress to renal failure. The renal involvement can vary in severity, and systemic clinical signs include lethargy, malaise, fever, polydypsia, polyuria, vomiting and diarrhoea.[1] Other clinical findings include anaemia and thrombocytopenia.

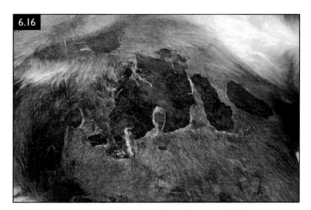

Fig. 6.16 Severe necrosis, sloughing and ulceration on the medial thigh of a Greyhound with cutaneous and renal glomerular vasculopathy (CRGV).

Differential diagnoses
- Drug reactions.
- Erythema multiforme–toxic epidermal necrolysis.
- Immune-mediated vasculitis and other immune-mediated ulcerating diseases.
- Staphylococcal toxic shock syndrome.
- Necrotising fasciitis.
- Leptospirosis and other causes of acute kidney injury.
- Venomous snake or spider bite.

Diagnosis
The diagnosis is based on the history and clinical findings. Skin biopsies can be performed, although in many cases history and physical exam are sufficient to make the diagnosis. There is a characteristic thrombotic microangiopathy in the skin and kidneys, although treatment should be started immediately while waiting for the results and antemortem renal biopsy is not normally performed. A complete blood count, serum chemistry and urinalysis should be performed to determine whether the patient has concomitant renal impairment, thrombocytopenia or anaemia. Other tests may be necessary to eliminate other conditions

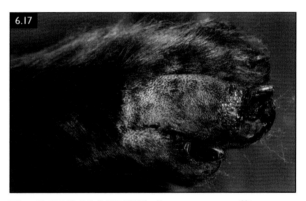

Fig. 6.17 Initial CRGV lesion – severe swelling, necrosis and haemorrhage of a forelimb digit in a Flat Coat Retriever.

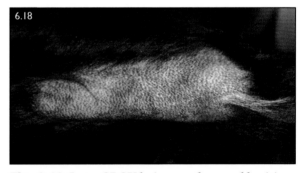

Fig. 6.18 Later CRGV lesion – oedema and bruising on the ventral chest of a Flat Coat Retriever.

(such as leptospirosis). Renal function tests and symmetrical dimethylarginine (SDMA) assays can be used to monitor dogs that present with skin lesions without renal failure.

Treatment

The cause of Alabama rot is unknown and there is no specific treatment. Washing and drying dogs after exercise in cold, wet and muddy ground has been advised, but it is not known if this helps prevent the disease. Treatment is initially based on wound care and monitoring kidney function; dogs with kidney failure need specialist care and support.

The ulcerated skin can be slow to heal and should be cleansed daily with a solution containing chlorhexidine or other effective antimicrobial. Silver sulfadiazine cream should be applied every 12 hours until healed. Systemic antibacterial therapy based on cytology and culture (generally a cephalosporin) should be given for treatment and control of secondary infection. However, antibiotics are controversial in the absence of infection because treatment may alter the local or systemic microbiome and encourage toxin production. Supportive treatment includes intravenous fluid and electrolyte therapy, analgesia, antiemetics, gastroprotection and renal dialysis. Intravenous immunoglobulins, dexamethasone and other immunomodulating drugs have not been effective. The risk of death in affected dogs that progress into kidney failure (azotaemia) is very high, and early detection and treatment to reduce damage to kidneys are considered essential to improve the outcome for the dog.[2]

Key points

- Ulcerative skin disease is often accompanied by concomitant renal disease.
- Potentially fatal.[2]

Prompt recognition and treatment are vital, and dogs may need rapid referral to a specialist centre for intensive care of the skin wounds and kidney failure.

References

1 Cowan LA, Hertzke DM, Fenwick BW, Andreasen CB. Clinical and clinicopathologic abnormalities in greyhounds with cutaneous and renal glomerular vasculopathy: 18 cases (1992–1994). *J Am Vet Med Assoc* 1997; **210**: 789–793.
2 Holm LP, Hawkins I, Robin C *et al*. Cutaneous and renal glomerular vasculopathy as a cause of acute kidney injury in dogs in the UK. *Vet Record* 2015; **176**: 384.

VESICULAR CUTANEOUS LUPUS ERYTHEMATOSUS OF THE SHETLAND SHEEPDOG AND COLLIE

Definition

Vesicular cutaneous lupus erythematosus (VCLE) is an autoimmune blistering disease that primarily affects middle-aged to older, female Shetland Sheepdogs and Collies.[1]

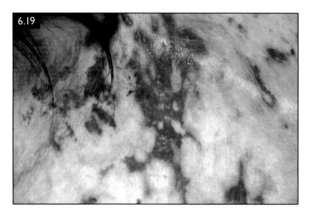

Fig. 6.19 Serpiginous ulcers on the abdomen of a Border Collie with vesicular cutaneous lupus erythematosus.

Aetiology and pathogenesis

It is likely that autoantibodies against nuclear antigens in the basal epidermis lead to T-cell infiltration and subepidermal clefting, and subsequent vesiculation. Exposure to ultraviolet light may be a contributing factor to the development of the disease because it is more common in the summer months.

Clinical features

VCLE is characterised by transient vesicles that develop into coalescing crusted ulcers with serpiginous borders. The groin and axilla are most frequently affected (**Fig. 6.19**), although lesions may also occur on the mucocutaneous junctions and oral cavity. The disease generally occurs in the spring and summer months,[1] and sparsely haired areas of the skin are most typically affected.

Differential diagnoses

- Erythema multiforme/Stevens–Johnson syndrome.
- Drug reaction.
- Systemic lupus erythematosus.
- Pemphigus vulgaris.
- Severe dermatomyositis.
- Bullous pemphigoid and other autoimmune subepidermal blistering diseases.

Diagnosis

The clinical signs in a Shetland Sheepdog or Collie are highly suggestive. The diagnosis is achieved with history, breed, physical examination, impression smears and skin biopsy. The skin should not be clipped or cleaned before sampling with a punch biopsy. Vesicles or epidermis adjacent to a fresh ulcer are the ideal lesions to sample.[1] Lesions devoid of epithelium have less diagnostic value.

Treatment

Treatment involves immunosuppression using prednisone or methylprednisolone combined with azathioprine, pentoxifylline, vitamin E, ciclosporin, hydroxychloroquine, topical glucocorticoids and/or topical tacrolimus[2] (see Immunosuppressive Drug Therapy Table, page 289, for dosages). Multi-modal therapy is generally most successful.[2] Sun avoidance is potentially important because sun exposure may be part of the pathogenesis of the disease. The ulcers should be kept clean using topical antimicrobials to prevent secondary infection. If necessary, topical and/or oral antibiotics can be considered.

Complications may include secondary pyoderma and even septicaemia. Prognosis is generally good to guarded.

Key points

- VCLE can have seasonal variation in clinical signs.[3]
- This disease can generally be controlled, but not cured.

References

1 Jackson HA. Vesicular cutaneous lupus. *Vet Clinics North Am Small Anim Pract* 2006; **36**(1): 251–255.
2 Lehner GM, Linek M. A case of vesicular cutaneous lupus erythematosus in a Border collie successfully treated with topical tacrolimus and nicotinamide–tetracycline. *Vet Dermatol* 2013; **24**: 639–e160.
3 Olivry T, Jackson HA. Diagnosing new autoimmune blistering skin diseases of dogs and cats. *Clin Techniques Small Anim Pract* 2001; **16**: 225–229.

SYSTEMIC LUPUS ERYTHEMATOSUS

Definition

Systemic lupus erythematosus (SLE) is an uncommon autoimmune disease of dogs and cats[1] that affects multiple body systems. This disease affects the skin in about half the cases.

Aetiology and pathogenesis

SLE is characterised by dysfunction of multiple aspects of the immune system that leads to the presence of autoantibodies and subsequent formation of immune complexes. The immune complexes may accumulate in any body organ, but the most common are joints,[2] skin, kidneys, blood, lymph nodes and spleen. Less frequently affected organs are the mucosa, pleura, pericardium, eyes and nerves. Genetics, hormones and environmental factors (such as ultraviolet light) may influence the development of SLE and drugs may be a trigger. German Shepherd dogs appear to be predisposed.[3]

Clinical features

The clinical features depend on which body organs are affected. When the skin is involved, individuals may exhibit pain when the skin is touched, ulcers, erythema (**Figs. 6.20–6.23**), mucocutaneous ulcerations (**Fig. 6.24**), loss of pigment (particularly from the nose and mucocutaneous junctions) and footpad ulcerations.[4] The skin lesions can be classified as cutaneous lupus erythematosus (generalised discoid lupus erythematosus [DLE] or exfoliative cutaneous lupus erythematosus [ECLE] of German Short-haired Pointers) or non-lupus-specific dermatoses (vasculitis, panniculitis and bullous SLE). Other clinical signs include polyarthritis and/or polymyositis,

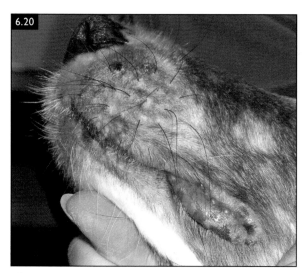

Fig. 6.20 Erythema and erosions on the muzzle of a dog (courtesy of Edda Hoffmann).

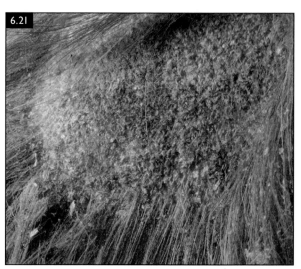

Fig. 6.21 Cutaneous erythema and scaling in a dog (courtesy of Valerie Fadok).

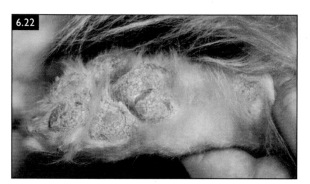

Fig. 6.22 Footpad hyperkeratosis and erosions (courtesy of Valerie Fadok).

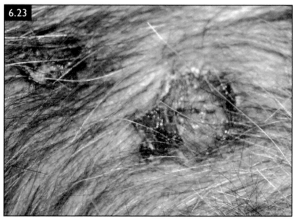

Fig. 6.23 Ulceration and crusting on the ventral abdomen in a dog.

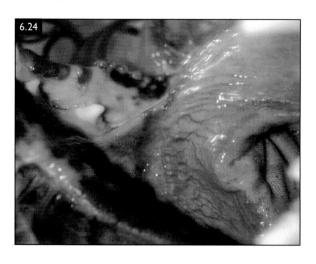

Fig. 6.24 Oral ulceration in a dog.

pyrexia of unknown origin, glomerulonephritis and proteinuria, haemolytic anaemia, thrombocytopenia, neutropenia, myocarditis, pleuritis/pericarditis, thyroiditis, splenomegaly, lymphadenopathy and central nervous system (CNS) disorders. Cats usually present with an autoimmune haemolytic anaemia, pyrexia, thrombocytopenia and renal failure.

Differential diagnoses (for skin lesions)

- Discoid lupus erythematosus.
- Cutaneous lupus erythematosus (VCLE, MCLE and ECLE).
- Epitheliotrophic cutaneous lymphoma.
- Vasculitis.
- Superficial necrolytic dermatitis (metabolic epidermal necrosis).
- Leishmaniasis.
- Tick-borne diseases (including *Rickettsia*, *Babesia* and *Borrelia* spp.).
- Erythema multiforme.
- Drug eruption.
- Infectious or sterile (immune-mediated) panniculitis, polyarthritis and/or glomerulonephritis.
- Pemphigus vulgaris.
- Pemphigus foliaceus.
- Mucous membrane pemphigoid.
- Epidermolysis bullosa acquisita and other AISBDs.

Diagnosis

A thorough exam of body systems is required to determine treatment and prognosis.[1,2,4] A minimum database including a complete blood count, serum chemistry and urinalysis is required. Further laboratory tests, imaging and/or joint aspirates may be necessary, depending on clinical signs and presence of abnormalities in the minimum database. A skin biopsy shows characteristic changes and is useful to rule out other causes of skin disease. *Table 6.1* summarises the criteria for diagnosis of canine SLE.

A diagnosis of SLE can be made if the patient has four of the above clinical signs or polyarthritis accompanied by a positive antinuclear antibody (ANA).[4]

The ANA test is variably helpful in the diagnosis of SLE. Certain drugs (griseofulvin, penicillin, sulphonamides, tetracyclines, phenytoin and procainamide) can cause false-positive ANA titres. Other immune-mediated, infectious and neoplastic diseases may also cause false-positive ANA titres. Glucocorticoid administration may cause false-negative ANA titres.[1]

Treatment

Treatment involves immunosuppression with glucocorticoids combined with azathioprine and/or ciclosporin, chlorambucil, hydroxychloroquine or tetracycline/niacinamide. Steroids should be

Table 6.1 Criteria for diagnosis of canine systemic lupus erythematosus[4]

CRITERION	DEFINITION
Erythema	Redness in the skin, particularly the face
Discoid rash	Depigmentation, erythema, erosions, ulcerations, crusts and scaling of the face, particularly the nasal planum
Photosensitivity	Erythematous skin as a result of sunlight exposure
Oral ulcers	Oral or nasopharyngeal ulceration
Arthritis	Non-erosive arthritis involving two or more peripheral joints
Serositis	Non-septic inflammation of pleura or pericardium
Renal disorders	Persistent proteinuria
Haematological disorders	Haemolytic anaemia, leukopenia, lymphopenia or thrombocytopenia
Immunological disorders	Antihistone, anti-Sm or antitype 1 antibodies, or decreased CD8+ population
Antinuclear antibodies (ANAs)	Abnormal ANA titres

administered at a high dose until lesions have improved (7–10 days), and then tapered eventually to an alternate-day dose. Multi-drug therapy (e.g. azathioprine or other immunomodulators combined with steroids) increases the likelihood of successful outcome. (See Immunosuppressive Drug Therapy Table, page 289, for more details and dosages.)

Additional therapy depends on the body systems that are affected (i.e. uveitis or nephropathy). Additional monitoring is required after the SLE has been controlled to determine if secondary health issues have developed (i.e. hypertension secondary to nephropathy).

Key points
- A potentially fatal disease that affects multiple body organs.
- A thorough diagnostic work-up is indicated to identify the extent of disease.

- SLE cannot be cured, but it can be controlled with continuous treatment.

References
1   Vitale C, Ihrke P, Gross TL, Werner L. Systemic lupus erythematosus in a cat: fulfillment of the American Rheumatism Association criteria with supportive skin histopathology. *Vet Dermatol* 1997; **8**: 133–138.
2   Stull JW, Evason M, Carr AP, Waldner C. Canine immune-mediated polyarthritis: clinical and laboratory findings in 83 cases in western Canada (1991–2001). *Can Vet J* 2008; **49**: 1195.
3   Soulard M, Della Valle V, Larsen CJ. Autoimmune antibodies to hnRNPG protein in dogs with systemic lupus erythematosus: epitope mapping of the antigen. *J Autoimmun* 2002; **18**: 221–229.
4   Miller WH, Griffin CE, Campbell KL, Muller GH. In: *Muller and Kirk's Small Animal Dermatology* 7. New York: Elsevier Health Sciences, 2013.

SUPERFICIAL NECROLYTIC DERMATITIS
(Diabetic dermatopathy, hepatocutaneous syndrome, necrolytic migratory erythema and metabolic epidermal necrosis)

Definition
Superficial necrolytic dermatitis is an uncommon skin disorder of dogs and (rarely) cats that is associated with hepatopathy or glucagonoma.

Aetiology and pathogenesis
Superficial necrolytic dermatitis is associated with metabolic diseases such as a hepatopathy, hepatic tumour, diabetes mellitus and glucagon-secreting pancreatic tumours (glucagonomas). There are characteristic liver abnormalities including moderate-to-severe vacuolation of hepatocytes, parenchymal collapse and nodular regeneration in most cases. Some cases are associated with phenobarbital administration.

Most affected dogs have markedly decreased plasma amino acid levels, which may lead to epidermal protein depletion and necrolysis. Elevated plasma glucagon levels and decreased levels or altered metabolism of zinc and essential fatty acids may also play a role in the pathogenesis.

Clinical features
This condition is uncommon in dogs and very rare in cats.[1] Superficial necrolytic dermatitis is a disease of older dogs, and cutaneous changes generally precede systemic illness. No sex predisposition has been noted, although the condition may be more frequent in West Highland White Terriers and Shetland Sheepdogs. Some dogs may have a history of weight loss.

Hyperkeratosis, scaling, crusting and cracking of the digital pads are the most consistent clinical findings (**Figs. 6.25, 6.26**) and may result in lameness.[2] In addition to footpad lesions, dogs may develop erythema, scaling, erosion, ulceration and crusting on the muzzle (**Fig. 6.27**), mucocutaneous junctions, ears, pressure points, genitalia, abdomen and axillae. Ulcerations of the oral cavity are seen in some cases. Dullness, inappetence and polyuria/polydipsia may occur in the later stages, with overt hepatic failure and/or diabetes mellitus. Rarely, animals may present in a ketoacidotic crisis. Secondary bacterial

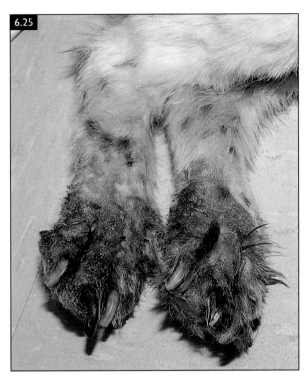

Fig. 6.25 Superficial necrolytic dermatitis: erythema, erosions, crust and alopecia on the distal limbs of a Springer Spaniel.

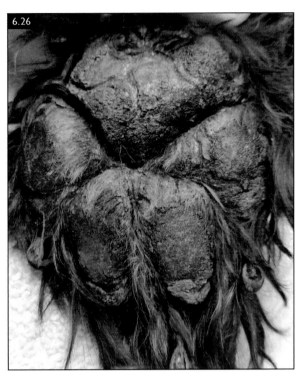

Fig. 6.26 Superficial necrolytic dermatitis: pedal lesions characterised by severe scaling, crusting and ulceration of the footpads.

infections, demodicosis and malassezia dermatitis are common.

Differential diagnoses
- Pemphigus foliaceus.
- Cutaneous or SLE.
- Zinc-responsive dermatosis.
- Superficial bacterial or fungal infections.
- Epitheliotrophic lymphoma.

Diagnosis
The history and physical exam findings are highly suggestive. Skin biopsy of a crusted lesion is necessary to confirm the diagnosis. The key histological signs are in the epidermis, so care should be taken to include the epidermis in the biopsy sample.

Additional testing should be done to determine whether the patient has diabetes mellitus and whether a hepatopathy or a glucagonoma is present. It is useful for treatment and prognosis to further characterise hepatopathy as neoplastic, cirrhotic, etc. Testing may include complete blood count, serum

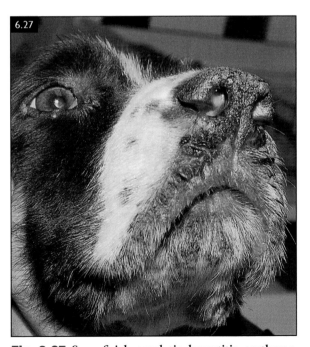

Fig. 6.27 Superficial necrolytic dermatitis: erythema, erosions, crust and alopecia on the face of a Springer Spaniel (photo courtesy of Sheila Torres).

chemistry, bile acids, urinalysis, abdominal ultrasound with fine-needle aspirates as indicated by the clinical findings, computed tomography or magnetic resonance imaging. Some cases may benefit from measurement of plasma amino acid levels and glucagon levels, although determination of these levels is not prerequisite to initiating treatment.

Surface cytology (i.e. impression smears) and skin scrapings are necessary to identify concurrent pyoderma, yeast dermatitis and/or demodicosis.

Treatment

Superficial necrolytic dermatitis is associated with serious internal disease and the prognosis is poor, with most dogs dying or being euthanised within 5 months of the development of cutaneous lesions. Despite this, aggressive therapy can result in prolonged survival times for a year or more in some dogs.

Nutritional therapy is critical for amelioration of the clinical signs. The patient should be fed high-quality protein supplements such as three to six whole eggs per day, powdered casein or proprietary amino acid combinations. Zinc (see Zinc-responsive dermatosis, page 139) and essential fatty acid supplements can also be given. S-Adenosylmethionine and silybin (Denamarin®) may reduce oxidative damage in the liver, and appear to be useful as adjunctive therapy. Colchicine may aid dogs with hepatic cirrhosis.

In addition to nutritional therapy, intravenous (IV) amino acid infusions can be administered to encourage faster resolution of skin lesions.[3] Some dogs need infusions every 2 weeks to maintain resolution of clinical signs. Some dogs need an infusion initially, and then the clinical signs can be kept in remission with nutritional therapy. Most infusion protocols use 8–10% amino acid solutions given at 25 ml/kg over 6–8 h using a jugular catheter. Peripheral catheters may also be used, but the catheter site must be monitored for phlebitis. Dogs should be monitored for signs of anaphylaxis and hepatic encephalopathy during the infusion.

Glucagonomas can be surgically resected, although the surgery can be difficult and associated with significant postoperative mortality. If IV amino acid therapy does not lead to improvement of skin lesions, then octreotide (2 µg/kg subcutaneous injection q12 h), which inhibits glucagon release, is indicated.[4]

Topical therapy is necessary to treat and prevent pyoderma. Antibacterial shampoos, such as those containing 3–4% chlorhexidine should be used to cleanse the skin as frequently as daily until resolution of pyoderma. Topical antibiotics such as mupirocin or gentamicin can be used every 12 h on focal areas of pyoderma. Systemic antimicrobials may be necessary in some cases, but care should be taken to avoid drugs that require hepatic metabolism and excretion (see Superficial pyoderma, page 70). Topical steroids can be used every 12 h on focal areas of inflammation.

Key point

- The long-term prognosis is guarded to poor, but prolonged survival times can be achieved with aggressive therapy.

References

1 Asakawa MG, Cullen JM, Linder KE. Necrolytic migratory erythema associated with a glucagon-producing primary hepatic neuroendocrine carcinoma in a cat. *Vet Dermatol* 2013; **24**: 466–e110.

2 Cellio LM, Dennis J. Canine superficial necrolytic dermatitis. *Compend Contin Educ Vet* 2005; **27**: 820.

3 Bach JF, Glasser SA. A case of necrolytic migratory erythema managed for 24 months with intravenous amino acid and lipid infusions. *Can Vet J* 2013; **54**: 873.

4 Oberkirchner U, Linder KE, Zadrozny L, Olivry T. Successful treatment of canine necrolytic migratory erythema (superficial necrolytic dermatitis) due to metastatic glucagonoma with octreotide. *Vet Dermatol* 2010; **21**: 510–516.

GERMAN SHEPHERD DOG PYODERMA

Definition

German Shepherd dog (GSD) pyoderma is a disease syndrome characterised by recurrent, deep ulceration and draining sinus tracts.

Aetiology and pathogenesis

Although *Staphylococcus pseudintermedius* is the primary infectious agent isolated, this disease is not a primary bacterial infection.[1] A bacterial infection typically starts because of some other factor such as atopic dermatitis or external parasites. The bacterial infection triggers a destructive cell-mediated inflammatory response that causes ulceration and necrosis of the skin.

Clinical features

GSD pyoderma occurs most commonly in middle-aged animals, but may be seen at any age. There appears to be no sex predisposition. Lesions generally start over the lateral thighs and dorsal lumbosacral areas, but any area of the body may be affected. Typical lesions include erythematous-to-violaceous papules, pustules, haemorrhagic bullae, erosions, deep ulcers, crusts and draining tracts (**Figs. 6.28–6.30**). The skin has a characteristic necrotic, 'melting' and underrun appearance, distinct from a typical folliculitis/furunculosis. Varying degrees of alopecia and

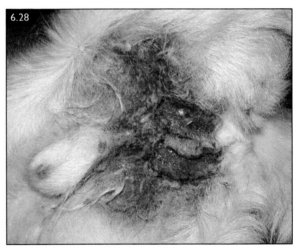

Fig. 6.28 German Shepherd dog pyoderma with ulceration, purulent discharge and crusting in the groin.

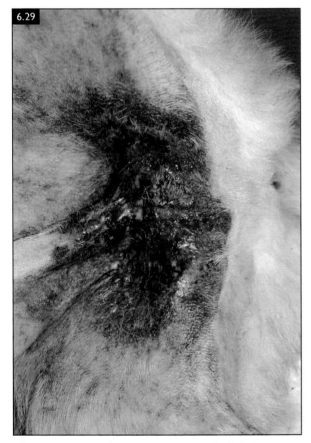

Fig. 6.29 Same dog as in Fig. 6.28; the hair has been clipped to show the extent of the lesions. Note the ill-defined margin, hyperpigmentation and scarring.

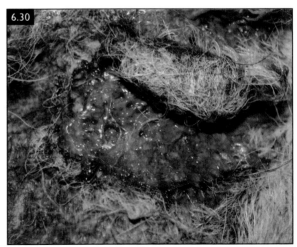

Fig. 6.30 Close-up of the dog in Fig. 6.28 showing the typical 'melting' necrosis and underrunning of affected skin.

hyperpigmentation may be noted and the peripheral lymph nodes are generally enlarged. Lesions are often pruritic and/or painful, and dogs may also be febrile and lethargic. Affected dogs may also have perianal fistulae (see page 211), metatarsal fistulation (see page 212) or symmetrical lupoid onychodystrophy (see page 222), suggesting that these may be clinical manifestations of a similar aetiology.

Differential diagnoses
- Panniculitis (sterile or infectious).
- Deep fungal infection, especially sporotrichosis.
- Demodicosis.
- Cutaneous foreign body.
- Epitheliotrophic lymphoma (late stage).
- Autoimmune bullous ulcerative disease.

Diagnosis
The signalment, history and physical exam are highly suggestive, but not necessarily conclusive. The diagnosis requires a deep skin scraping, surface cytology and cytology of draining tracts (if present). A skin biopsy with special stains should be performed to rule out other differential diagnoses. A bacterial

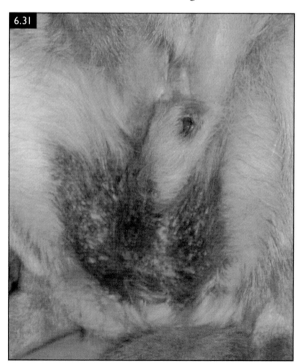

Fig. 6.31 Same dog as in Figs. 6.28–6.30; there has been a complete response to oral ciclosporin.

culture and sensitivity should be performed because a long course of antibiotics is needed. A thyroid panel can be considered; total thyroxine (T_4) will often be depressed due to systemic illness.

Treatment
Concurrent conditions should be ruled out and controlled (see pruritic dog diagnostic flow chart [**Fig. 2.17**], and canine atopic dermatitis treatments, page 25). Atopic dermatitis and flea allergy dermatitis are common triggers, and specific therapy that controls these underlying conditions will control the recurrent pyoderma. If underlying causes are not controlled, the condition will recur.

The pyoderma should initially be treated with an antibiotic for 4–8 weeks, depending on how deep the pyoderma is. Cephalexin 25–30 mg/kg po q12 h or cefpodoxime proxetil 5–10 mg/kg q24 h are the best empirical antibiotics while waiting for culture results (see Superficial pyoderma, page 74 for other drug doses). The pyoderma will return unless treatment is started to prevent recurrence.

Topical therapy with 3–4% chlorhexidine shampoo, benzoyl peroxide shampoo, salicylic acid shampoo or selenium sulphide shampoo should be performed daily to weekly. Chlorhexidine tends to be most effective, although there is variation among individuals. These products can be alternated throughout the week or month if needed (see Superficial pyoderma, page 72).

Modified ciclosporin (Atopica®) is effective in some cases (**Fig. 6.31**), and may control all conditions if the patient has concurrent perineal or metatarsal fistulae. The dose is 4–7 mg/kg po q24 h for 4–8 weeks beyond the end of antibiotic therapy, then tapered to the lowest frequency as needed to maintain remission.

If treatments for underlying conditions are not helpful, or if an underlying cause cannot be found, staphage lysate (SPL) can be tried. SPL is sterile-mix staphylococcal proteins and other products. It may act as an immunostimulant or, conversely, induce tolerance to staphylococci in dogs with aberrant immune responses. Several dosing protocols are available, but SPL is generally given twice weekly for 10–12 weeks, then every 7–30 days for maintenance. Adverse effects are rare, but can include injection site reactions, pyrexia, malaise and anaphylaxis. Due to the safety, efficacy and possible ability to avoid oral antibiotics, this treatment option should be strongly considered for long-term use.

Key points
- The genetic predisposition means that affected dogs should not reproduce.
- This condition can be controlled, but not cured.

- This is a secondary condition.
- Skin biopsy is important to rule out other causes of draining tracts.

Reference
1   Rosser EJ. German Shepherd dog pyoderma. *Vet Clinics North Am Small Anim Pract* 2006; **36**: 203–211.

DECUBITAL ULCERS
(Pressure sores)

Definition
Decubital ulcers (pressure sores) occur mainly over bony prominences because of continual localised pressure to the skin (see also Callus, page 152).

Aetiology and pathogenesis
Animals that are recumbent due to neurological deficits or musculoskeletal problems are predisposed to decubital ulcers. Compression of the skin and subcutaneous tissue collapses blood vessels, resulting in ischaemia, necrosis and subsequent ulceration. Laceration, friction, burns from heating pads, irritation from urine or faecal material, malnutrition secondary to inadequate diet, anaemia or hypoproteinaemia may also be contributing factors. In addition cutaneous atrophy due to spontaneous or iatrogenic hyperadrenocorticism, including topical drugs, may predispose to ulcers. Non-healing wounds commonly result from attempts to surgically remove calluses at pressure points.

Clinical features
The initial clinical finding is hyperaemia. Tissue necrosis (evidenced by whitening of the skin) and ulceration with or without crusting follow if the pressure is not relieved. Lesions most frequently occur in skin overlying the scapular acromion, lateral epicondyle of the humerus, tuber ischii, tuber coxae, trochanter major of the femur, lateral condyle of the tibia (**Figs. 6.32, 6.33**), and the lateral sides of the fifth digits of the forelimbs and hindlimbs. Secondary bacterial infection can lead to undermining of the skin beyond the ulcer edges. Osteomyelitis can develop in bone underlying the ulcer.

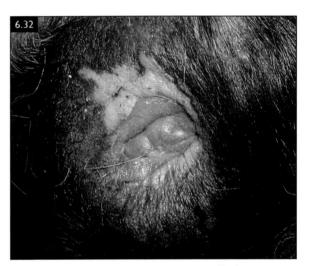

Fig. 6.32 Decubital ulcer and a non-healing wound on the lateral elbow of a Rottweiler; the dog was subsequently diagnosed with hyperadrenocorticism.

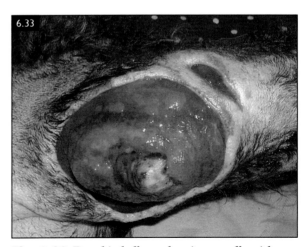

Fig. 6.33 Decubital elbow ulcer in a poodle with hyperadrenocorticism.

Differential diagnoses

- Cutaneous neoplasia (squamous cell carcinoma).
- Primary deep bacterial infection (*Actinomyces*, *Actinobacillus* and *Nocardia* spp., and mycobacteria).
- Deep mycotic infection.

Diagnosis

The diagnosis is based primarily on history and clinical findings; cultures and histopathological examination of biopsy samples will help rule out other causes. Additional testing may be necessary to characterise underlying predisposing diseases.

Treatment

The key to successful healing of a decubital ulcer is relief of pressure over the affected area. Non-ambulatory patients need to lie on a padded surface such as a mattress or egg carton foam. They need to be turned every 2 hours. These patients also require adequate nutrition and daily bathing with an antiseptic shampoo or rinse, such as chlorhexidine or hypochlorous acid. Ulcerated skin may need to be cleansed two to three times a day. Particular attention should be paid to protecting the skin from urine scald and applying petrolatum to areas of skin that urine is likely to contact. High standards of wound care and dressings with non-adherent absorbent materials will be necessary in severe cases.

Ambulatory patients can wear special padding to aid the healing of decubital ulcers. Effective padding options include DogLeggs® (customised joint pads), doughnut-shaped pads or pads containing beanbag beans. The affected joint may also need to be splinted to stop movement and alleviate pressure necrosis. Feminine hygiene pads are useful to place against the ulcer inside the padding. This keeps the padding clean and is easy to change frequently. Topical antibacterial therapy such as medical honey, silver sulfadiazine or mupirocin will treat and prevent secondary infections. RediHeal®, a borate-based, biological glass material that aids in re-epithelialisation, can be applied once or twice daily.

Surgical repair should be attempted with caution. The goal of surgery is to debride necrotic and infected tissue and close the wound. If the pressure necrosis persists postoperatively, the surgical site will most certainly dehisce, causing an even larger lesion[1] (see Callus, page 152).

Key points

- Pressure must be relieved in order for skin to heal.
- Pressure necrosis will lead to dehiscence of surgical incisions.

Reference

1 Swanson EA, Freeman LJ, Seleem MN, Snyder PW. Biofilm-infected wounds in a dog. *J Am Vet Med Assoc* 2014; **244**: 699–707.

MUCOCUTANEOUS LUPUS ERYTHEMATOSUS

Definition

Mucocutaneous lupus erythematosus (MCLE) is a recently described condition with mucocutaneous erosive lesions and lupus-specific histopathology.

Aetiology and pathogenesis

MCLE is an autoimmune condition that targets the basal epidermis at the mucocutaneous junctions. The aetiology is unknown, but the strong breed predisposition in German Shepherd dogs suggests a genetic susceptibility. There is a lymphocyte and plasma cell-rich interface dermatitis with basal keratinocyte apoptosis, loss and/or hydropic change.

There is also a lupus band along the epidermal basement membrane zone with immunoglobulin and complement deposition.[1]

Clinical features (Figs. 6.34, 6.35)

MCLE is characterised by symmetrical, well-demarcated erythema, erosion, ulceration, crusting, alopecia and eventual hyperpigmentation of the mucocutaneous junctions. Multiple mucocutaneous junctions are affected in most dogs. The lesions are often painful, which can result in dysphagia, dyschezia and dysuria, but specific systemic signs are not seen.

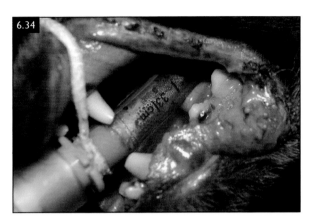

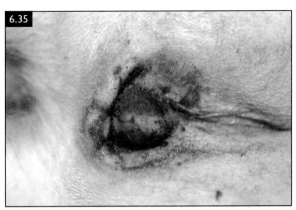

Fig. 6.34 Erosions, ulcers, crusts and hyperpigmentation on the lip margins of a Spaniel with MCLE.

Fig. 6.35 Severe perivulval ulceration in dog with MCLE. The lesions were painful and associated with licking and dysuria.

Differential diagnoses
- Mucous membrane pemphigoid.
- Erythema multiforme.
- Pemphigus foliaceus.
- Pemphigus vulgaris.
- Drug reaction.
- Discoid lupus erythematosus.
- Cutaneous lymphoma.
- Zinc-responsive dermatosis.
- Mucocutaneous pyoderma.

Diagnosis
The diagnosis is based on the history, signalment, physical exam and biopsy. Superficial cytology must be performed to identify secondary bacterial colonisation and infection. Biopsies should be obtained ideally when infections are resolved. Most dogs are ANA negative.

Treatment
- Exudate and crust should be removed by soaking the lesion with warm water or a solution containing chlorhexidine or an appropriate antimicrobial.
- Treatment options reported to be effective include: niacinamide with tetracycline or doxycycline; oral glucocorticoids alone or combined with topical glucocorticoids or other treatments; topical tacrolimus; and/or oral ciclosporin.[1] (See Immunosuppressive Drug Therapy Table, page 289, for more details.)

The prognosis is usually good, and oral glucocorticoids may result in more rapid remission. Most dogs require maintenance therapy to maintain remission.

Key point
- MCLE is a condition that is controlled but not cured.

Reference
1   Olivry T, Rossi MA, Banovic F, Linder KE. Mucocutaneous lupus erythematosus in dogs (21 cases). *Vet Dermatol* 2015; **26**: 256–e55.

VASCULITIS AND VASCULOPATHY

Definition

Vasculitis is inflammation of blood vessel walls. Vasculopathy refers to tissue changes consistent with poor blood flow and ischaemia in the absence of demonstrable vasculitis. There are well-recognised breed predispositions to certain types of vasculitis in dogs.

Aetiology and pathogenesis

Vasculitis may be caused by a wide variety of infectious agents, toxins, drugs and immune-mediated mechanisms, although most cases are idiopathic.[1-3] The blood vessels may be damaged by immune-complex deposition (type 3 hypersensitivity or Arthus reactions) and complement activation or direct antibody binding with activation of neutrophils. This results in endothelial damage, fibrin exudation, microhaemorrage, oedema, thrombosis and ischaemia.

Clinical signs

The clinical signs depend on the location, size and depth of the vessels affected and can therefore be very varied.[1-3] Damage to capillaries can result in petechiae, ecchymoses and cutaneous and follicular atrophy (**Fig. 6.36**). Damage to venules and arterioles results in purpura, haemorrhagic wheals and oedema. These lesions can be differentiated from erythema by diascopy – pressing a glass slide against the skin will blanch erythema but not vascular lesions. Using a dermatoscope identifies non-blanching lesions as well as revealing capillary stasis and thrombosed vessels. Damage to larger vessels leads to ulceration and necrosis. Other clinical signs can include ulcerated nodules and panniculitis. Ischaemic scarred skin is strikingly alopecic, thin and smooth, and may be hyper- or hypopigmented.

Lesions most commonly affect the extremities and pressure points, but can occur anywhere on the body or mucosal surfaces.[1-3] Lesions are usually multiple and often symmetrical, although they can also be multi-focal. The pinnae often have necrotic tips and or scalloped margins (**Fig. 6.37**). Lesions can also be seen on the medial (i.e. concave) surface. The footpads typically have well demarcated ('punched out') ulcers, often in the centre of the pads (**Fig. 6.38**).

Systemic involvement leads to other clinical signs depending on the organ involved. These can include malaise, pyrexia, anorexia, glomerulonephritis, polyarthropathies, myopathy, ocular disease, neuropathies, gastrointestinal signs and/or peritoneal and pleural effusions.

Injection site vasculitis

Injection site vasculitis is characterised by alopecia following subcutaneously administered drugs, including vaccines.[4] Lesions may occur at the site of injection or be remote and usually occur within 3–6 months (**Fig. 6.39**). Rarely, animals may show systemic signs, oedema, lesions on the extremities, mucocutaneous ulceration and muscular atrophy.

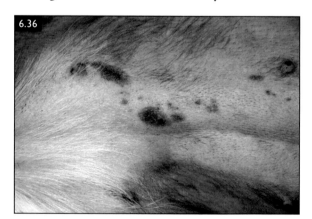

Fig. 6.36 Petechiae, ecchymoses and erosions on the ventral abdomen of a dog with a drug-induced vasculitis.

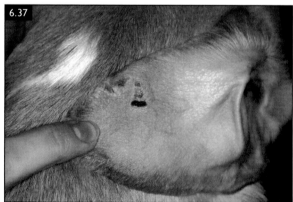

Fig. 6.37 Early vasculitis lesion on the pinna – there is a well-demarcated wedge-shaped area of discoloured skin with central necrosis and crusting.

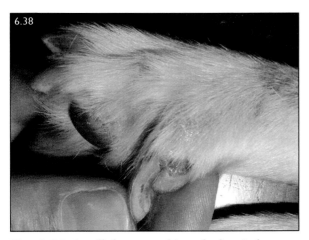

Fig. 6.38 A well-demarcated 'punched out' ulcer on the lateral digit of a dog with idiopathic vasculitis.

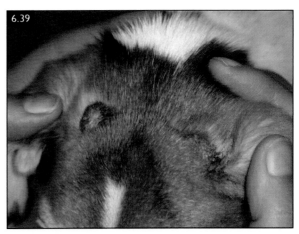

Fig. 6.39 Vaccine-associated vasculopathy in a dog with symmetrical alopecia, scarring and hyperpigmentation of the head.

Dermatomyositis and juvenile- or adult-onset ischaemic dermatopathies

Canine familial dermatomyositis is most often seen in Rough Collies, Shetland Sheepdogs and Beauceron.[5,6] Clinical signs include papules, erosions, ulcers and crusts affecting the face, limbs, extremities and pressure points. Multi-focal well-demarcated alopecia and scarring is seen at affected sites (**Fig. 6.40**). The myositis most commonly affects the temporal and masseter muscles causing profound muscle atrophy around the head, but may be more widespread.

Familial cutaneous vasculopathies of Jack Russell Terriers, German Shepherd dogs and Scottish Terriers

Lesions usually occur in puppies, which develop depigmentation, oedema and ulceration of the footpads.[7] The nasal planum, dorsal muzzle, ear tips and tail tips may also be affected, particularly in Scottish Terriers and Jack Russell Terriers (**Fig. 6.41**).[8] Jack Russell Terriers can show nail base haemorrhage and sloughing (symmetrical lupoid onychodystrophy is an important differential – see page 222). The condition usually resolves spontaneously in German Shepherd dogs.

See also Idiopathic ear margin vasculitis (page 85), Vasculopathy of Greyhounds (page 168), Vasculitis of the footpads (page 221), and Nasal arteritis (page 228).

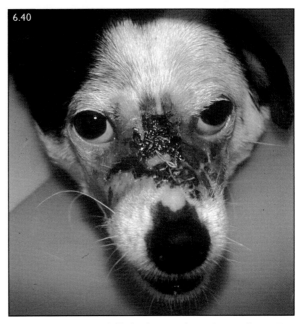

Fig. 6.40 Severe full-thickness ulceration and scarring in a Jack Russell Terrier with familial vasculitis.

Differential diagnoses

The differential diagnosis for vasculitis is very wide and depends on the clinical presentation (see above). Important differentials include:

- Deep ulcerating bacterial or fungal infections.
- Bacterial toxic shock syndrome.
- Demodicosis.
- Dermatophytosis.

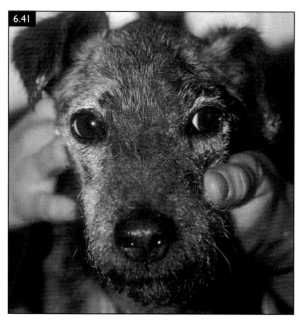

Fig. 6.41 Ear tip necrosis, multi-focal scarring alopecia and temporal muscle atrophy in a Border Terrier with dermatomyositis.

- Sterile immune-mediated panniculitis.
- Pemphigus vulgaris.
- Bullous pemphigoid and other immune-mediated subepidermal blistering diseases.
- Systemic lupus erythematosus.
- Discoid lupus erythematosus.
- Symmetrical lupoid onychodystrophy.
- Epitheliotropic lymphoma.
- Squamous cell carcinoma.
- Disseminated intravascular coagulation.
- Coagulopathies.
- Thermal or chemical burns.
- Frostbite.

Diagnosis

The diagnosis is based on suggestive clinical signs and compatible histopathology. The breed may be suggestive of some breed-associated syndromes. Because of the problems in identifying the lesions on histopathology and the transient nature of the specific pathology, multiple biopsies from different lesions should be submitted. Deep wedge biopsies should be taken where the disease affects the deep dermis or subcutis.

A detailed history should be taken to identify possible trigger factors. Haematology, biochemistry and urinalysis should be performed to identify possible systemic involvement and/or underlying conditions including systemic disease, neoplasia and infections. Any chronic infectious disease can cause vasculitis, and work-up should include testing for tick-borne infections (such as rickettsial diseases, *Borrelia* and *Anaplasma* spp.) and *Leishmania*. It is very important to check the history for any possible drug associations. If ongoing therapy is unavoidable (e.g. antibiotics, analgesics, antiepileptics, etc.) a different class of drug should be used.

Treatment

The mainstay of treatment has been systemic glucocorticoids. Prednisolone or methyl-prednisolone are normally used at 1–2 mg/kg po q12–24 h to achieve remission. The dose is then slowly reduced to the lowest every other day dose that maintains remission. Topical glucocorticoids (e.g. betamethasone, flucinolone +/– DMSO, or hydrocortisone aceponate) can be used as adjunct or sole therapy in appropriate cases. Steroids may also be combined with other immune-modulating or cytotoxic drugs in more severe and/or recalcitrant cases (see Immunosuppressive Drug Therapy Table, page 289). Pentoxifylline also promotes peripheral blood flow and oxygenation, making it particularly useful in vasculopathies. Supportive care may include removing crusts, managing wound healing, controlling infection and surgery to control haemorrhage and/or remove necrotic tissue.

Necrotic tissues heal by scar formation and do not grow back. Ear and tail tips may therefore be permanently lost, and other tissues may have punched out areas, irregular margins or depressed scars. Atrophic hair loss may also be permanent.

References

1   Innera M. Cutaneous vasculitis in small animals. *Vet Clin N Am Small An Pract* 2013; **43**: 113–124.
2   Nichols PR, Morris DO, Beale KM. A retrospective study of canine and feline cutaneous vasculitis. *Vet Dermatol* 2001; **12**: 255–264.
3   Swann JW, Priestnall SL, Dawson C *et al*. Histologic and clinical features of primary and secondary

vasculitis: a retrospective study of 42 dogs (2004–2011). *J Vet Diag Invest* 2015; **27**: 489–496.

4 Medleau L, Hnilica KA. Injection reaction and post-rabies vaccination alopecias. In: *Small Animal Dermatology: A Color Atlas and Therapeutic Guide.* Elsevier, St. Louis. 2006: p. 267.

5 Hargis AM and Mundell AC. Familial canine dermatomyositis. *Compend Contin Educ Vet* 1992; **14**: 855–64.

6 Wahl JM, Clark LA, Skalli O *et al.* Analysis of gene transcript profiling and immunobiology in shetland

sheepdogs with dermatomyositis. *Vet Dermatol* 2008; **19**: 52–58.

7 Weir JAM, Yager JA, Caswell JL *et al.* Familial cutaneous vasculopathy of german-shepherds – clinical, genetic and preliminary pathological and immunological studies. *Canadian Veterinary Journal-Revue Veterinaire Canadienne* 1994; **35**: 763–769.

8 Parker WM, Foster RA. Cutaneous vasculitis in five Jack Russell terriers. *Vet Dermatol* 1996; **7**: 109–115.

ERYTHEMA MULTIFORME COMPLEX

Definition

Erythema multiforme (EM) complex is a group of uncommon, immune-mediated dermatoses with varied clinical signs. These include EM minor, EM major, Stevens–Johnson syndrome (SJS), SJS-toxic epidermal necrolysis (TEN) overlap syndrome and TEN (*Table 6.2*).[1–5] It is very rare in cats.[4]

Aetiology and pathogenesis

The pathogenesis involves a specific immune-mediated assault on keratinocytes causing widespread, confluent keratinocyte apoptosis and epidermal necrosis.[1–3,5] EM minor and EM major are most commonly idiopathic or associated with infections and systemic illness, whereas SJS, SJS–TEN overlap and TEN are more commonly associated with drug eruptions.[1,4] Feline EM has been associated with feline herpesvirus-1.

The classification of EM diseases is controversial. One study[1] split cases into five distinct groups: EM minor, EM major, SJS, SJS-TEN overlap syndrome and TEN. However, histopathology alone could not

be relied upon to differentiate them.[1–3,5] Apoptosis, furthermore, is widely observed in many immune-mediated and inflammatory dermatoses and is not specific for EM.

Clinical features

EM usually presents with variable erythematous macules, papules, plaques, wheals, scaling and crusts, often arranged in annular, arcuate or polycyclic shapes (**Figs. 6.42–6.44**).[1–5] The typical target lesions consist of a flat to raised erythematous central disk and outer ring, separated by a zone of pale, occasionally oedematous skin, but are not seen in all cases. Some dogs present with marked scaling and crusting overlying the lesions. Mucosal lesions are similar, although more usually bullous or vesicular and quickly rupture to form ulcers. Rarely, lesions may be restricted to the oral cavity.[5]

Polycyclic and target lesions are unusual in SJS-TEN, which presents with an erythematous macular dermatitis, and focal to widespread mucocutaneous vesicles, epithelial detachment and

Table 6.2 Classification of erythema multiforme (EM) diseases

	EM MINOR	EM MAJOR	SJS	SJS–TEN	TEN
Flat or raised, erythematous polycyclic to target lesions	Y	Y	N	N	N
Mucosal surfaces involved	N (or 1)	>1	>1	>1	>1
Erythematous or purpuric macules/patches (%BSA)	<50%	<50%	>50%	>50%	>50%
Epidermal ulceration (%BSA)	<10%	<10%	<10%	10–30%	>30%

BSA, body surface area; SJS, Stevens–Johnson syndrome; TEN, toxic epidermal necrolysis.

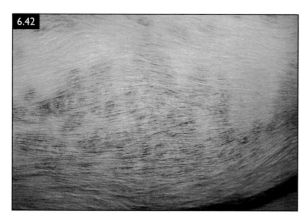

Fig. 6.42 Polycyclic erythema and target lesions with erosions and crusting of the ventral abdomen in a Boxer dog with erythema multiforme major.

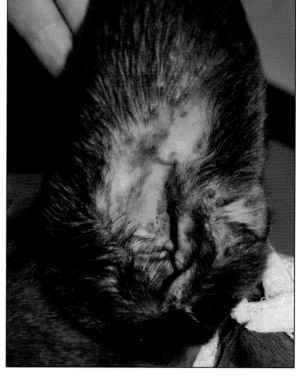

Fig. 6.43 Polycyclic erythema, erosions and crusting of the pinna in a Boxer dog with erythema multiforme major.

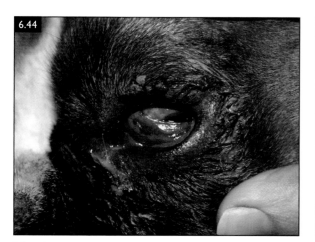

Fig. 6.44 Conjunctival ulceration in a Boxer dog with erythema multiforme major.

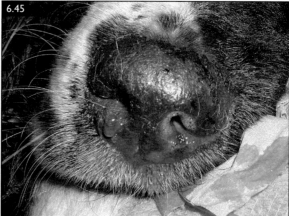

Fig. 6.45 Full-thickness ulceration of the nasal planum in a dog with drug-induced Stevens–Johnson syndrome.

ulceration (**Figs. 6.45–6.47**).[1–3] The skin lesions are often painful, especially with widespread necrosis and ulceration. Other clinical signs include loss of nails, corneal ulceration and ulcerative otitis. Internal involvement can include mild to severe loss mucosal ulcers, renal failure, hepatopathy and blood dyscrasias.

EM typically has a chronic, insidious history, whereas SJS–TEN usually has an acute onset and is one of the few genuine dermatological emergencies.

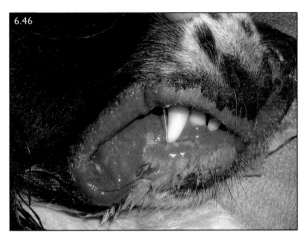

Fig. 6.46 Ulceration of the mucocutaneous junctions and oral cavity in a dog with drug-induced Stevens–Johnson syndrome.

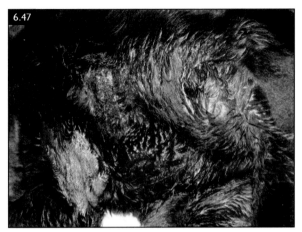

Fig. 6.47 Widespread full-thickness necrosis of the skin in a dog with drug-induced toxic epidermal necrolysis.

Differential diagnosis

- Vasculitis.
- Superficial and deep bacterial or fungal infections.
- Demodicosis.
- Pemphigus foliaceus and vulgaris.
- Bullous pemphigoid.
- Systemic lupus erythematosus.
- Epitheliotropic lymphoma.
- Thermal or chemical burns.
- Gnat and midge bites (Simuliidae and Ceratopogonidae) can cause EM-like target lesions in some dogs.

Adverse drug reactions are the most commonly identified trigger for SJS/TEN. However, adverse drug reactions are less commonly implicated in EM minor and major, and drug-associated non-EM immune-mediated dermatoses should be considered as a differential for EM.

Diagnosis

The history and clinical signs are highly suggestive, and the diagnosis can be confirmed by histopathology of early lesions. However, histopathology does not reliably differentiate between the various forms of EM, as there is extensive overlap in the changes between the different stages of disease and clinical manifestations.[1-3] A final diagnosis relies on careful evaluation of the clinical signs and history.

Treatment

EM can be a challenging condition to manage. The prognosis is better if the inciting cause can be identified and removed. It is very important to check the history for any possible drug association. Where ongoing therapy is unavoidable (e.g. antibiotics, analgesics, antiepileptics, etc.) treatment should be switched to a different class of drug.

Some cases of EM spontaneously resolve or wax and wane, but progression to SJS–TEN does not appear to occur. Treatment options include glucocorticoids, ciclosporin and pentoxifylline (see Immunosuppressive Drug Therapy Table, page 289, for more details). Long-term maintenance treatment may be necessary in idiopathic cases.

The prognosis for SJS–TEN is poor, with mortality rates exceeding 50%. Severe cases with widespread ulceration should receive intravenous fluid therapy to combat dehydration and shock. The ulcers should be cleaned and protected, taking measures to encourage healing and prevent infection. Consideration should also be given to analgesia and antibiotics to prevent sepsis. The role of glucocorticoids alongside supportive treatment is controversial but high-dose short-term therapy may be beneficial. Intravenous therapy with human immunoglobulin (ivHIG) (0.5–1.5 g/kg IV over 6–12 hours) has been helpful in few cases of SJS and TEN in dogs and cats.[6]

References

1 Hinn AC, Olivry T, Luther PB, Cannon AG, Yager JA. Erythema multiforme, Stevens-Johnson syndrome and toxic epidermal necrolysis in the dog: Classification, drug exposure and histopthological correlations. *J Vet Allergy Clinical Immunol* 1998; **6**: 13–20.

2 Banovic F, Olivry T, Bazzle L *et al*. Clinical and microscopic characteristics of canine toxic epidermal necrolysis. *Vet Pathol* 2015; **52**: 321–330.

3 Yager JA. Erythema multiforme, Stevens-Johnson syndrome and toxic epidermal necrolysis: a comparative review. *Vet Dermatol* 2014; **25**: 406–413.

4 Scott DW, Miller WH. Erythema multiforme in dogs and cats: literature review and case material from the Cornell University College of Veterinary Medicine (1988–96). *Vet Dermatol* 1999; **10**: 297–309.

5 Nemec A, Zavodovskaya R, Affolter VK *et al*. Erythema multiforme and epitheliotropic T-cell lymphoma in the oral cavity of dogs: 1989 to 2009. *J Small Anim Pract* 2012; **53**: 445–452.

6 Trotman TK, Phillips H, Fordyce H *et al*. Treatment of severe adverse cutaneous drug reactions with human intravenous immunoglobulin in two dogs. *J Am Anim Hosp Assoc* 2006; **42**: 312–320.

GENERAL APPROACH TO DRAINING TRACTS

Draining tracts may indicate deep infection, foreign body or autoimmune disease. They indicate that the subcutis is affected, and the prognosis may be guarded.

Draining tracts almost always require a biopsy for diagnosis and additional tests may be indicated if systemic disease is possible (especially in the case of deep fungal infections).

Draining tracts are preceded by bullae. Fine-needle aspirates of bullae may be diagnostic, especially if a deep fungal infection is present. If organisms cannot be detected by fine-needle aspirate, then a biopsy should be taken. The skin should not be shaved or cleansed before biopsy. The erythematous skin adjacent to a draining tract should be biopsied. The biopsy should include abnormal epidermis, dermis and subcutis, which will normally need a deep wedge excision. Special stains are needed to check for mycobacteria, *Actinomyces* and *Nocardia* spp., and fungal organisms.

A culture from a bulla or from deep within a draining tract will help guide antibiotic choices (see Deep pyoderma, page 195).

PANSTEATITIS
(Yellow fat disease)

Definition
Pansteatitis is a sterile inflammatory condition of the adipose tissue in cats, caused by a nutritional imbalance.

Aetiology and pathogenesis
Pansteatitis is a sterile, inflammatory condition of the fat that is caused by insufficient dietary vitamin E and/or excessive dietary unsaturated fatty acids. The inadequate vitamin E:unsaturated fatty acid ratio results in oxidative damage to adipocytes and subsequent lipid peroxidation.[1] Cats that eat a fish-only diet are at increased risk of developing this disease. Other unbalanced, meat-based diets have also been implicated in the development of pansteatitis.[1,2]

Clinical features
Clinical signs include subcutaneous nodules, draining tracts, lethargy, inappetence, fever, pain and reluctance to move. Haematological abnormalities may also be present. Affected adipose tissue has an unusual yellow–orange colour.[1] Some cats in the household may develop pansteatitis whereas others will not, even when fed the same diet.

Differential diagnoses
- Mycobacteriosis.
- Nocardiosis, actinobacillosis, actinomycosis.
- Neoplasia.
- Deep fungal infection.

Diagnosis

The dietary history and clinical signs will strongly suggest pansteatitis. However, a skin biopsy (being careful to include adipose tissue in the biopsy) with special stains for infectious agents is necessary to confirm the diagnosis and rule out infectious causes of inflammation of the fat. Plasma tocopherol levels of <300 mg/100 ml further confirm the diagnosis.[1]

Treatment

Affected cats should receive supportive care including pain medication and parenteral fluid therapy, depending on the severity of their condition. Affected cats should be fed a high-quality, properly balanced diet. Additional α-tocopherol supplementation (50 mg/kg po q24 h) may also be helpful to speed recovery. Full recovery may take several weeks. It is imperative that affected cats continue to consume a balanced diet even after resolution of clinical signs.

Key point

- Cats have different abilities to tolerate diets high in unsaturated fatty acids and/or deficient in vitamin E. Some cats will develop pansteatitis and others will not.

References

1 Niza MMRE, Vilela CL, Ferreira LMA. Feline pansteatitis revisited: hazards of unbalanced home-made diets. *J Feline Med Surg* 2003; **5**: 271–277.
2 Schlesinger DP, Joffe DJ. Raw food diets in companion animals: a critical review. *Can Vet J* 2011; **52**: 50.

FELINE MYCOBACTERIAL INFECTIONS

Definition

An infection of the skin and subcutis with mycobacteria.

Aetiology and pathogenesis

Three manifestations of mycobacterial infection are recognised in cats: cutaneous tuberculosis (CT), feline leprosy syndrome (FLS) and non-tuberculous mycobacterial infections (NTMs).

CT is caused by *Mycobacterium microti*, *M. bovis* and *M. tuberculosis*. The bacteria spread to cats when they have contact, particularly bite wounds, with an infected rodent (especially voles). Cattle or badgers are also sources of mycobacterial infection for cats. Zoonotic transmission has not been reported in cases of *M. microti*.[1] *M. bovis* and *M. tuberculosis* may pose a zoonotic risk.

FLS is most commonly caused by *M. lepraemurium*, although other types of mycobacteria have also been implicated. The bacteria spread to cats when they have contact with an infected rodent, especially rats. This syndrome has two histological patterns. Briefly, one pattern reveals large numbers of bacteria and the other has low numbers of bacteria. Immunocompromised cats are more likely to have large numbers of mycobacteria on histopathology. This is not a zoonotic disease.

NTMs are caused by a variety of mycobacteria including *M. chelonae*, *M. phlei*, *M. thermoresistible* and others. This type of infection is contracted through bite wounds from rodents and exposure of wounds to contaminated soil or plant matter. Zoonoses are unlikely.[2]

Clinical features

CT is characterised by cutaneous nodules with or without draining tracts and ulceration (**Fig. 7.1**). Lesions most often occur on the head, neck and limbs. Local lymphadenopathy may occur. Pulmonary lesions, anorexia, gastrointestinal signs and weight loss may also be present. The alimentary tract can become infected if the cat drinks tuberculous milk. In addition, the eyes, liver, spleen, neurological system and bones may be affected.

FLS is characterised by single or multiple nodules on the head and limbs, and sometimes the trunk. The nodules may or may not be ulcerated and draining (**Fig. 7.2**). Lymphadenopathy may be present, but systemic disease is rare.

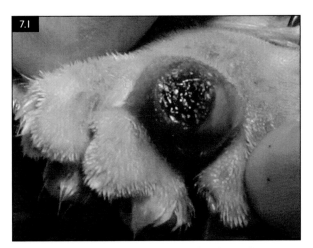

Fig. 7.1 Ulcerated nodule on the forefoot of a cat with an *M. microti* infection.

NTM is characterised by single or multiple subcutaneous nodules, diffuse panniculitis and draining tracts (**Fig. 7.3**). Lesions are variably painful. The inguinal fat pad, flanks and tail base are most frequently affected. Systemic involvement is possible, but rare. Affected cats may display fever, anorexia and reluctance to move.[2]

Differential diagnoses
- Nocardiosis.
- Actinomycosis.
- Deep mycoses.
- *Cuterebra* spp. (for nodular lesions).
- Foreign body.
- Neoplasia.
- Pansteatitis.

Diagnosis
Cytology will usually show a granulomatous to pyogranulomatous dermatitis. Mycobacteria will not stain with standard stains (**Figs. 7.4, 7.5**). Histopathology of affected skin is the most common way to diagnose mycobacterial infections. Care should be taken to include the epidermis, dermis and subcutis in the biopsy sample. Multiple skin biopsies should be collected, as the organisms can be present in affected skin in low numbers. Ziehl–Neelsen (ZN) staining is required to identify the organisms as mycobacteria; several sections may be required to detect the organisms and some samples may be persistently ZN negative.[3]

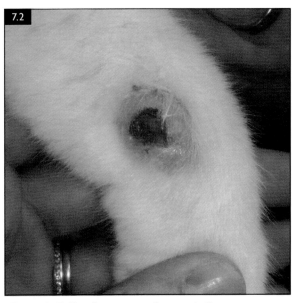

Fig. 7.2 Feline leprosy syndrome. A discrete, erythematous, eroded and crusted nodule on the forelimb of a cat (photo courtesy of Danielle Gunn-Moore).

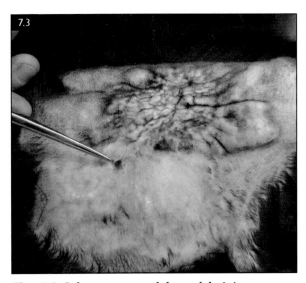

Fig. 7.3 Subcutaneous nodules and draining tracts on the ventro-lateral abdomen of a cat with mycobacteriosis (photo courtesy of Danielle Gunn-Moore).

Mycobacteria cannot be cultured with traditional laboratory techniques. Tissue samples should be submitted to laboratories with special capabilities for culturing this organism, but sensitivity testing does not always correlate with in-vivo results.

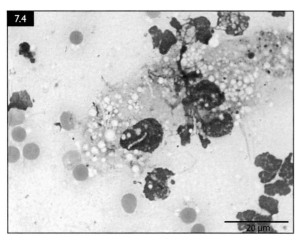
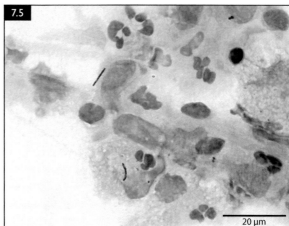

Figs. 7.4, 7.5 Cytology from a mycobacterial infection in a cat showing pyogranulomatous inflammation with non-staining rod-shaped vacuoles (Fig. 7.4). The mycobacterial are only visible using a Ziehl–Neelsen stain (Fig. 7.5) (courtesy of Dr Paola Cazzini).

Polymerase chain reaction (PCR) testing of affected tissue can detect some species of mycobacteria but may be limited, e.g. in the UK the available tests will distinguish *M. tuberculosis* complex from *M. avium* complex but will not distinguish species within these complexes (e.g. *M. microti* from *M. bovis*) or other types of mycobacteria. A whole-blood interferon γ (IFN-γ) release assay (IGRA) can be used to help distinguish infections with environmental mycobacteria, avian TB (*Mycobacterium avium*), *M. microti* and *M. bovis* or *M. tuberculosis*.

Affected animals should be screened for systemic disease and possible immunosuppressive factors such as concurrent illness, feline leukaemia virus (FeLV) or feline immunodeficiency virus (FIV). These mycobacteria are not normally zoonotic, but veterinary staff and owners should observe hygienic precautions and guard against inoculation into deep tissues, ingestion, splashing and inhalation.

Treatment[2]

Treatment of CT has an initial phase and a continuation phase. The initial phase involves administration of three antibiotics for 2 months and the continuation phase administration of two antibiotics for a subsequent 4–6 months. If three antibiotics cannot be administered in the initial phase, then two antibiotics should be administered for at least 6–9 months. An antibiotic protocol to consider is rifampicin–fluoroquinolone–clarithromycin as the initial treatment, followed by a continuation of rifampicin and a fluoroquinolone or clarithromycin (*Table 7.1*).

Surgical excision or CO_2 laser excision/ablation of small, superficial lesions may be considered, but debulking larger lesions risks wound dehiscence and recurrence of infection.

FLS may be treated with surgical excision of small cutaneous lesions, and spontaneous remission has been reported. Some patients require antibiotic therapy. Concurrent use of two or three antibiotics increases the odds of successful resolution. Antibiotics should be administered for 2 months beyond clinical resolution of lesions (*Table 7.1*).

NTM should be treated with a combination of two or three antibiotics for 2 months beyond clinical resolution of lesions. If lesions become static after 1–2 months of antibiotic therapy, then surgical excision of the lesion should be considered. In addition, tissue culture should be attempted. Mycobacteria can develop antibiotic resistance over time, and the antibiotics may have to be periodically changed.

For all but the smallest of lesions, the prognosis is guarded to poor. Some cases never resolve, whereas others may go into remission only to relapse when therapy is withdrawn. Unsuccessful surgery worsens the prognosis.

Table 7.1 Antibiotic therapy for feline mycobacterial infections[2]

USES	DRUG	DOSE	SIDE EFFECTS
First-line treatment for CT and NTM	Marbofloxacin Moxifloxacin	2 mg/kg po q24 h 10 mg/kg po q24 h	GI signs GI signs
First-line treatment for CT and NTM	Rifampicin	10–15 mg/kg po q24 h (maximum 600 mg/day)	Potentially fatal hepatotoxicity, discoloration of body fluids
First-line treatment for CT, FLS and NTM	Clarithromycin Azithromycin	5–15 mg/kg po q12 h 5–15 mg/kg po q24 h	Hepatotoxicity GI signs
Second-line treatment for CT	Isoniazid	10–20 mg/kg po q24 h (maximum 300 mg/day)	Hepatotoxicity, peripheral neuritis, nephrotoxicity
Second-line treatment for CT	Dihydrostreptomycin	15 mg/kg im q24 h	Ototoxicity
Second-line treatment for CT	Pyrazinamide (not effective against *M. bovis*)	15–40 mg/kg po q24 h	Hepatotoxicity, GI signs
Second-line treatment for FLS and NTM	Clofazamine	4–8 mg/kg po q24 h	Hepatoxicity, GI signs, discoloration of body fluids, photosensitisation, corneal lesions
Second-line treatment for NTM	Doxycycline	5–10 mg/kg po q12 h	GI signs, oesophagitis

CT, cutaneous tuberculosis; FLS, feline leprosy syndrome; GI, gastrointestinal; im, intramuscularly; NTM, non-tuberculous mycobacterial infection; po, by mouth.

Key points

- Tuberculosis (*M. bovis* and *M. tuberculosis*) is a reportable disease in some countries – clinicians should be aware of local regulations for reporting and treatment.
- Although a zoonosis is unlikely, immunocompromised people may be at risk.

References

1 Laprie C, Duboy J, Malik R, Fyfe J. Feline cutaneous mycobacteriosis: a review of clinical, pathological and molecular characterization of one case of *Mycobacterium microti* skin infection and nine cases of feline leprosy syndrome from France and New Caledonia. *Vet Dermatol* 2013; **24**: 561–e134.
2 Gunn-Moore D, Dean R, Shaw S. Mycobacterial infections in cats and dogs. *In Practice* 2010; **32**: 444–452.
3 Davies JL, Sibley JA, Myers S, Clark EG, Appleyard GD. Histological and genotypical characterization of feline cutaneous mycobacteriosis: a retrospective study of formalin-fixed paraffin-embedded tissues. *Vet Dermatol* 2006; **17**: 155–162.

POSTGROOMING FURUNCULOSIS

Definition

A pyoderma that occurs because of harsh grooming.

Aetiology and pathogenesis

Two forms of postgrooming furunculosis are recognised. The first, superficial suppurative necrolytic dermatitis (SSND), is a severe contact reaction to herbal or tar shampoo.[1] Secondary pyoderma develops because the skin is inflamed and ulcerated. The second form is associated with grooming techniques[2] such as using shampoos that have been contaminated with bacteria and/or back-combing, back-clipping and aggressive bathing. The grooming techniques cause hairs to rupture through follicles and inoculate the skin with bacteria such as *Pseudomonas* or *Staphylococcus* spp.

Clinical features

SSND is typically characterised by severe, diffuse erythema, papules, pustules, plaques, erosions, crusts, necrosis, purulent exudate and haemorrhage affecting multiple areas of the skin.[1] Lesions are very painful, and systemic signs include fever, lethargy and anorexia. Severe cases can be fatal. Lesions develop within several days of bathing with the offending shampoo. In some cases, the animal can be exposed to the shampoo several times before a reaction occurs.

Grooming technique-associated furunculosis is typically characterised by pustules, haemorrhagic bullae, papules, cellulitis, ulcers, erosions and draining tracts on the dorsal trunk (**Fig. 7.6**). Other areas of the skin may also be affected depending on how the grooming was performed. In addition, dogs may present with pain, lethargy and reluctance to move. No breed or sex predilection has been noted. Lesions occur with 1–2 days of the grooming.[2]

Differential diagnoses
- Pemphigus foliaceus.
- Superficial pustular drug reaction.
- Toxic shock syndrome.
- Erythema multiforme.
- Canine sterile neutrophilic dermatosis (Sweet's syndrome).
- Demodicosis.
- Dermatophytosis.
- Flea-allergic dermatitis.
- German Shepherd dog pyoderma.

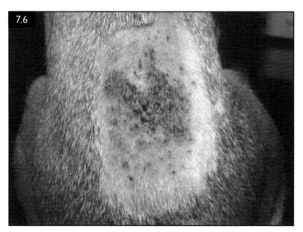

Fig. 7.6 Postbathing pseudomonas furunculosis in a dog (courtesy of Jan DeClercq).

Diagnosis
A presumptive diagnosis can be made with history, physical exam findings, skin scraping and superficial cytology. Cytology should be collected from each different lesion on the skin, because the bacterial counts and types of cells present may vary. Skin biopsy (including crust or pustule, epidermis, dermis and subcutis) is diagnostic, but treatment must be initiated before receiving the biopsy results.

Treatment
Both types of skin disease require immediate treatment while culture and sensitivity testing and skin biopsies are pending. The clinician should presume that *Pseudomonas* sp. is present in either condition and should start treatment with a fluoroquinolone such as marbofloxacin (2.75–5.5 mg/kg po q24 h).

In addition to antibiotics, SSND requires treatment with prednisone (1.1 mg/kg po q24 h until lesions improve, and then taper) and pain medication (tramadol 2–4 mg/kg po q8–12 h). Severely affected patients may require hospitalisation with intravenous fluids and wound care.

Grooming technique-associated furunculosis should also be treated with prednisone (0.5–1 mg/kg po q24 h until lesions improve, and then taper) and may need analgesia in addition to the antibiotics.

Antibiotic therapy should be continued for 2 weeks beyond clinical resolution of lesions (see Deep pyoderma, page 195). Steroids can be discontinued when the skin is no longer inflamed.

Key point
- Both types of postgrooming furunculosis are very painful.

References
1 Murayama N, Midorikawa K, Nagata M. A case of superficial suppurative necrolytic dermatitis of miniature schnauzers with identification of a causative agent using patch testing. *Vet Dermatol* 2008; **19**: 395–399.
2 Hillier A, Alcorn JR, Cole LK, Kowalski JJ. Pyoderma caused by *Pseudomonas aeruginosa* infection in dogs: 20 cases. *Vet Dermatol* 2006; **17**: 432–439.

DEEP PYODERMA
(Furunculosis)

Definition
Deep pyoderma is a bacterial infection that affects the epidermis, dermis and subcutaneous tissues.

Aetiology and pathogenesis
Deep pyoderma is almost always secondary to an underlying disease, and commonly occurs as a result of furunculosis. Bacteria from ruptured hair follicles inoculate the dermis and subcutis causing a deep infection. Common causes of furunculosis include dermatophytosis, demodicosis, allergic skin disease and skin-fold irritation. Deep pyoderma can also result from extension of severe, chronic, superficial pyoderma. Common causes of superficial pyoderma include hypothyroidism, hyperadrenocorticism, allergic skin disease and ectoparasites. Finally, deep pyoderma can occur as a result of a penetrating wound. Examples of this include foreign body, bite wounds and other trauma.

The agents involved in deep pyoderma include staphylococci, *Escherichia coli*, *Pseudomonas aeruginosa* and, less commonly, other types of bacteria.[1] Mixed bacterial populations may be present. The site and cause of the infection will influence the most likely bacteria, although this will also depend on prior antibiotic therapy. Antimicrobial-resistant organisms are not uncommon after multiple broad-spectrum antibiotic courses. The organisms on the surface may not be representative of the infection in the deeper tissues.

Clinical features
The clinical lesions of deep pyoderma are more severe than superficial infections, and they are usually more painful than pruritic. Clinical signs include erythema, swelling, haemorrhagic bullae, bleeding, draining sinus tracts, ulceration, crusts, abscesses and cellulitis (**Figs. 7.7, 7.8**). Lesions may be focal, multi-focal or generalised. Several distinct clinical variants of deep pyoderma are recognised as follows:

- Localised deep folliculitis and furunculosis (**Fig. 7.9**).
- Nasal pyoderma.

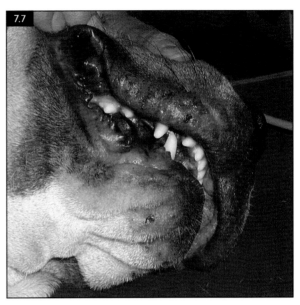

Fig. 7.7 Muzzle of a Mastiff-cross with swelling, erythema, haemorrhage, folliculitis, furunculosis, ulcers, sinus tracts and crusts typical of deep pyoderma.

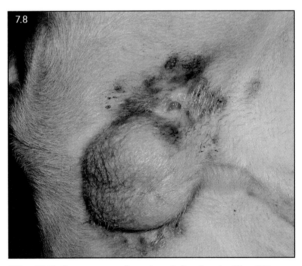

Fig. 7.8 Scrotum and groin of the dog in Fig. 7.7.

- Foreign body sinus (**Figs. 7.10, 7.11**).
- Muzzle furunculosis or canine acne (see page 75).
- Callus pyoderma (see page 152).
- Interdigital furunculosis or interdigital cysts (see page 216).
- Bite wounds and subsequent abscessation (**Figs. 7.12, 7.13**).
- German Shepherd dog pyoderma (see page 177).
- Acral lick dermatitis (see page 13).

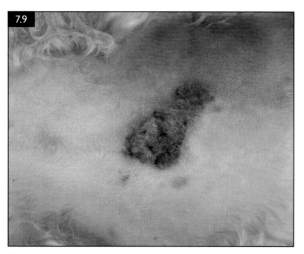

Fig. 7.9 Localised furunculosis with draining sinus tracts and a haemo-purulent discharge in a dog at a prior venepuncture site.

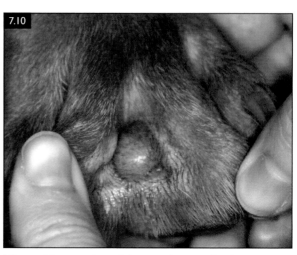

Fig. 7.10 Interdigital furunculosis and a draining tract caused by a penetrating foreign body.

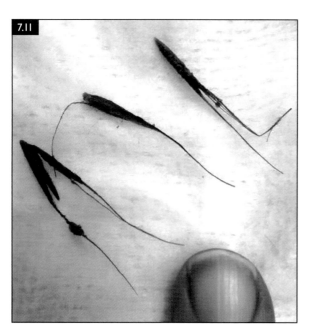

Fig. 7.11 Foxtails or grass awns; these are common foreign bodies in the interdigital skin and ears in dogs (courtesy of Dr Amy Haarstad).

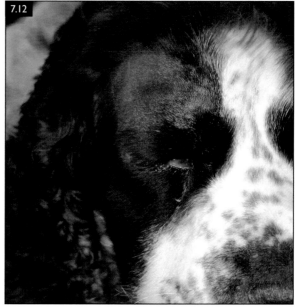

Fig. 7.12 Retrobulbar abscess following a penetrating bite in a Springer Spaniel (courtesy of Candace Sousa).

Localised deep folliculitis and furunculosis

This is thought to be a complication of pyotraumatic dermatitis or superficial pyoderma. Affected animals present with pruritic, exudative, erythematous, thickened patches on their skin (**Fig. 7.9**). The major differential diagnosis is acute moist dermatitis (see page 68). Localised deep folliculitis and furunculosis may be differentiated from pyotraumatic dermatitis clinically by a thickened feel and the presence of satellite lesions with draining tracts. Localised deep pyoderma is often secondary to focal demodicosis, dermatophytosis and physical or chemical trauma.

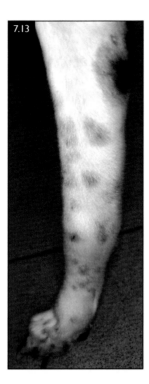

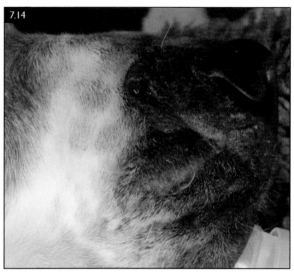

Fig. 7.13 Diffuse cellulitis following a bite to a dog's leg. The actual bites healed well and were difficult to find.

Fig. 7.14 Dorsal muzzle folliculitis and furunculosis; it is important to eliminate dermatophytosis and *Demodex* spp. in these cases. It may also be necessary to rule out eosinophilic furunculosis and immune-mediated disease.

Nasal pyoderma

This affects the dorsal muzzle but not the nasal planum. The peracute form presents as inflammatory papules, which rapidly coalesce and progress to an erythematous, eroded, granulomatous, proliferative plaque that is extremely painful. Chronic infections are characterised by crusted papules and occasionally by sinus formation (**Fig. 7.14**). These lesions have been traditionally associated with rooting behaviour, possibly where trauma drives hairs into the skin, initiating the formation of hair granulomas. Additional causes of deep pyoderma of the dorsal muzzle include eosinophilic folliculitis and furunculosis and facial dermatophytosis (see page 85).

Differential diagnoses

- Demodicosis.
- Deep fungal infection.
- Dermatophytosis.
- Eosinophilic folliculitis and furunculosis (if on the muzzle).
- Mycobacterial infection.
- Nocardiosis or actinobacillosis.
- Sterile nodular panniculitis.
- Postgrooming furunculosis.

Diagnosis

Deep pyoderma is a secondary condition[1] except in the rarest of circumstances. Pyoderma is diagnosed via demonstration of intracellular bacteria on cytology of fresh exudates. It is important to obtain representative superficial and deep material for cytology and culture. Biopsy samples may be necessary to confirm the diagnosis and obtain deep tissue for culture in some cases. Thorough diagnostics (i.e. superficial cytology, deep skin scraping, skin culture, endocrine testing and skin biopsy) help to diagnose underlying causes or rule out other conditions.

Treatment

The hair on affected skin should be clipped to reveal the extent of the lesions, improve access for treatment and prevent matting. Whole body clips may be necessary with generalised disease, especially in long-haired animals. Daily or alternate-day bathing with antibacterial shampoos such as benzoyl peroxide and chlorhexidine is useful. Systemic antibiotics after culture and sensitivity testing are required until the lesions have resolved (which may take 8–12 weeks).[1] A cephalosporin[1] combined with topical mupirocin is generally a good antibiotic choice pending culture. Dramatic lesion improvement is generally seen within the first 2–4 weeks. Full resolution will require prolonged treatment because associated fibrosed pyogranulomas take more time to resolve. (See Superficial pyoderma, page 72, for more details of topical and systemic antibacterials.)

The prognosis is generally good if the primary cause is identified and managed. If the underlying cause is not managed, the condition will probably be recurrent.

Key points
- Treatment of deep pyoderma is much more successful if an underlying cause can be identified and concurrently treated.
- Culture and sensitivity testing are mandatory.
- Demodicosis is a common and sometimes overlooked aetiology.

Reference
1 Summers JF, Brodbelt DC, Forsythe PJ, Loeffler A, Hendricks A. The effectiveness of systemic antimicrobial treatment in canine superficial and deep pyoderma: a systematic review. *Vet Dermatol* 2012; **23**: 305–e61.

CANINE MYCOBACTERIOSIS
(Canine leproid granuloma and opportunistic [atypical] mycobacterial infections)

Definition
Canine mycobacterial infections of the skin usually manifest as two syndromes. Canine leproid granuloma (CLG) is a nodular infection of the cutaneous and/or subcutaneous tissues by mycobacteria.[1] Opportunisitic mycobacteria causes infection of the subcutis, resulting in draining tracts. Systemic and cutaneous tuberculosis is rare but can result from exposure to infected animals and contaminated carcasses.

Aetiology and pathogenesis
The mycobacterial agent for CLG has not been fully characterised. The mode of inoculation is believed to be biting flies and other insects.[1] Traumatic wounds and fomites may also be sources for infection.

Many species of opportunistic mycobacteria exist, including *Mycobacterium fortuitum*, *M. chelonae*, *M. phlei*, *M. smegmatis* and others. These species are ubiquitous in soil, water and decaying vegetation. Infection generally follows a traumatic wound.

Clinical features
CLG presents as single to multiple, variably pruritic, firm, well-circumscribed nodules in the skin and/or subcutis (**Fig. 7.15**).[1] Short-coated breeds, Boxer dogs, Foxhounds,[2] Doberman Pinschers and their crosses are overrepresented. Boxer dogs are particularly susceptible to this infection.[1] Lesions are most often located on the head and pinnae, although limbs and trunk may also be affected. Lesions may become ulcerative.[2] Systemic involvement is unlikely.

Opportunistic mycobacteria cause lesions typical of panniculitis, including multiple punctate ulcers, draining tracts, ulcerated nodules and subcutaneous granulomas. The ventral abdomen and inguinal region are most commonly affected. No breed or sex predilection has been identified. Lethargy, pyrexia, lymphadenopathy, anorexia and weight loss may also be present.

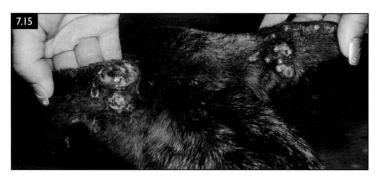

Fig. 7.15 Multiple leproid granulomas on the dorsal ears and neck of a dog (photo courtesy of Candace Sousa).

Differential diagnoses

CLG
- Mast cell tumour or other neoplasia.
- Histiocytic disease.
- Sterile pyogranuloma/granuloma syndrome.
- Actinomycosis.
- Nocardiosis.
- Pseudomycetoma.
- Mycetoma or nodular dermatophytosis.
- Leishmaniasis.

Opportunistic mycobacteria
- Foreign body.
- Sterile panniculitis.
- Nocardiosis.
- Deep mycoses.
- Cutaneous haemangiosarcoma or other neoplasia.

Diagnosis

Cytology will reveal granulomatous to pyogranulomatous inflammation. Mycobacteria do not stain with standard stains but may be demonstrated by ZN staining (although some samples will be ZN negative). The diagnosis relies on a skin biopsy (including epidermis, dermis and subcutis), with ZN staining to identify the organisms histopathologically. The number of organisms present on histopathology may vary based on the stage of infection. Multiple biopsies should be collected to increase likelihood of achieving an accurate diagnosis. Several sections may be required and some biopsies will be persistently ZN negative. Culture of the mycobacteria in CLG is not possible.[1] Culture of opportunistic mycobacteria is possible, albeit difficult. IGR assays can be used to confirm infection and identify the species in cases of atypical and tuberculous mycobacterial infections (see Feline mycobacterial infections, page 192).

Treatment

Lesions may become secondarily infected with staphylococci, especially if ulceration is present. Superficial cytology is necessary to identify secondary pyoderma.

CLG is generally self-limiting and lesions will spontaneously resolve within 1–3 months.[1] Immunosuppressive drugs or concurrent disease processes may delay or prevent spontaneous resolution. Some cases require antimicrobial therapy. The prognosis is good.

Opportunistic mycobacterial infections require systemic treatment with antimicrobials. The prognosis is guarded to poor (see Feline mycobacterial infections, page 190).

Severe, progressive or persistent lesions should be treated with antimicrobials. A combination of rifampicin (10–15 mg/kg po q24 h) and clarithromycin (7.5–12.5 mg/kg po q8–12 h) is recommended for severe or refractory CLG and opportunistic mycobacteria. Rifampicin can cause fatal hepatotoxicity. Doxycycline (5–7.5 mg/kg po q12 h) or oral fluoroquinolones are also effective in some cases.[3]

Silver sulfadiazine (or silver sulfasalazine) compounded with clofazamine and dimethyl sulfoxide (DMSO) can be applied topically q12–24 h as a sole treatment for small lesions (CLG), and as an adjunctive treatment for larger lesions.

Surgical resection or CO_2 laser excision/ablation can be useful for lesions that are large or poorly responsive to antimicrobials. Surgical resection alone may not be curative because the infection may be present in tissue surrounding the nodule. Concurrent antimicrobials are recommended. Surgical resection of lesions may decrease the length of time antimicrobials are needed, which is significant in patients where treatment with rifampicin is being considered.

Key point
- Biopsy with special stains is mandatory for diagnosis of either syndrome.

References

1   Malik R, Smits B, Reppas G, Laprie C, O'Brien C, Fyfe J. Ulcerated and nonulcerated nontuberculous cutaneous mycobacterial granulomas in cats and dogs. *Vet Dermatol* 2013; **24**: 146–e33.
2   Smits B, Willis, R, Malik R *et al*. Case clusters of leproid granulomas in foxhounds in New Zealand and Australia. *Vet Dermatol* 2012; **23**: 465–e88.
3   Bennie CJM, To JLK, Martin PA, Govendir M. In vitro interaction of some drug combinations to inhibit rapidly growing mycobacteria isolates from cats and dogs and these isolates' susceptibility to cefovecin and clofazimine. *Aust Vet J* 2015; **93**: 40–45.

NOCARDIOSIS/ACTINOMYCOSIS

Definition
Nocardiosis and actinomycosis are pyogranulo-matous infections with the filamentous bacteria *Nocardia* and *Actinomyces* spp., respectively. They are included together in this chapter because the clinical signs and work-up are very similar, although the treatments are not.

Aetiology and pathogenesis
Nocardia spp. are saprophytic aerobic bacteria that enter the body through soil contamination of wounds or inhalation.[1,2] *Actinomyces* spp. are normal inhabit-ants of the oral cavity.[1,2] Plant awns may also serve as a means of introducing both organisms into tissues.[1] Immunosuppression predisposes animals to infec-tion.[1,3] When a *Nocardia* sp. is the causative agent, *N. asteroides* and *N. nova* are the species most often associated with lesions in dogs, whereas *N. nova* is most common in cats.[2]

- *Nocardia*: aerobic, gram-positive, partially acid fast, with filaments that branch at right angles. Staining may produce beading. Culture easily with minimal to no other bacteria.
- *Actinomyces*: anaerobic, gram-positive, non-acid fast, and often form tissue granules. Staining may also produce beading. Difficult to culture, and often a mixed bacterial population grows.

Clinical features
Cutaneous infection typically occurs after a wound is contaminated with soil, or in the case of *Actinomyces* spp., from a bite wound. There may be systemic signs. Draining fistulous tracts, ulcers, abscesses and subcutaneous nodules are the most common clinical findings, and the lesions may be singular or multiple (**Figs. 7.16, 7.17**). *Actinomyces* spp. may produce yel-lowish granules in the tissue or discharge.

Differential diagnoses
- Deep bacterial infection with other species.
- Cutaneous manifestation of systemic fungal infections.
- Cutaneous infections of opportunistic fungi, *Pythium* or *Lagenidium* spp.
- Mycobacterial infection.
- Penetrating foreign bodies.
- Sterile nodular panniculitis.

Diagnosis
Cats or dogs with multiple draining lesions of the skin should have the following performed:

- Cytology with Diff-Quik® type and Gram stains (**Fig. 7.18**).
- Biopsies from multiple locations, extending the biopsy very deeply into the subcutis to reach the heart of the lesion and not just the draining tract. Histopathological special stains

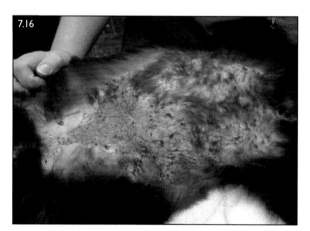

Fig. 7.16 Nocardiosis of the abdomen of a cat with nodules, draining sinus tracts and scarring (courtesy of Candace Sousa).

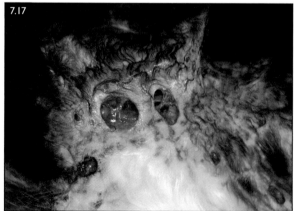

Fig. 7.17 Actinomycosis of the axilla of a cat with ulceration, necrosis and draining sinus tracts.

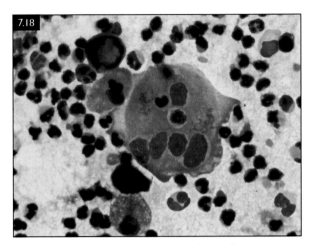

Fig. 7.18 Cytology showing a multi-nucleate giant cell with intracellular beaded filamentous rods typical of *Nocardia* or *Actinomyces* (in this case).

(e.g. Brown–Brenn Gram, Gomori methenamine silver and Fite's modified acid fast) should be requested.
- Aerobic and anaerobic (may take 2–4 weeks) cultures of exudate and tissue; labs should be informed that actinomycosis and nocardiosis are rule outs.
- Mycobacterial culture (takes months).
- Fungal culture of tissue (not just dermatophytes).
- Complete blood count, serum biochemistry, urinalysis, FIV/FeLV (cats), thyroid function tests and, if in an endemic area, mycobacterial, fungal or oomycete serology or PCR tests.
- Consider chest radiographs and abdominal ultrasonography for systemic disease.

Treatment[1]
The prognosis is guarded because many pets do not respond to treatments and many others relapse after therapy. Surgical debulking and drainage may be helpful, especially for *Actinomyces* spp.

Nocardia spp. in dogs or cats
Trimethoprim/sulfamethoxazole (15–30 mg/kg q12 h) or sulfadiazine (80 mg/kg po q8 h) are the treatments of choice, although animals should be monitored for myelosuppression and keratoconjunctivitis sicca. Alternatives include minocycline (5–25 mg/kg po q12 h), erythromycin (10 mg/kg po q8 h) and ampicillin (20–40 mg/kg po q6 h), among others. Injectable formulations of the above as well as amikacin (8–12 mg/kg im or sc q8 h) are also effective if orals are not tolerated.[1] Treatment will generally take at least 6 weeks and should be continued 1 month beyond clinical cure. Some animals need treatment indefinitely to maintain remission.

Actinomyces spp. in dogs or cats
Benzylpenicillin or phenoxymethylpenicillin at 40 mg/kg po q8 h is the treatment of choice, and injectable penicillins can be given if pets do not tolerate oral treatment.[1] Alternatives include erythromycin 10 mg/kg po q8 h, minocycline 5–25 mg/kg po q12 h or chloramphenicol 50 mg/kg po q8 h for dogs or q12 h for cats, among others.

Key points
- *Nocardia* and *Actinomyces* infections are very similar in clinical appearance and diagnostic work-up but their treatments are very different.
- The prognosis is guarded.

References
1   Edwards DF. Actinomycosis and nocardiosis. In: Greene E (ed.), *Infectious Diseases of the Dog and Cat.* St Louis, MO: Saunders Elsevier, 2006: pp. 451–461.
2   Malik R, Krockenberger MB, O'Brien CR *et al. Nocardia* infections in cats: A retrospective multi-institutional study of 17 cases. *Aust Vet J* 2006; **84**: 235–245.
3   Siak MK, Burrows AK. Cutaneous nocardiosis in two dogs receiving ciclosporin therapy for the management of canine atopic dermatitis. *Vet Dermatol* 2013; **24**: 453–e103.

SPOROTRICHOSIS

Definition

Sporotrichosis is a subacute or chronic pyogranulomatous infectious disease of dogs and cats caused by the dimorphic fungus *Sporothrix schenckii*.

Aetiology and pathogenesis

The organism is found worldwide and grows as a saprophytic mycelial fungus in moist organic debris. Infection occurs via inoculation of the fungus into the skin by thorns or plant material, or by contamination of open wounds or broken skin with exudates from infected animals.[1,2] In a host the organism establishes infection in the yeast form. The number of organisms found in draining fluids is much greater in cats than in other species, which increases the risk of transmission to other animals or humans. Motile organisms have been found to penetrate intact human skin.

Clinical features

The typical papular or nodular swellings appear 3–5 weeks after inoculation. Lesions become alopecic, crusted and ulcerated, draining a reddish-brown serosanguineous fluid. They are more common on the dorsal aspects of the head and trunk, but the extremities may also be involved (**Figs. 7.19, 7.20**). Regional lymphadenopathy is common and affected lymph nodes may fistulate. Occasionally, lesions may extend along the lymphatics or become disseminated to bone, eyes, gastrointestinal (GI) tract, central nervous system (CNS) and other visceral organs.[1,2]

Differential diagnoses

- Cutaneous infections with systemic fungi.
- Subcutaneous mycoses or algal infections.
- Demodicosis.
- Deep pyoderma.
- Opportunistic mycobacterial infection.
- Penetrating foreign bodies.
- Panniculitis.
- Histiocytic or sterile pyogranuloma or granuloma syndrome lesions.

Diagnosis

Impression smears or biopsies may reveal the round, oval or cigar-shaped yeast, which may be extracellular or within macrophages or inflammatory cells (**Fig. 7.21**).[1] Organisms are often present in small numbers and may be difficult to demonstrate with routine stains. The preferred stains to demonstrate the organisms are periodic acid–Schiff (PAS) or Grocott's methenamine silver (GMS). Fluorescent

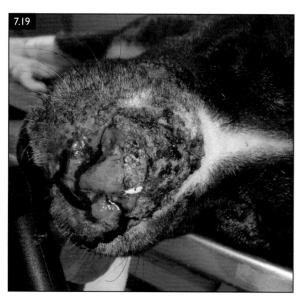
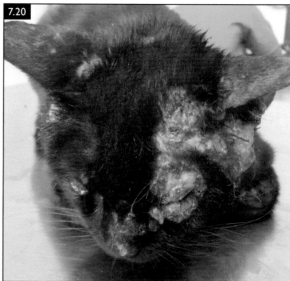

Figs. 7.19, 7.20 Sporotrichosis: generalised cutaneous lesions in a dog (Fig. 7.19); nodular form on the face of a cat (Fig. 7.20) (photos courtesy of Mariana Bezerra Mascarenhas).

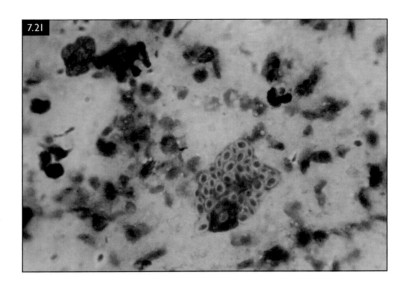

Fig. 7.21 Impression smear showing the characteristic small cigar-shaped organisms of *Sporothrix schenckii*, with a thick, refractile and non-staining cell wall (photo courtesy of Clarissa Pimentel de Souza).

antibody techniques also help to detect the organisms. Enzyme-linked immunosorbent assay (ELISA) testing for *S. schenckii* antibodies is a useful screening tool in cats. The test has >90% sensitivity and specificity.[1]

The diagnosis can also be made by culture or inoculation of laboratory animals. The culture and/or inoculation method of diagnosis is not recommended for routine cases due to the public health risk.

Treatment

A systemic antifungal should be administered for 1 month beyond clinical resolution of signs.

Itraconazole (10 mg/kg po q24 h) is the treatment of choice in cats.[1] Terbinafine (30 mg/cat po q24 h) and fluconazole (50 mg/cat po q24 h) may be used alone or in combination with itraconazole. Terbinafine and fluconazole have fewer data to support their use compared with itraconazole. Potassium iodide (20 mg/kg po q24 h) may also be used. Potassium iodide has greater potential for adverse events compared with itraconazole.[1] Side effects include: hepatotoxicity, fever, ptyalism, ocular and nasal discharges, anorexia, hyperexcitability, dry hair coat with excess scaling of the skin, vomiting or diarrhoea, depression, twitching, hypothermia and cardiovascular failure.

Itraconazole (10 mg/kg po q24 h) and ketoconazole (5–15 mg/kg po q12 h)[2,3] have been used successfully in dogs. Sodium iodide solution (44 mg/kg of a 20% solution po q8 h) may also be used.[1] Side effects of iodides in dogs are similar to those in cats.

Public health significance

As there are documented cases of humans acquiring sporotrichosis by contact with ulcerated wounds or fluids from lesions, extreme care should be taken in handling infected animals, exudates or contaminated materials. There is a greater risk associated with cats.

Key points
- Zoonotic potential.[1,4]
- Cats may serve as asymptomatic carriers.

References
1 Lloret A, Hartmann K, Pennisi MG *et al*. ABCD guidelines on prevention and management. *J Feline Med Surg* 2013; **15**: 619–623.

2 Crothers SL, White SD, Ihrke PJ, Affolter VK. Sporotrichosis: a retrospective evaluation of 23 cases seen in northern California (1987–2007). *Vet Dermatol* 2009; **20**: 249–259.

3 Plumb DC. *Plumb's Veterinary Drug Handbook*. Oxford: Wiley-Blackwell, 2008.

4 Chomel BB. Emerging and re-emerging zoonoses of dogs and cats. *Animals* 2014; **4**: 434–445.

BLASTOMYCOSIS

Definition
Blastomycosis is a deep fungal infection that can affect multiple organ systems in dogs and cats.[1]

Aetiology and pathogenesis
Blastomycosis usually occurs after haematological spread following inhalation of spores.[1] Therefore, in addition to cutaneous lesions, most cases have internal granulomas, especially in the lungs. However, primary cutaneous infection may occur after inoculation of wounds. Large, adult, male hunting and sporting dogs are predisposed to blastomycosis,[2] presumably because of the risk of traumatic cutaneous inoculation. *Blastomycosis dermatitidis* is presumed to be a soil saprophyte associated with moist, acidic or sandy soil containing decaying wood, animal faeces or other organic matter.[1] The disease has a geographical distribution within river valleys of southern Canada and the midwestern USA.[1,2] Humans may be infected from the same sources as animals, but the disease is not zoonotic.[1]

Clinical features
Cutaneous signs of blastomycosis include multifocal subcutaneous nodules and draining tracts (**Figs. 7.22, 7.23**). The lesions may be subtle initially, but progress with time or if glucocorticoids are administered. The lesions are generally minimally painful and are not pruritic. Additional clinical signs are variable and dependent on which body organs are also affected. Pulmonary lesions are common.[1] Blastomycosis may also affect the lymph nodes, GI tract, bones, CNS, heart, urogenital system and eyes.[1]

Differential diagnoses
* Foreign body.
* Sterile nodular panniculitis.
* Other deep mycoses.
* Mycobacteria.
* Actinomycosis.
* Nocardiosis.
* Demodicosis.
* Cuterebriasis or dracunculiasis.
* Cutaneous neoplasia.
* Sterile nodular granuloma and pyogranuloma.

Diagnosis[1]
Diagnosis is made by identification of the organism (5–20-µm, refractile double-walled, broad-based budding yeast) (**Fig. 7.24**), through histopathology, surface cytology and/or fine-needle aspirate.

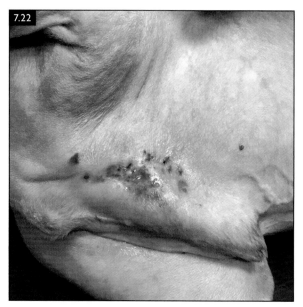

Fig. 7.22 Blastomycosis in a dog with swelling and draining sinus tracts in its groin (photo courtesy of Sheila Torres).

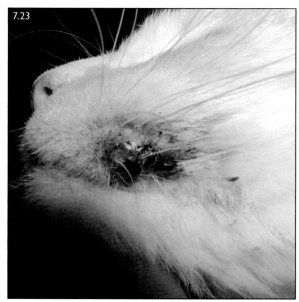

Fig. 7.23 Blastomycosis in a cat with an ulcerated nodule on its lower jaw (photo courtesy of Sheila Torres).

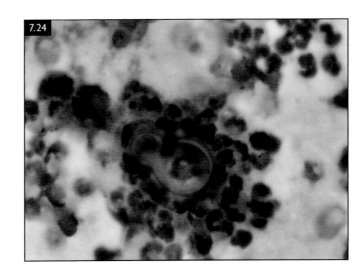

Fig. 7.24 Impression smear showing characteristic large, refractile, spheroid and thin-walled blastomyces organisms (photo courtesy of Sheila Torres).

A fine-needle aspirate of a subcutaneous nodule generally yields more organisms than an impression smear of a draining tract.

Thoracic radiographs, abdominal ultrasonography, magnetic resonance imaging and lymph node aspirates will help determine the extent of the fungal infection.

Serum and/or urine rBAD-1 antibody testing via enzyme immunoassay (EIA) is also useful for diagnosing blastomycosis. One study indicated 100% sensitivity in affected dogs;[3] however, up to 30% of dogs lack detectable antibody at the time of presentation.[1] Urine antigen testing via EIA is 93% sensitive,[1] and recommended for patients where the yeast organisms are not demonstrated.

Treatment[1]

Itraconazole (5–10 mg/kg po q24 h) is the treatment of choice.[4] Fluconazole (5–10 mg/kg po q24 h) or ketoconazole (10 mg/kg po q24 h) is also a treatment option, but may be less efficacious in some patients.[4] If significant pulmonary lesions are present, amphotericin B (1–10 mg/kg q24 h) is recommended along with itraconazole for the first 4–7 days. Corticosteroids should be administered if the patient experiences dyspnoea after initiation of antifungal therapy. Patients may require hospitalisation and oxygen therapy.

Systemic mycoses always require systemic medication, and clinical cure may take 2–10 months. Treatment should be continued for 30 days beyond clinical and radiological resolution of the lesions. In general, up to 25% of patients fail to respond to treatment.

Urine antigen testing can be useful when considering stopping treatment or if relapse of infection is suspected.[5]

Key points

- Blastomycosis is usually a systemic disease.
- Administration of corticosteroids without concurrent use of systemic antifungals leads to rapid progression of infection.

References

1   Werner A, Norton F. Blastomycosis. *Compend Contin Educ Vet* 2011; **33**: E1–E5.
2   Davies JL, Epp T, Burgess HJ. Prevalence and geographic distribution of canine and feline blastomycosis in the Canadian prairies. *Can Vet J* 2013; **54**: 753.
3   Mourning AC, Patterson EE, Kirsch EJ *et al.* Evaluation of an enzyme immunoassay for antibodies to a recombinant *Blastomyces* adhesin-1 repeat antigen as an aid in the diagnosis of blastomycosis in dogs. *J Am Vet Med Assoc* 2015; **247**: 1133–1138.
4   Mazepa ASW, Trepanier LA, Foy DS. Retrospective comparison of the efficacy of fluconazole or itraconazole for the treatment of systemic blastomycosis in dogs. *J Vet Intern Med* 2011; **25**: 440–445.
5   Foy DS, Trepanier LA, Kirsch EJ, Wheat LJ. Serum and urine *Blastomyces* antigen concentrations as markers of clinical remission in dogs treated for systemic blastomycosis. *J Vet Intern Med* 2014; **28**: 305–310.

SAPROPHYTIC DEEP FUNGAL INFECTIONS
(Eumycotic mycetoma, chromomycosis [phaeohyphomycosis and chromoblastomycosis], hyalohyphomycosis, zygomycosis)

Definition
- Eumycotic mycetomas are pyogranulomatous nodules with draining tracts and tissue granules.
- Chromomycoses are infections caused by dematiaceus (darkly pigmented) fungi of the class Deuteromycetes, which have thick walls with yeast-like swellings.
- Hyalohyphomycoses are caused by non-dematiaceous (non-pigmented) fungi.
- Zygomycoses are caused by members of the orders Mucorales, Mortierellales and Etomophthorales.

Aetiology and pathogenesis
Subcutaneous infection results from traumatic implantation from a bite, scratch or foreign material and local infection. Systemic involvement is rarely reported.[1] Granulomatous inflammation ensues and nodules, ulcerative or fistulous lesions may develop. German Shepherd dogs[2] and immunosuppressed animals[3] are most predisposed.

Clinical features
Animals present with cutaneous papules or subcutaneous nodules, which may develop ulceration or discharging tracts. Lesions typically are located on the feet, limbs or head (**Fig. 7.25**), but the abdomen and trunk may be affected. There may be local lymphadenopathy, but animals are not usually pyrexic unless there is systemic involvement. The lesions are refractory to antibacterial therapy. Disseminated disease is possible.

Differential diagnoses
- Deep bacterial infection (*Staphylococcus*, *Actinomyces* and *Nocardia* spp., bite wound, etc.).
- Cutaneous manifestation of systemic fungal infections (blastomycosis, sporotrichosis, etc.).
- Cutaneous infections of *Pythium* or *Lagenidium* spp.
- Mycobacterial infection.
- Penetrating foreign bodies.
- Sterile nodular panniculitis.

Diagnosis
Cats or dogs with multiple nodules or draining lesions of the skin should have the following performed:

- Complete blood count, serum biochemistry, urinalysis, FIV/FeLV (cats), thyroid function tests and, if in an endemic area, serology or PCR tests for mycobacteria, fungi and oomycetes antigen.
- Consider chest radiographs and abdominal ultrasonography for systemic disease.
- Cytology with Diff-Quik® type and Gram stains.
- Aerobic and anaerobic (may take 2–4 weeks) cultures of exudate and tissue; labs should be warned if zoonotic organisms are suspected (**Fig. 7.26**).
- Fungal culture of tissue (not just dermatophytes) and, if culture and histopathology support a primary saprophytic fungal infection of tissue, antifungal susceptibility testing should be performed if possible.
- Biopsies from multiple locations (or complete surgical resection of the lesion with wide margins if localised), extending the biopsy very deeply into the subcutis to reach the heart of the lesion and not just the draining tract.

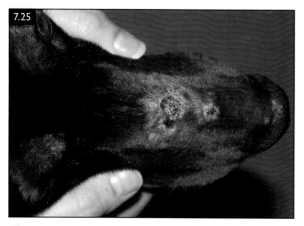

Fig. 7.25 Ulcerated and crusted nodules on the nose of a Doberman with an *Altenaria* infection.

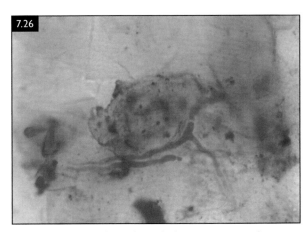

Fig. 7.26 Branching fungal elements on cytology from the lesions.

Histopathological special stains (e.g. Brown–Brenn Gram, GMS and Fite's modified acid fast) should be requested.

- Mycobacterial culture (takes months) and other diagnostic techniques (see pages 190 and 198).

Treatment

If localised, wide surgical excision of affected tissue is often curative with or without systemic antifungal therapy. In areas where complete excision may be difficult (e.g. the nasal region or disseminated disease), systemic antifungal agents such as fluconazole, ketoconazole (do not use in cats), itraconazole, terbinafine or amphotericin B may be prescribed at the upper end of the dose range, although their use has met with variable success. Treatment should be continued for months beyond apparent clinical cure, and relapses have been reported. There are no reports of consistently favourable outcomes using a certain treatment protocol for disseminated disease, and owners should be warned of the poor prognosis. For more detailed information, see Greene.[1]

Key points

- A rare infection in the USA and Europe.
- Disseminated disease has a poor prognosis.

References

1 Greene CE. *Infectious Diseases of the Dog and Cat*. New York: Elsevier Health Sciences, 2013.
2 Krockenberger MB, Swinney G, Martin P, Rothwell TR, Malik R. Sequential opportunistic infections in two German Shepherd dogs. *Aust Vet J* 2011; **89**(1–2): 9–14.
3 Dowling SR, Webb J, Foster JD *et al*. Opportunistic fungal infections in dogs treated with ciclosporin and glucocorticoids: eight cases. *J Small Anim Pract* 2016; **57**: 105–109.

STERILE NODULAR PANNICULITIS

Definition

Panniculitis is a reaction pattern characterised by inflammation of the subcutaneous fat.

Aetiology and pathogenesis

Panniculitis may result from several different aetiologies:

- Postinjection panniculitis occurs infrequently in cats and rarely in dogs. It may be underdiagnosed because clinical signs may not be obvious or may seem inconsequential. This condition has been associated with various vaccines[1] and injection of other medications, including antibiotics. The reaction may result from a combination of foreign body and hypersensitivity reactions.[1]

- Traumatic panniculitis occurs when blunt trauma, chronic pressure or decreased blood supply induces focal ischemia.[2]

- Infectious panniculitis occurs when bacteria or deep mycotic agents become established in the subcutaneous tissue.

- Foreign material deep under the skin may cause a draining panniculitis and be difficult to find on surgical exploration. These lesions are usually solitary and may be near an area of previous trauma.

- Nutritional panniculitis includes feline pansteatitis, which results from a severe, absolute or relative deficiency of vitamin E, often a result of a diet rich in oily fish[3] (see page 189).

Sterile nodular panniculitis is a diagnosis of exclusion. It is an immune-mediated deep granulomatous to pyogranulomatous disease, which causes nodules and draining tracts, that responds to immunomodulatory therapy and usually has no known trigger. Some underlying diseases include systemic lupus erythematosus, rheumatoid arthritis and pancreatitis. It has also been associated with drug reactions, infectious agents or with visceral malignancy.[2–5]

Clinical features

Lesions may be solitary or multiple (**Figs. 7.27, 7.28**). The lesions are initially often firm and deep, and eventually become more soft and superficial.[3] Some nodules regress without draining whereas others form single to multiple draining tracts that discharge an oily serosanguineous liquid. With multiple deep lesions, dogs are often lethargic, pyrexic and anorexic.[3] There is no age or sex predisposition, but Dachshunds are more frequently affected than other breeds of dogs.

Differential diagnoses

- Abscess.
- Deep cutaneous and/or systemic bacterial infection (mycobacteria, nocardiosis, actinobacillosis, etc.).
- Deep bacterial folliculitis and furunculosis.
- Deep cutaneous and/or systemic fungal infection (blastomycosis, histoplasmosis, sporotrichosis, cryptococcosis, etc.).
- Follicular inclusion cysts.
- *Cuterebra* spp. infestation.
- Cutaneous neoplasia.
- Foreign body reactions.
- Trauma.
- Injection site reaction.

Diagnosis

Systemic causes or other underlying diseases should be eliminated by performing a full work-up for internal disease. Excision or wedge biopsy of nodules should be submitted for both histopathological examination with special stains and culture and sensitivity to help rule out infectious agents. Single lesions warrant a surgical search for foreign material, removing the nodule and submitting for pathology, special stains and tissue cultures.

Treatment

Panniculitis secondary to systemic diseases should resolve when appropriate treatment is instituted. Solitary lesions often do not recur after surgical removal.

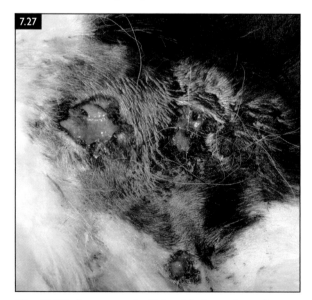

Fig. 7.27 Acute panniculitis with deep ulceration and draining sinus tracts in a Papillion.

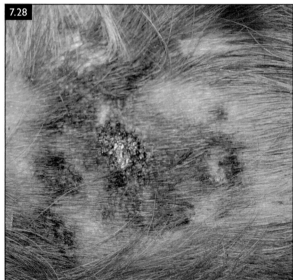

Fig. 7.28 Chronic panniculitis with erythematous nodules, hyperpigmentation, erosions and scarring.

- Animals with idiopathic sterile nodular panniculitis often require long-term or permanent remission after the lesions have resolved.
- Most cases respond well to systemic glucocorticoids. Methylprednisolone (0.3–1.0 mg/kg po) or prednisone (1–2 mg/kg po) may be given daily until lesions resolve (usually 3–6 weeks), before tapering the dose. Fever and other systemic signs generally resolve rapidly.
- The combination of doxycycline or minocycline antibiotic (5 mg/kg po q12 h) and niacinamide (250 mg po q12 h in dogs <10 kg and 500 mg po q12 h in dogs >10 kg) often works well, although it may take a month or so of treatment for effectiveness to be seen, so starting initially with glucocorticoids will hasten resolution.
- Daily supplementation with vitamin E (300 IU) may have a steroid-sparing action in some cases.
- Ciclosporin (modified) given at 5 mg/kg po q24 h to remission and then tapering the frequency is also often effective,[6] but the onset of improvement is sometimes slow, so initial treatment with steroids can be used to hasten remission in severe cases.
- Intralesional injection of dexamethasone has also been reported.
- Other therapies may need to be used in refractory cases, particularly those associated with other immune-mediated diseases (see Immunosuppressive Drug Therapy Table, page 289).

Key point

- There are many diseases that cause panniculitis. Sterile nodular panniculitis is a diagnosis of exclusion.

References

1   Hendrick MJ, Dunagan CA. Focal necrotizing granulomatous panniculitis associated with subcutaneous injection of rabies vaccine in cats and dogs: 10 cases (1988–1989). *J Am Vet Med Assoc* 1991; **198**: 304–305.
2   Shanley KJ, Miller WH. Panniculitis in the dog: a report of five cases. *J Am Anim Hosp Assoc* 1985; **21**: 545–550.
3   Hagiwara MK, Guerra JL, Maeoka MRM. Pansteatitis (yellow fat disease) in a cat. *Feline Pract* 1986; **16**: 25–27.
4   Scott DW, Anderson WI. Panniculitis in dogs and cats: a retrospective analysis of 78 cases. *J Am Anim Hosp Assoc* 1988; **24**: 551–559.
5   Gross TL, Ihrke PJ, Walder EJ. Diseases of the panniculus. In: *Veterinary Dermatopathology*. St Louis, MO: Mosby Year Book, 1992: pp. 316–326.
6   Contreary CL, Outerbridge CA, Affolter VK, Kass PH, White SD. Canine sterile nodular panniculitis: a retrospective study of 39 dogs. *Vet Dermatol* 2015; **26**: 451–e105.

DERMOID SINUS

Definition

A dermoid sinus is a persistent congenital connection between the dura and the skin of the dorsal midline.

Aetiology and pathogenesis

A dermoid sinus results from incomplete separation of the ectoderm and the neural tube during embryogenesis.[1] Rarely, similar cysts and connections may be seen on the head, connecting with the dura via a skull defect. Accumulation of keratinaceous debris and sebum may result in inflammation and secondary bacterial infection.[2] Neurological signs may accompany inflammation or infection.

Clinical features

There is no sex predisposition, but Rhodesian Ridgebacks are predisposed, with an autosomal dominant mode of inheritance.[1] Rarely, other breeds may be affected such as Boxers, Shih Tzus, Bull Terriers, Golden Retrievers, Huskies, Springer Spaniels and Yorkshire Terriers.[2–5]. Cats are very rarely affected.[6] The clinical signs may be minimal, e.g. a whorl of hair on the dorsal midline. Sometimes, hairs or even discharge may be apparent emerging from the sinus (**Figs. 7.29–7.31**). Closed sinus tracts may present as non-painful, soft-to-fluctuating nodules in the midline. Neurological signs vary from non-existent to dramatic.

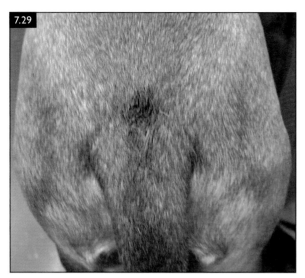

Fig. 7.29 Dermoid sinus in a dog with a crusted lesion on the midline of its tailbase (photo courtesy of Silvia Rufenacht).

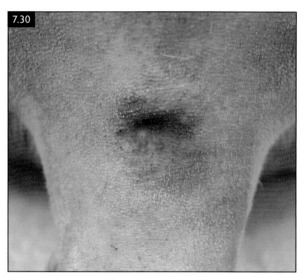

Fig. 7.30 The area in Fig. 7.29 has been clipped to show the opening to the sinus (photo courtesy of Silvia Rufenacht).

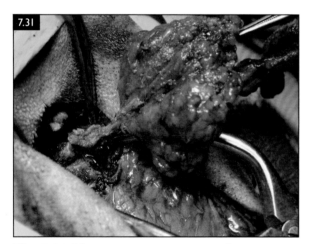

Fig. 7.31 The sinus tract in Fig. 7.30 is being dissected away from the surrounding tissues (photo courtesy of Silvia Rufenacht).

Differential diagnoses
- Foreign body penetration.
- Injection reaction.
- Neoplasia, particularly keratoacanthomas or follicular tumours.
- Cysts.
- Naevi.

Diagnosis
The clinical signs are very suggestive, especially if neurological signs are present. Radiography and contrast radiography may be necessary to delineate the sinus tract and confirm the diagnosis.[2]

Treatment
Surgical excision of the tract and associated debris is the treatment of choice.[2]

Key point
- Pathognomonic presentation in Rhodesian Ridgebacks.

References
1   Salmon Hillbertz NHC, Andersson G. Autosomal dominant mutation causing the dorsal ridge predisposes for dermoid sinus in Rhodesian Ridgeback dogs. *J Small Anim Pract* 2006; **47**: 184–188.

2   Burrow RD. A nasal dermoid sinus in an English bull terrier. *J Small Anim Pract* 2004; **45**: 572–574.

3   Cornegliani L, Ghibaudo G. A dermoid sinus in a Siberian Husky. *Vet Dermatol* 1999; **10**: 47–49.

4   Cornegliani L, Jommi E, Vercelli A. Dermoid sinus in a golden retriever. *J Small Anim Pract* 2001; **42**: 514–516.

5   Pratt JNJ, Knottenbelt CM, Welsh EM. Dermoid sinus at the lumbosacral junction in an English springer spaniel. *J Small Anim Pract* 2000; **41**: 24–26.

6   Fleming JM, Platt SR, Kent M, Freeman AC, Schatzberg SJ. Cervical dermoid sinus in the cat: case presentation and review of the literature. *J Feline Med Surg* 2011; **13**: 992–996.

PERIANAL FISTULAE
(Anal furunculosis)

Definition
Perianal fistulae are ulcerations and sinus tracts involving the perianal and perirectal tissues, due a chronic inflammatory process that often extends into the anal mucosa.

Aetiology and pathogenesis
Perianal fistulae are immune mediated with a genetic predisposition, but the true aetiology is unknown.[1] Perianal fistulae in dogs share many similarities with the anal fistulation seen in Crohn's disease in humans.[1]

Clinical features
The condition is most common in German Shepherd dogs (**Fig. 7.32**), but has also been diagnosed in other breeds. The most common clinical signs are pain and straining while defecating, narrowed or ribbon-like stools, diarrhoea, weight loss, matting of hair with faecal material surrounding the anus, foul odour, not wanting to sit and frequent licking of the anal area. The perineum is often very painful and many animals must be sedated to evaluate the extent of the lesions. Erythema with raw tracts and ulcers vary from pinpoint solitary lesions to 360° deep fistulation of the perianal area.[2] The tracts may have a slit-like appearance and extend deeply into the anus or anal sacs. Rectal palpation often reveals firm, granulomatous change to the anal lining. Affected German Shepherd dogs frequently have a concurrent colitis and may have concurrent lesions of German Shepherd dog pyoderma.

Differential diagnoses
- Anal sac abscess.
- Anal or rectal neoplasia.
- Rectal foreign bodies.
- Rectal fistula.

Diagnosis
Diagnosis is based on history and clinical findings. Biopsy may be helpful in more equivocal cases. A careful history will help identify dogs with concurrent GI disease that will benefit from a trial

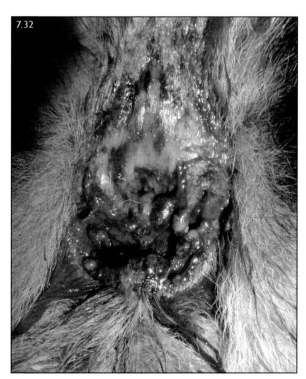

Fig. 7.32 Perianal fistulas in a German Shepherd dog with severe ulceration, under running of the skin, and draining sinus tracts.

with a novel limited ingredient or hydrolysed diet (see page 18).

Treatment
- The treatment of choice is modified ciclosporin at 5 mg/kg po q12–24 h, which results in clinical improvement in almost all cases and resolution of lesions in 50–100% of cases. Clinical improvement is generally seen by 4 weeks, although resolution may take months. Lesions often recur upon discontinuing medications and so long-term therapy is needed in most cases. Some dogs require higher doses for full remission.
- Tacrolimus ointment 0.1% applied twice daily may prevent recurrence or can be used for mild or superficial disease. Most pets are too painful initially for topical therapy.
- Dietary management with or without sulfasalazine (1 g po q8 h for at least 4 months, or 1 month after cessation of prednisone therapy) is helpful in cases with concurrent colitis.

- Dogs that fail to respond to or cannot tolerate ciclosporin can be treated with prednisone/prednisolone (1–2 mg/kg po q24 h until resolution of lesions, and then tapered to 0.5 mg/kg po q24 h for an additional 6–8 weeks) and/or other immunosuppressive agents (see Immunosuppressive Drug Therapy Table, page 289) with or without 0.1% tacrolimus ointment q12 h.
- Surgery is no longer recommended routinely due to complications. The only exception may be if the anal sacs are chronically involved, where anal sacculectomy may be helpful.

Key points
- Pathognomonic presentation.
- More likely to be a situation where the disease is controlled rather than cured.

References
1 Massey J, Short AD, Catchpole B *et al*. Genetics of canine anal furunculosis in the German shepherd dog. *Immunogenetics* 2014; **66**: 311–324.
2 Patterson AP, Campbell KL. Managing anal furunculosis in dogs. *Compend Contin Educ Vet* 2005; **27**: 339–355.

METATARSAL FISTULATION

Definition
Metatarsal fistulation is an uncommon condition where draining tracts occur in the skin of the plantar metatarsal area.

Aetiology and pathogenesis
The pathogenesis of this condition is unknown, but circulating antibodies to types I and II collagen were elevated in some affected dogs.[1]

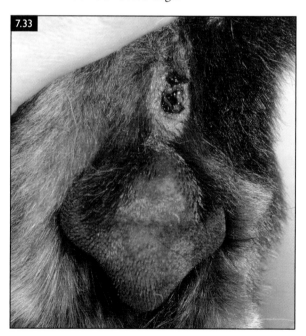

Fig. 7.33 Swelling, ulceration and a draining sinus tract just proximal to the metatarsal pad in a German Shepherd cross.

Clinical features
The condition is found in German Shepherd dogs (GSDs), crossbreeds of GSDs[1] and occasionally other breeds.[2] Initial lesions consist of a soft swelling in the skin, which progress to well-demarcated single or multiple tracts containing a serosanguineous discharge located on the plantar metatarsal skin surface, just proximal to the metatarsal pad (**Fig. 7.33**). Both hindlimbs are affected and occasionally lesions occur in the plantar metacarpal skin. Secondary bacterial infection can occur once sinus tracts develop. The affected skin of chronic lesions may become scarred. Pain is variable, but appears to be mild in most dogs.

Differential diagnoses
There would not be many differentials with bilaterally symmetrical disease with no systemic signs, but if asymmetrical or the pet is sick, consider the following:

- Foreign body.
- Puncture wound.
- Subcutaneous mycosis such as blastomycosis.
- Deep bacterial infection such as actinomycosis.

Diagnosis
Any case with fever or changes on blood work should have infectious causes more aggressively ruled out. When this disease is suspected, cytology, bacterial culture and biopsy with special stains to rule out other causes should be considered before empirical treatment.

Treatment

- Modified ciclosporin 5 mg/kg per day is the treatment of choice.
- Other options include topical 0.1% tacrolimus q12 h, topical fluocinolone/DMSO, prednisolone at 1 mg/kg per day and then tapered,[3] doxycycline or minocycline and niacinamide, or vitamin E.

Key point

- Be aware that this is a condition generally controlled but not cured, and it may need long-term medications and management to maintain remission.

References

1 Gross TL, Ihrke PJ, Walder EJ, Affolter VK. Metatarsal fistulation of German Shepherd Dogs. In: *Skin Diseases of the Dog and Cat: Clinical and Histopathologic Diagnosis*, 2nd edn. Oxford: Blackwell Publishing, 2005: pp. 553–555.
2 Oliveira AM. Focal metatarsal sinus tracts in a Weimaraner successfully managed with ciclosporin. *J Small Anim Pract* 2007; **48**: 161–164.
3 Paterson S. Sterile idiopathic pedal panniculitis in the German shepherd dog – clinical presentation and response to treatment of four cases. *J Small Anim Pract* 1995; **36**: 498–50.

CHAPTER 8

DISEASES OF THE PAWS AND NAILS

GENERAL APPROACH TO PAWS AND NAILS

Fig. 8.1 outlines the basic principles of the diagnostic work-up of nail and paw disease.

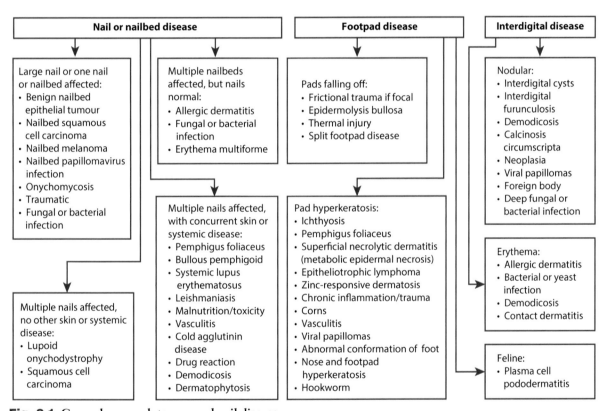

Fig. 8.1 General approach to paw and nail disease.

INTERDIGITAL CYSTS AND FURUNCULOSIS

Definition

Interdigital furunculosis is an inflammatory process that is usually multi-factorial. It is characterised by swelling and draining tracts between the toes.

Aetiology and pathogenesis

It is useful to think about these cases as having primary, predisposing and perpetuating causes, and secondary infections similar to chronic otitis. The recurrent interdigital 'cysts' on the dorsal surface of the interdigital web are often the first thing to be noticed, but it is important to realise that the condition originates on the underside of the feet.

Primary triggers include any abnormal pressure to the haired skin of the feet, which may be caused by flat-footed conformation, sideways walking on the foot pads, musculoskeletal problems (e.g. osteoarthritis, hip dysplasia or dysplasia of the elbows[1]), or housing on a slatted or wire-bottom cage.[2] Other primary causes of pedal inflammation and infection include atopic dermatitis, food allergies, contact dermatitis, *Demodex* spp. and hypothyroidism, particularly if the feet become swollen, thereby altering weight bearing and occluding interdigital spaces.

Predisposing factors include bent leg or splay foot conformation, short-hair coats and obesity. Underlying diseases that predispose to infection include endocrinopathies, hepatic disease, cancer or immunosuppressive therapy.[3,4]

Perpetuating problems arise when the hair follicles around the pads or in the interdigital skin become trapped in hyperplastic or callused skin and form cystic structures under the skin. Further trauma results in inflammatory foreign body reactions and will often drain from the dorsal interdigital web.[5] Scarring and swelling cause more of the haired interdigital skin to be exposed to pressure, thereby spreading the problem. Chronic problems include conjoined pads, new pad formation and deep tissue folds and pockets.

Secondary infections are common. Most involve staphylococci but *Escherichia coli* and other gram-negative bacteria can also be found. Mixed infections are not uncommon and the organisms in deep lesions may be different from those on the interdigital skin surface. Repeated use of antibiotics can select for antimicrobial-resistant bacteria.

Interdigital furunculosis may occur with or without cysts if there is deep inflammation or infection associated with a hair follicle. Interdigital furunculosis is common with demodicosis and staphylococcal infections. A subset of pododermatitis cases shows lymphocytic plasmacytic inflammation (without noted folliculitis or furunculosis) on biopsy and respond only to immune modulation.[6]

Clinical features (Figs. 8.2–8.6)

Interdigital cysts are most common in larger breeds of dogs with short hair, such as Pitbulls, American Bulldogs, English Bulldogs, Great Danes, Boxers, Mastiffs, Weimaraners and Vizslas. Dogs are

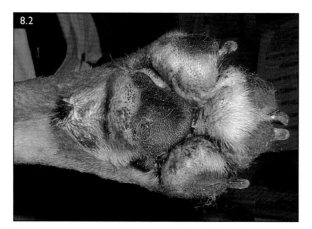

Fig. 8.2 Severe erythema, swelling, ulceration and sinus tracts in a dog with pedal deep pyoderma.

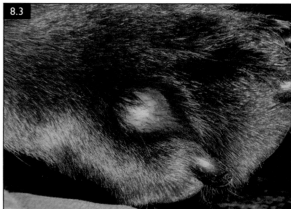

Fig. 8.3 Interdigital furunculosis ('cysts') in a Labrador with atopic dermatitis.

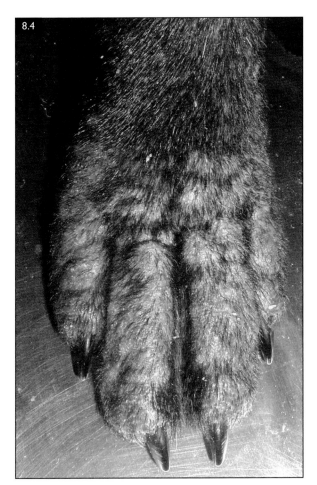

Fig. 8.4 Severe erythema, furunculosis, scarring and alopecia in a Staffordshire Bull Terrier with idiopathic sterile lymphocytic–plasmacytic pododermatitis.

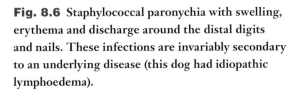

Fig. 8.6 Staphylococcal paronychia with swelling, erythema and discharge around the distal digits and nails. These infections are invariably secondary to an underlying disease (this dog had idiopathic lymphoedema).

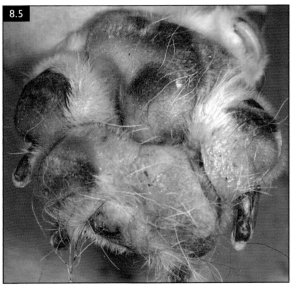

Fig. 8.5 Severe pododermatitis in an English Bulldog with new pad formation, conjoined pads, interdigital pockets, ingrown hairs, comedones, sinus tracts and secondary infection. Trigger factors in this dog included obesity and a food allergy.

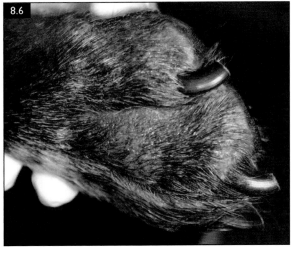

generally older than 1 year, with an average of approximately 4 years.[2] If a younger dog is presented, demodicosis should be strongly suspected. The front feet are often affected more severely than the hind feet. Interdigital furunculosis (without cysts) can be found in any breed or size pet. These conditions are usually more painful than pruritic, although secondary infections and allergies may also cause pruritus. Animals are usually presented for swelling or draining lesions on the dorsal aspect of the interdigital skin. Sometimes pets are presented for lameness or licking the feet. Thorough evaluation of the palmar aspect of the foot is vital to determine the extent and severity of the disease if cystic follicles are present. Comedones on weight-bearing skin are an early sign of cystic follicles.

Differential diagnoses

- Allergic dermatitis predisposes to interdigital inflammation and infections.
- Primary infections such as demodicosis, actinomycosis, mycobacteria or *Nocardia* spp. can cause interdigital nodular and draining lesions.
- Penetration of parasites such as *Pelodera* or *Ancylostoma* spp. may cause pododermatitis.
- Interdigital foreign bodies can cause interdigital swelling and draining tracts; usually only one foot is affected.
- Neoplasia usually affects only one foot.
- Calcinosis circumscripta is visually distinctive, and biopsy would rule it out.
- Viral papillomas are inflammatory and nodular, and are often interdigital.
- Systemic fungal infections such as blastomycosis can cause interdigital draining tracts, but the pet is also systemically ill.

The lesions of this condition are highly distinctive; the diagnostic challenge is often more in identifying all the potential triggers in an individual dog.

Diagnosis

- Cytology of interdigital skin may reveal yeast or bacterial infections, although these organisms may differ from those in deeper lesions.
- Cytology of draining lesions may reveal pyogranulomatous inflammation, hair fragments, bacteria or other organisms.
- Skin scrapings and hair plucks will help to rule out demodicosis.
- Bacterial culture and sensitivity should be performed of any draining lesions; biopsy may be necessary to obtain representative material.
- Pets should be evaluated for osteoarthritis, hip dysplasia, elbow dysplasia and other musculoskeletal problems.
- With systemic signs or suspicion of parasites, complete blood counts, serum biochemistry, thyroid tests, faecal flotation and urinalysis should be performed.
- Biopsy and histopathology may be needed to confirm the diagnosis.

Treatment

- It is critical to address all the triggers in each case. The condition is otherwise likely to recur as the pet walks on new areas of haired skin. Underlying conditions such as allergies, arthritis or immunosuppression need to be addressed.
- Primary infectious causes such as demodicosis need to be treated.
- Weight-loss programmes should be started to maintain dogs at or slightly under their ideal body weight.
- The animal should not be kept on slatted, wire or rough flooring.
- Secondary bacterial or yeast infections need to be treated. If draining tracts are present, then antibiotic treatment, based on culture, needs to be prolonged. Often 4–8 weeks of antibiotic are needed.
- When draining lesions are present, magnesium sulphate (Epsom salt) soaks for 10 minutes twice daily can be helpful.
- Anti-inflammatory doses of steroids (prednisone 1 mg/kg per day until resolution, then taper) are an effective way to alleviate pain and inflammation. The clinician must rule out primary infection before starting steroid therapy.
- Ciclosporin (modified) at 5 mg/kg per day, perhaps eventually tapering to every other day (see Immunosuppressive Drug Therapy Table, page 289), can be used in cases that need constant long-term management. Other steroid-sparing options include azathioprine, chlorambucil, mycophenolate and methotrexate.
- Complete surgical fusion podoplasty, by surgical removal of all interdigital skin and suturing the pads together to form a complete weight-bearing surface, may be useful in select cases.[7] Surgical or CO_2 laser removal of large areas of interdigital skin is sometimes helpful. Conservative surgical approaches often result in cyst recurrence.

Key points

- Rule out infectious primary causes, treat underlying diseases, and look for and treat secondary infections.
- Bacterial culture and sensitivity of deep draining lesions are critically important to diagnose secondary infections.
- Lifelong management may be needed.

References

1   Paterson S. Elbow dysplasia as a cause of interdigital cysts in 20 dogs *Vet Dermatol* 2012; **23**: 90–91.
2   Kovacs MS, McKiernan S, Potter DM, Chilappagari S. An epidemiological study of interdigital cysts in a research beagle colony. *J Am Assoc Lab Anim Sci* 2005; **44**: 17–21.
3   Breathnach RM, Fanning S, Mulcahy G, Bassett HF, Jones BR. Canine pododermatitis and idiopathic disease. *Vet J* 2008; **176**: 146–157.
4   Duclos D. Canine pododermatitis. *Vet Clin North Am Small Anim Pract* 2013; **43**: 57–87.
5   Duclos DD, Hargis AM, Hanley PW. Pathogenesis of canine interdigital palmar and plantar comedones and follicular cysts, and their response to laser surgery. *Vet Dermatol* 2008; **19**: 134–141.
6   Breathnach RM, Baker KP, Quinn PJ, McGeady TA, Aherne CM, Jones BR. Clinical, immunological and histopathological findings in a subpopulation of dogs with pododermatitis. *Vet Dermatol* 2005; **16**: 364–372.
7   Papazoglou LG, Ellison GW, Farese JP *et al*. Fusion podoplasty for the management of chronic pedal conditions in seven dogs and one cat. *J Am Anim Hosp Assoc* 2011; **47**: e199–e205.

NEOPLASIA OF THE NAILBEDS AND FEET

Squamous cell carcinoma, melanoma, mast cell tumour, keratoacanthoma, inverted papilloma, lymphosarcoma, eccrine adenocarcinoma, neurofibrosarcoma, haemangiopericytoma, fibrosarcoma, metastatic pulmonary adenocarcinoma and osteosarcoma have all been reported to occur in the nailbed. Animals are presented for swelling of the claw or digit, and variable degrees of onychomadesis, paronychia, onychodystrophy, erosion and ulceration.

Squamous cell carcinomas are the most common digital tumours in dogs; 75% of those affected are large breeds, 70% are black in colour. Multiple digits may be involved over a course of 2–6 years.[1]

In dogs, **melanomas** of the digits and footpads carry a worse prognosis than melanomas on other areas of the skin. At digital melanoma presentation, metastatic lesions are found in 30–40% of patients. Of the patients in which melanoma metastases were not found at presentation and the digit was amputated, only 42–57% were alive at 1 year and 11–13% at 2 years.[2]

Dark pigmentation of a digital mass or radiographic bony destruction of bone strongly indicates a cancerous process. In dogs, surgical removal of the affected digit or digits with histopathology is the treatment of choice. If cancer is suspected, the lung fields should be radiographed and local lymph nodes aspirated before surgery to look for metastases. The local lymph node should be excised during surgery and submitted for histopathological examination as well.

In cats, the most common digital tumour is **metastatic pulmonary adenocarcinoma**. Most cats present for lameness rather than respiratory signs. Chest radiographs show lung masses. Removal of the affected digits is not helpful.

Calcinosis circumscripta (see page 220) can be nodular, light coloured, firm masses on the footpads and feet.

Viral papillomas (see page 252) are commonly seen as rapidly appearing masses interdigitally or on the lower legs; they are often painful especially when foot lesions result in a keratin horn or nail-like structure. Viral papillomas usually resolve on their own in a few weeks to months. If non-resolving, these can progress to squamous cell carcinoma.

Sebaceous adenomas (see page 250) are common on the feet of dogs; complete removal is curative.

References

1   MG, Berg J, Engler SJ. Treatment by digital amputation of subungual squamous cell carcinoma in dogs: 21 cases (1987–1988). *J Am Vet Med A* 1992; **201**(5):759–761.
2   Nishiya A, Massoco C, Felizzola C, Perlmann E, Batschinski K, Tedardi M *et al*. Comparative aspects of canine melanoma. *Vet Sci* 2016; **3**(1): 7.

CALCINOSIS CIRCUMSCRIPTA

Definition

Calcinosis circumscripta is a tumour-like nodule of the skin resulting from dystrophic calcification.

Aetiology and pathogenesis

Lesions appear at sites of repetitive or previous trauma such as pressure points, footpads or sites of injury.[1-3] The specific mechanism of the calcium salt deposition is not understood. Hypercalcaemia is not present in most dogs.

Clinical features

Lesions occur more frequently in young, rapidly growing dogs, with German Shepherd dogs (**Fig. 8.7**), Boston Terriers and Boxers predisposed.[2] Firm, well-circumscribed, generally single nodules ranging from 0.5 cm to 7 cm occur in the subcutaneous tissue at sites of pressure points, footpads, chronic injury or the tongue.[1-3] Ulceration may occur in larger lesions or with repeated trauma. Lesions are non-painful, except for those occurring

in the footpads. White gritty or pasty material may extrude from the lesions.[2]

Differential diagnoses

- Metastatic calcification secondary to chronic renal failure.
- Calcinosis cutis.
- Viral papillomatosis.
- Granulomatous disease due to an infectious agent.

Diagnosis

- Cytology may show calcium fragments and granulomatous inflammation.
- Biopsy and histopathology are diagnostic; special stains help to rule out infectious agents.
- Radiology, if necessary, to demonstrate deposits of calcium if the nodules are deep within the metacarpal or metatarsal pads.
- Further investigation including complete blood counts, serum biochemistry and ionised calcium may be necessary in individual cases, but most affected animals are otherwise normal.

Treatment

Surgical excision is curative.

Key point

- This disease is idiopathic in most cases; surgical excision is curative.

References

1. Gross TH, Ihrke PJ, Walder EJ, Affolter VK. Calcinosis circumscripta. In: *Skin Diseases of the Dog and Cat: Clinical and Histopathologic Diagnosis*, 2nd edn. Oxford: Blackwell Publishing, 2005: pp. 378–380.
2. Scott DW, Buerger RG. Idiopathic calcinosis circumscripta in the dog: a retrospective analysis of 130 cases. *J Am Anim Hosp Assoc* 1988; **24**: 187–189.
3. Tafti AK, Hanna P, Bourque AC. Calcinosis circumscripta in the dog: a retrospective pathological study. *J Vet Med A* 2005; **52**(1): 13–17.

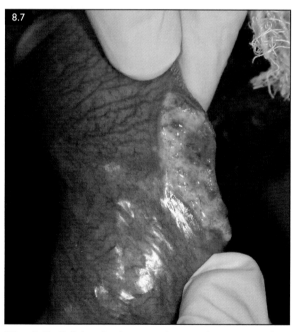

Fig. 8.7 Calcinosis circumscripta in the tongue of a German Shepherd dog; note the characteristic white deposits.

VASCULITIS OF THE FOOTPADS

Definition

Vasculitis, or inflammation of the blood vessels, can affect multiple organs of the body including the skin. This section focuses on the appearance of vasculitis when it affects the footpads. Vasculitic lesions may be limited to the footpads, or may affect many parts of the skin including the footpads (see page 182).

Aetiology and pathogenesis

Vasculitis is caused by antigen–antibody complexes that deposit in blood vessel walls.[1] The resultant damage to blood vessels impairs blood flow and causes ischaemic lesions in associated tissue.

Vasculitis may be triggered by any number of infectious, neoplastic or inflammatory conditions. Tick-borne disease, feline leukaemia virus (FeLV), feline immunodeficiency virus (FIV), adverse reaction to food, vaccination (especially rabies vaccines) and drugs are some of the more commonly implicated causes. However, it is not uncommon to see idiopathic vasculitis.[1]

Clinical features

Vasculitis of the paw pads is characterised by acute onset, variable pain, variable erythema and oedema. Characteristic, well-demarcated, circular erosions or ulcerations ('punched-out ulcers') occur in the central portion of one or more pads.[2]

Differential diagnoses

- Contact dermatosis.
- Pemphigus foliaceus.
- *Leishmania* spp.
- Split-pad disease.
- Corns.
- Viral papillomas.

Diagnosis

Clinical signs typically lead to a high index of suspicion for vasculitis. A thorough history, physical exam, complete blood count, serum chemistry, urinalysis, viral panel (for cats) and tick-borne disease screening are necessary to rule in or out underlying causes of the vasculitis. These tests also help determine if other body organs are affected.[1]

Skin biopsy will also aid in the diagnosis. The clinician should be certain to include epithelium in the biopsy sample. Where possible, multiple biopsies should be selected to maximise the chances of finding diagnostic changes.

Treatment

Underlying causes should be removed or treated if possible. If vaccination is suspected as the trigger for the vasculitis, the pet should avoid further exposure to the vaccine in question. Repeat vaccination could cause a recurrence of vasculitis that is more severe than the initial presentation. Alternative vaccination strategies (e.g. fewer vaccines, different vaccines and/or serological testing) based on the risk of exposure should be discussed with the owners.

If other body organs are affected, treatment should be directed based on the organ affected (e.g. glomerulonephritis).

Skin lesions can be managed with a variety of medications. Skin lesions that have an identifiable underlying cause may be curable. Skin lesions due to idiopathic vasculitis typically require lifelong medication. Glucocorticoids (1–2 mg/kg po q24 h until lesions are in remission, then taper to q48 h dosing) can be used to induce quick remission of lesions. They can be used concurrently with medications that are more appropriate for chronic therapy. Medications appropriate for chronic therapy include doxycycline and niacinamide, pentoxifylline or ciclosporin. (See Immunosuppressive Drug Therapy Table, page 289, for dosages.)

Doxycycline and niacinamide can take 2–3 months to reach maximum effect. Pentoxifylline and ciclosporin can take 4–6 weeks to reach maximum effect. If these lesions are used concurrently with glucocorticoids, the glucocorticoids should be discontinued when the drug being used for chronic therapy is expected to be at maximum effect. Sulfasalazine (10–20 mg/kg po q8–12 h) can be quite effective for vasculitis in dogs, and lesions tend to resolve within 4–6 weeks. Many dogs tolerate this medication well; however, keratoconjunctivitis sicca and hepatotoxicity are possible. Schirmer tear tests, complete blood count and serum chemistry should be checked after 1 month of treatment, and then repeated at least every 6 months for dogs receiving sulfasalazine.

No treatment is uniformly effective for vasculitis. If one therapy does not work, then another therapy should be tried.[2]

Key points

- Vasculitis is often a condition that can be controlled but not cured.
- It is important to determine if vasculitis is systemic or isolated to the skin.

References

1 Innerå, M. Cutaneous vasculitis in small animals. *Vet Clin North Am Small Anim Pract* 2013; **43**: 113–134.
2 Nichols PR, Morris DO, Beale KM. A retrospective study of canine and feline cutaneous vasculitis. *Vet Dermatol* 2001; **12**: 255–264.

SYMMETRICAL LUPOID ONYCHITIS
(Onychodystrophy)

Symmetrical lupoid onychodystrophy, symmetrical onychomadesis, lupoid onychodystrophy

Definition

Symmetrical onychitis is an idiopathic condition affecting only the nails in dogs, where nail plates separate from the underlying quick and dry, brittle, misshapen nails regrow.

Aetiology and pathogenesis

Symmetrical lupoid onychitis is an immune-mediated disease that is characterised by a lymphoplasmacytic subepidermal infiltrate and necrosis of the basal epidermal cells of the claw, causing the nail plate to loosen and break free from the quick. This inflammatory pattern is similar to what is seen in lupus,

hence the term 'lupoid' often used in the literature. There is no evidence that this is related to the disease of lupus: antinuclear antibody testing is always negative and dogs have no other (known) systemic disease or skin lesions related to this condition.[1]

Clinical features (Figs. 8.8–8.11)

Certain medium/large breed dogs are predisposed including Schnauzers, German Shepherds,[1,2] Gordon Setters,[3] English Setters[3] and Rottweilers. The reported age range is broad – 6 months to 12 years.[2]

Onychomadesis (nails loosening and falling off) with exudate under the claw plate of one or a few claws is the most common clinical presentation, although sometimes the loss of a nail is not noticed and only the dry, brittle nails (onychodystrophy) are questioned by

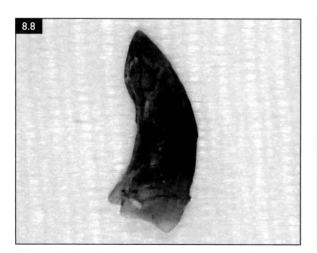

Fig. 8.8 Sloughed nail from an acute case of symmetrical lupoid onychodystrophy.

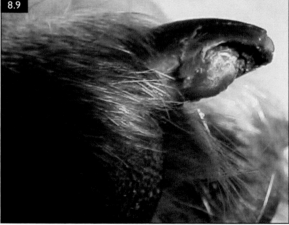

Fig. 8.9 Early symmetrical lupoid onychodystrophy with swelling, subungual haemorrhage and early lifting of the claw nail plate.

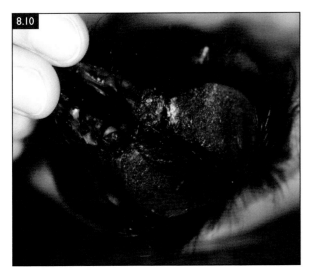

Fig. 8.10 Acute symmetrical lupoid onychodystrophy with separation and lifting of the claws, claw loss and secondary infection with a haemopurulent discharge; this stage is very painful.

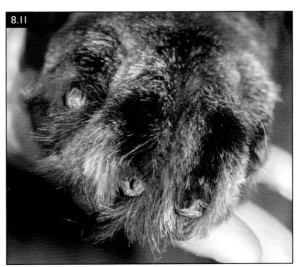

Fig. 8.11 Chronic symmetrical lupoid onychodystrophy with friable and dystrophic claws; this stage is less painful but the claws are vulnerable to fracture, loss and infection.

the owner. In some cases, involvement will initially occur in only one to three nails, but slowly over a 9-week period (sometimes longer) many, if not all, of the claws will become involved. After sloughing, dry, brittle, misshapen nail plates regrow. If untreated, resloughing may occur, although some dogs self-resolve. Pain is pronounced at the time of nail plate sloughing. Secondary infection is common.

Differential diagnoses

- Trauma is a common reason for nails to fall off; however more than two nails being affected within a few months, or abnormally brittle, short, cracked nails in an otherwise healthy dog, should raise suspicion of lupoid onychitis.
- Neoplasia of the nailbed may cause a nail to fall off, and neoplasia may affect multiple nails at the same time. Often the nailbeds are infiltrated and enlarged more than what would be typical of just an inflamed quick.
- Immune-mediated disease – vasculitis, epidermolysis bullosa, drug reaction, systemic lupus erythematosus and pemphigus, can all affect the nails but systemic signs or other skin symptoms would typically be present. It would be extremely unusual for these diseases to affect only the nails.

- Any disease that affects the claw fold and claw bed may cause nail abnormalities; however, concurrent skin or systemic signs would also be observed (leishmaniasis, larval migrans, demodicosis, dermatophytosis, hypothyroidism, diabetes, superficial necrolytic dermatitis and zinc-responsive dermatosis).

Diagnosis

- Clinical appearance with absence of other skin or systemic symptoms is diagnostic.
- Blood work should be normal, other than perhaps mild inflammatory changes.
- Cytology will help reveal if secondary bacterial overgrowth is present, and culture and sensitivity may be required to select an appropriate antibiotic. Repeated antibiotic use can select for antibiotic resistance in these cases.
- It is not easy to obtain a definitive diagnosis without amputation and histopathology of the third phalanx (P3). However, this is not recommended as a diagnostic test unless there is a high suspicion of cancer.
- Radiographs rarely reveal bony changes unless the onychitis has progressed to osteomyelitis in severe cases or neoplasia is present.

Treatment

- Treatments require up to 3 months to be helpful, because the entire new nail must regrow while on the treatment.
- Throughout the treatment, loose nails may need to be periodically removed. As the abnormal nails grow out, they need to be kept well trimmed to help prevent traumatic splitting.
- The claws should be kept trimmed short. Owners should use a nail file or an electric disc-sanding tool designed for use on nails, because (unlike nail clippers) they do not split or crack the nails. Tough nail varnish may help reduce splitting and cracking of the nails
- The loose, cracked nail plates are prone to infection and repeated flexing as the dog walks may be painful. For severe, painful cases, anaesthesia and removal of all loose or inflamed nail plates give the most rapid pain relief. With removal of the nail plate, it is important to preserve the quick for the best nail regrowth. The bare quicks rapidly dry out and become non-painful in 2–3 days. Residual pain suggests that not all of the nail plate has been removed.
- Spontaneous remission has been reported.[1,2] In addition, once initial disease has been controlled, some dogs remain in remission long term without further treatment.[2,4]
- This disease usually needs to be treated lifelong although, after 3–4 months with no nail breakage and if the nails look fairly normal, doses of medications may be able to be slowly decreased. In some cases, omega 3-fatty acids alone are effective to prevent recurrence of disease.
- The goal of therapy is to prevent nails from painfully breaking, separating and sloughing, and not the regrowth of normal looking nails. Although some dogs do regrow visually normal nails, most dogs regrow nails that are mildly abnormal in some way.
- The most typical therapy for this condition is one of the following tetracycline class drugs with niacinamide:
  - 250 mg tetracycline and 250 mg niacinamide for dogs <15 kg, and 500 mg each for dogs >15 kg po q8 h;
  - doxycycline 5–10 mg/kg q12 h with niacinamide as above;
  - minocycline 5–10 mg/kg q12 h with niacinamide as above;
  - ciclosporin 5 mg/kg po q24 h is also effective (see Immunosuppressive Drug Therapy Table, page 289).
- High doses of omega 3-fatty acids should always be used in combination with any therapy given; diets high in omega 3-fatty acids may be helpful.[4]
- Biotin (0.05 mg/kg po q24 h) may be beneficial as adjunct therapy in many cases.
- Gelatin (10 grains [600 mg] po q12 h) has also been reported to be beneficial.
- Severe cases can also be treated with prednisone 0.5–1 mg/kg/day and tapered over 2–3 weeks, in addition to tetracycline/niacinamide treatment.[2]
- Pentoxifylline at 15–25 mg/kg q8–12 h can be helpful if tetracyclines/niacinamide is not tolerated or not helpful.[2]
- Dietary elimination trials may be helpful for some patients.[1]
- Some dogs appear recalcitrant to therapy and require treatment as for immune-mediated diseases (see Immunosuppressive Drug Therapy Table, page 289, for dosages).

Key points

- History and appearance are diagnostic.
- Treatment may require 2–3 months before improvement is evident.

References

1 Mueller RS, Friend S, Shipstone MA, Burton G. Diagnosis of canine claw disease – a prospective study of 24 dogs. *Vet Dermatol* 2000; **11**: 133–141.

2 Mueller RS, Rosychuk RA, Jonas LD. A retrospective study regarding the treatment of lupoid onychodystrophy in 30 dogs and literature review. *J Am Anim Hosp Assoc* 2003; **39**: 139–150.

3 Ziener ML, Bettenay SV, Mueller RS. Symmetrical onychomadesis in Norwegian Gordon and English setters. *Vet Dermatol* 2008; **19**: 88–94.

4 Ziener ML, Nødtvedt A. A treatment study of canine symmetrical onychomadesis (symmetrical lupoid onychodystrophy) comparing fish oil and cyclosporine supplementation in addition to a diet rich in omega-3 fatty acids. *Acta Vet Scand* 2014; **56**: 66.

FELINE PLASMA CELL PODODERMATITIS

Definition

Plasma cell pododermatitis is a rare disorder of cats associated with plasma cell infiltration into one or more footpads.

Aetiology and pathogenesis

The cause of the disease is not known, although the lack of demonstrated infectious agents, dermoepidermal immune complex deposition and response to immunosuppressive agents suggest an immune-mediated disorder.[1–3] The gradual accumulation of plasma cells and granulation tissue results in soft, poorly-defined swelling of the affected pad. Ulceration and secondary infection of the protruding tissue usually follow.

Clinical features

There is no breed, age or sex predisposition. Usually only a single pad is affected, typically the central metacarpal or metatarsal pad. Occasionally, a digital pad or several pads may be affected. Initially, there is a soft, painless swelling of the affected pad, accompanied by hyperkeratotic, interlacing striae. A pale blue or violet discoloration may be apparent (**Fig. 8.12**). If the pad ulcerates, a mound of haemorrhagic granulation tissue protrudes. There may be local lymphadenopathy, but discomfort and pain are rare. Secondary infection or bleeding may occur. Affected cats are generally reported to be negative for FeLV and FIV. However, in one report, 50% of the cats were FIV positive.[4]

Differential diagnoses

The clinical presentation is almost unique. Other causes to consider include:

* Bacterial or fungal granuloma.
* Eosinophilic granuloma.
* Neoplasia (squamous cell carcinoma) or foreign body if only one pad is affected.

Diagnosis

* Stained impression smears may reveal plasma cells.
* Biopsy and histopathological examination are diagnostic.

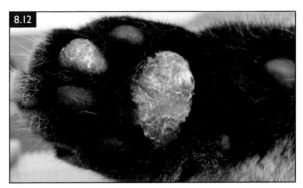

Fig. 8.12 Plasma cell pododermatitis prior to ulceration. Note the swelling, violet hue and scaling.

* Consider testing for FIV, because some studies have shown 44–62% of cats with plasma cell pododermatitis are infected.

Treatment

* Doxycycline monotherapy at 10 mg/kg po q24 h for 4–8 weeks will result in improvement or resolution in 80% of cases. A liquid formulation should be considered to prevent oesophagitis.[5]
* Prednisolone 4.4 mg/kg per day, other steroids or ciclosporin (modified) at 5–7 mg/kg per day may also be helpful.

Key point

* Almost pathognomonic appearance.

References

1 Bettenay SV, Lappin MR, Mueller RS. An immunohistochemical and polymerase chain reaction evaluation of feline plasmacytic pododermatitis. *Vet Pathol* 2007; **44**: 80–83.

2 Taylor JE, Schmeitzel LP. Plasma cell pododermatitis with chronic footpad ulceration in two cats. *J Am Vet Med Assoc* 1990; **197**: 375–377.

3 Medleau L, Kaswan RL, Lorenz MD *et al*. Ulcerative pododermatitis in a cat: immunofluorescent findings and response to chrysotherapy. *J Am Anim Hosp Assoc* 1982; **18**: 449–451.

4 Guaguere E, Declercq J. Viral dermatoses. In: Guaguere E, Prelaud P (eds), *A Practical Guide to Feline Dermatology*. Oxford: Blackwell Science, 2000: pp. 7.1–7.11.

5 Bettenay SV, Mueller RS, Dow K *et al*. Prospective study of the treatment of feline plasmacytic pododermatitis with doxycycline. *Vet Rec* 2003; **152**: 564–566.

FOOTPAD CORNS
(Keratomas)

Definition
Corns are hard protuberances that occur on the digital footpads of Greyhound dogs.

Aetiology and pathogenesis
Footpad corns are most commonly seen in Greyhounds, in both racing and non-racing animals. They are occasionally seen in other breeds. Possible causes include chronic trauma or pressure, abnormalities in the underlying fatty pad cushion or phalangeal bone, scar tissue, foreign bodies and papillomavirus infections.[1,2] There are anecdotal reports of possible transmission between Greyhounds in households. A recent study revealed DNA from canine papillomavirus type 12 and an unknown papillomavirus in four corns from two Greyhounds.[3]

Clinical features
Affected dogs develop small, well-demarcated, hard, slightly raised areas of hyperkeratosis on their pads[1,2] (**Fig. 8.13**). Most occur in the centre of the pads of digits 3 and 4, but they can also be found on the pads of other digital, metacarpal and metatarsal pads. Corns can be painful, leading to significant lameness, especially on rough ground.

Differential diagnoses
- Viral papillomatosis (see page 252).
- Histiocytic lesions.
- Sterile nodular granuloma and pyogranuloma.
- Split-pad syndrome.

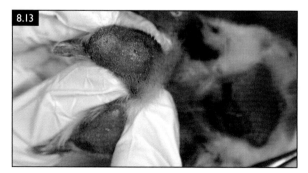

Fig. 8.13 Foot corn in a Greyhound; there is a well-demarcated area of raised hyperkeratotic tissue in the centre of the digital pad.

Diagnosis
The diagnosis is usually based on the clinical appearance. Histopathology reveals well-defined conical hyperkeratosis projecting above the skin surface, with minimal evidence of infection or inflammation.[1]

Treatment[1,2]
There is no one ideal treatment, and options include:

- Using boots to relieve pressure and pain.
- Using nail files, pumice stone or craft tools to remove the protruding hyperkeratinised tissue; this may relieve pressure and pain but needs to be frequently repeated.
- Topical therapy with keratolytics and emollients for shallow lesions.
- Some corns can be expressed by digital pressure, especially if the pad is thoroughly soaked first; this can be painful in some dogs.
- Excision using dental elevators, curettes, scalpel blades or biopsy punches; the corns usually shell out easily. This can be done in the conscious animal or using sedation and digital nerve blocks.
- Cryosurgery under sedation and digital nerve blocks.
- CO_2 laser ablation or cautery under sedation and digital nerve blocks; anecdotally ablating the base and walls of the defect may help reduce the recurrence rate.
- Deep excision or CO_2 laser ablation/cautery seem to be the most effective options, although up to 50% of the lesions will recur.

Key points
- There is a high recurrence rate.
- Treatment can be frustrating.

References
1 Balara JS, McCarthy RJ, Kiupel M *et al*. Clinical, histologic, and immunohistochemical characterization of wart-like lesions on the paw pads of dogs: 24 cases (2000–2007). *J Am Vet Med Assoc* 2009; **234**: 1555–1558.
2 Guilliard MJ, Segboer I, Shearer DH. Corns in dogs; signalment, possible aetiology and response to surgical treatment. *J Small Anim Pract* 2010; **51**: 162–168.
3 Anis EA, Frank LA, Francisco R, Kania SA. Identification of canine papillomavirus by PCR in Greyhound dogs. *Peer J* 2016; **4**: e2744.

NASAL DERMATOSES

GENERAL APPROACH TO NASAL DERMATOSES

When performing a biopsy of conditions that affect the skin as well as the nasal planum, it can be useful to sample affected skin rather than the actual nasal planum. Histopathology of inflamed nasal planum may look 'lupus-like' (lymphoplasmacytic interface inflammation, basal cell apoptosis and pigmentary incontinence) in many conditions in the absence of discoid lupus erythematosus. Biopsies of the nasal planum should target primary lesions, as inflamed and ulcerated areas can be non-diagnostic. Areas of non-ulcerated loss of pigment are likely to be most diagnostic in immune-mediated diseases. **Fig. 9.1** outlines the general approach to nasal dematoses.

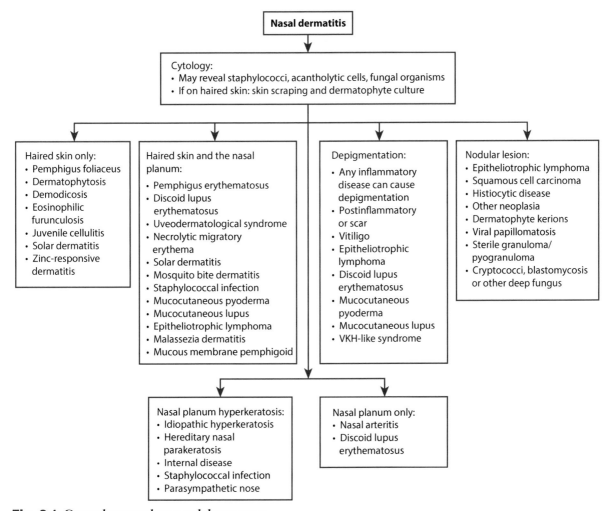

Fig. 9.1 General approach to nasal dermatoses.

NASAL ARTERITIS

Definition
Proliferative arteritis of the nasal philtrum is a disease that results in deep fissures and ulcers of the nasal philtrum. It is often associated with extensive haemorrhage.

Aetiology and pathogenesis
Arteritis is an immune-mediated disease. It is speculated that inflammation of the arterial walls leads to progressive thickening, resulting in partial occlusion, local tissue ischaemia, necrosis and ulceration.[1]

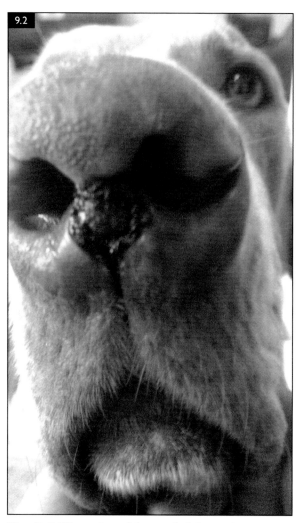

Fig. 9.2 Ulceration of the nasal philtrum in a Weimaraner dog.

Clinical features
Four of five dogs in the original report were Saint Bernard's and one was a Giant Schnauzer.[1] It has also been reported in a Newfoundland.[2] Linear ulcers varying from 3 cm to 5 cm in length and 2 mm to 5 mm in width are found spanning the nasal philtrum (**Fig. 9.2**). Arterial bleeding from the ulcers is often noted and may be so severe that it requires surgical repair.

Differential diagnoses
- The lesions are distinctive, but early lesions may have some features of discoid lupus erythematosus or parasympathetic nasal dermatitis.
- Trauma.
- Neoplasia (particularly squamous cell carcinoma and epitheliotrophic lymphoma).

Diagnosis
Diagnosis is based on history and clinical findings. Biopsy is not recommended unless the lesion is surgically resected because severe bleeding is possible.

Treatment
- Most cases can be managed medically.
- For mild cases, treat topically with tacrolimus 0.1% q12 h and orally with doxycycline or minocycline 5 mg/kg q12 h with niacinamide. (See Immunosuppressive Drug Therapy Table, page 289 for dosages.)
- Other options are pentoxifylline at 15–25 mg/kg q8–12 h, vitamin E, fish oil and topical steroids.
- For cases that are bleeding, start topical tacrolimus 0.1% q12 h and prednisone 1mg/kg per day until lesion is stable (14 days or so) and then taper off slowly.
- Ciclosporin (modified) at 5 mg/kg per day can also be used alone or in combination with the above measures.
- Treatment will probably be lifelong, but the doses and frequency of medication can be decreased and some medications stopped without recurrence. Ideally, the disease would be kept in remission with topical and/or non-steroid systemic medication.
- Surgical intervention may be necessary if there is severe haemorrhage. Surgical cases should be treated medically as well.[3]

Key points
- Arterial bleeding from the ulcer can be severe.
- Lifelong treatment is often required.

References
1 Torres SM, Brien TO, Scott DW. Dermal arteritis of the nasal philtrum in a Giant Schnauzer and three Saint Bernard dogs. *Vet Dermatol* 2002; **13**: 275–281.

2 Gross TH, Ihrke PJ, Walder EJ, Affolter VK. Proliferative arteritis of the nasal philtrum. In: *Skin Diseases of the Dog and Cat: Clinical and Histopathologic Diagnosis*, 2nd edn. Oxford: Blackwell Publishing, 2005: pp 255–256.

3 Vuolo S, Peters L, Licari L. Successful medical and surgical treatment of dermal arteritis of the nasal philtrum in a Saint Bernard dog. *Vet Med Res Rep* 2014; **5**: 115—118.

DISCOID LUPUS ERYTHEMATOSUS

Definition
Discoid lupus erythematosus (DLE) is an autoimmune, photoaggravated skin disease predominantly characterised by nasal lesions.

Aetiology and pathogenesis
Solar radiation induces an inflammatory cascade that damages dermal and epidermal components and provokes a chronic, immune-mediated reaction. Certain individuals may be genetically susceptible to DLE.

Clinical features (Figs. 9.3, 9.4)
There is no age predilection, but females and some breeds of dogs (e.g. Shetland Sheepdogs, Rough Collies, German Shepherd dogs and Siberian Huskies) may be predisposed. Lesions are characterised by depigmentation and loss of cobblestone architecture of the nasal planum. Scaling, erythema and light crusting may also be present. In addition to the nasal planum, the periocular skin, pinnae and muzzle may be affected. Erosions of the buccal mucosa may be present in severe cases. Very rarely, generalised, truncal lesions may be present (with generalised DLE).[1,2]

DLE is very rare in cats.[3] The most common sites for lesions are the nose and planum nasale. Interestingly, the pinnae are more commonly affected in cats.[3]

Differential diagnoses
- Actinic dermatitis.
- Dermatophytosis (if haired skin is also involved).
- Epitheliotrophic lymphoma.
- Pemphigus complex.
- Drug eruption.
- Systemic lupus erythematosus.

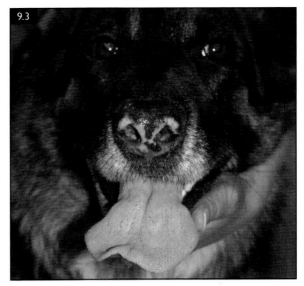

Fig. 9.3 Classical discoid lupus erythematosus with depigmentation and erosion of the nasal planum.

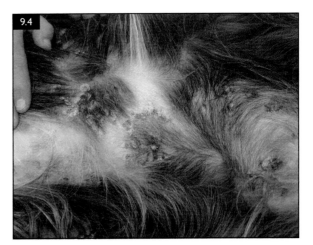

Fig. 9.4 Generalised discoid lupus erythematosus with multiple lichenified, hyperpigmented and scaling plaques on the ventral abdomen.

- Uveodermatological syndrome.
- Vasculitis.
- Mucocutaneous pyoderma.
- Parasympathetic nasal dermatitis.
- Idiopathic nasal depigmentation.
- Vitiligo.
- Hereditary nasal parakeratosis.
- Neoplasia (particularly squamous cell carcinoma and epitheliotrophic lymphoma).
- Mucous membrane pemphigoid.

Diagnosis

Loss of pigmentation and cobblestone architecture on the nose should raise a high index of suspicion for DLE. Surface cytology can identify secondary yeast or bacterial infections. Secondary infections can be treated in a similar fashion as yeast dermatitis (see page 31) and superficial pyoderma (see page 70). Acantholytic keratinocytes on surface cytology should raise suspicion of the pemphigus complex (see page 83). A fungal culture should be performed if haired skin is involved.

If the lesions are generalised, appear infiltrative or are severe, a biopsy should be performed. Where possible, biopsies should be taken from affected skin that does not include the nasal planum. Biopsy samples of inflamed nasal planum almost always reveal a lupoid-type pattern no matter what type of disease is present. Biopsy of the planum should be used primarily to rule out conditions such as epitheliotrophic lymphoma and should target depigmented non-ulcerated sites. Immunofluorescence is the only way to absolutely confirm DLE, but this test is rarely necessary because the clinical signs, histopathology and other findings will be diagnostic. Antinuclear antibody tests are nearly always negative, and should not be pursued unless there are systemic signs (see Systemic lupus erythematosus, page 171).

Treatment

The goal of treatment should be to prevent the development of crusting, ulceration and new lesions. It is rare that normal pigmentation or cobblestone architecture will ever be restored. The avoidance of intense sun exposure is an important part of treatment. (See Immunosuppressive Drug Therapy Table, page 289, for dosages.)

The combination of a tetracycline antibiotic with niacinamide will control most cases. However, this therapy may take several weeks to take effect. If significant inflammation is present, systemic prednisolone at 1 mg/kg per day will usually induce remission of the lesions while waiting for the tetracycline antibiotic and niacinamide to take effect.

Topical 0.1% tacrolimus ointment applied twice daily and tapering to the lowest effective dose after remission may be used as an adjunct treatment. Cases that are less severe may respond to tacrolimus ointment as the sole therapy.[4] Some cases may be kept in remission with topical hydrocortisone cream or other topical glucocorticoids.

Vitamin E (400–800 IU daily) has been reported as useful in some cases, although there is a 1- to 2-month lag phase.

Ciclosporin[1] (modified; 4–7 mg/kg po q24 h to remission and then tapering for maintenance) and hydroxychloroquine[2] (5 mg/kg po q24 h) can also be effective in severe or refractory cases.

Key points
- Animals with classic DLE do not have systemic signs.
- Biopsy of inflamed nasal planum may look 'lupus like' no matter what the diagnosis.
- Cases generally respond well to treatment.

References

1   Banovic F, Olivry T, Linder KE. Ciclosporin therapy for canine generalized discoid lupus erythematosus refractory to doxycycline and niacinamide. *Vet Dermatol* 2014; **25**: 483–e79.
2   Oberkirchner U, Linder KE, Olivry T. Successful treatment of a novel generalized variant of canine discoid lupus erythematosus with oral hydroxychloroquine. *Vet Dermatol* 2012; **23**: 65–e16.
3   Willemse T, Koeman JP. Discoid lupus erythematosus in cats. *Vet Dermatol* 1989; **1**: 19–24.
4   Griffies JD, Mendelson CL, Rosenkrantz WS *et al*. Topical 0.1% tacrolimus for the treatment of discoid lupus erythematosus and pemphigus erythematosus in dogs. *J Am Anim Hosp Assoc* 2004; **40**: 29–41.

GENERAL APPROACH TO JUVENILE DERMATOSES

The flow chart shows the general approach to juvenile dermatoses (**Fig. 10.1**).

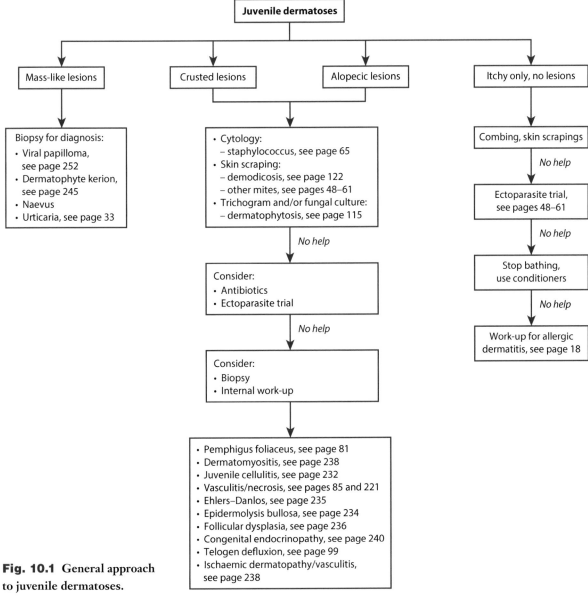

Fig. 10.1 General approach to juvenile dermatoses.

JUVENILE CELLULITIS
(Puppy strangles)

Canine juvenile cellulitis (juvenile sterile granulomatous dermatitis and lymphadenitis, juvenile pyoderma or puppy strangles)

Definition
Canine juvenile cellulitis is a granulomatous condition of puppies affecting the skin of the face, pinnae and submandibular lymph nodes.

Aetiology and pathogenesis
The aetiology and pathogenesis of this condition are unknown. An immunological abnormality appears to be involved, because immunosuppressive therapy results in resolution of lesions. There is some evidence for a hereditary factor, because some breeds, as well as particular lines within a breed, are predisposed.[1,2]

Clinical features (Fig. 10.2)
The condition most commonly develops in puppies from age 3 weeks to 16 weeks, but it has also been reported in young adult dogs. It occurs more frequently in Golden Retrievers, Dachshunds, Labrador Retrievers, Lhasa Apso and Gordon Setters.[1–3] Puppies are usually febrile, depressed, and anorexic with severe submandibular lymphadenopathy. There is acute swelling of the muzzle, lips and eyelids. Sterile pustules often develop in the affected

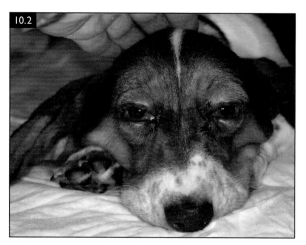

Fig. 10.2 Facial swelling, blepharitis, conjunctivitis and otitis in a 12-week-old Bassett Hound.

skin and on the inner surface of the pinnae. After the pustules rupture, small ulcers, draining tracts, seropurulent exudates or crusts can develop. Secondary otitis externa is fairly common. Nodules over the trunk, preputial and perineal areas (associated with a pyogranulomatous panniculitis), and sterile suppurative arthritis have been reported in a small number of cases.[2] Permanent areas of alopecia and scarring may result if the lesions are extensive.

Differential diagnoses
- Angio-oedema due to an insect bite reaction or vaccine.
- Dermatophytosis.
- Demodicosis.
- Bacterial folliculitis/furunculosis (most commonly staphylococci).
- Pemphigus foliaceus.
- Adverse drug reaction.

Diagnosis
The signalment and clinical signs are very suggestive. Skin scrapings and cytological examination of the contents of an intact pustule will help to identify demodicosis or staphylococcal folliculitis, respectively. Samples should be taken for dermatophyte culture. Lymph node aspirates usually show the characteristic pyogranulomatous inflammation. Biopsies should be obtained for definitive diagnosis.

Treatment
Prednisolone (1–2 mg/kg po q12 h) should be continued until the lesions resolve (7–14 days) and then be tapered over another 4 weeks. In most cases, significant improvement will be noted during the first 1–3 days of treatment. Appropriate topical or systemic antimicrobials can be used to treat secondary infections (see Superficial pyoderma, page 72). This regimen resolves most cases, but will occasionally have to be repeated if there is a relapse. If the lesions are chronic or recurrent, ciclosporin (modified; 5 mg/kg po q24 h) can be used. The dose and/or frequency can be tapered for long-term maintenance.[3,4]

Key point
- These cases require steroid or ciclosporin therapy. Be sure to rule out demodicosis.

References

1   Mason IS, Jones J. Juvenile cellulitis in Gordon Setters. *Vet Rec* 1989; **124**: 642.

2   White SD, Rosychuk RAW, Stewart LJ *et al.* Juvenile cellulitis in dogs: 15 cases (1979–1988). *J Am Vet Med Assoc* 1989; **195**: 1609–1611.

3   Miller WH, Griffin CE, Campbell KL, Muller GH. In: *Muller and Kirk's Small Animal Dermatology*. Amsterdam: Elsevier Health Sciences, 2013: pp. 573–617.

4   Park C, Yoo J-H, Kim H-J, Kang B-T, Park H-M. Combination of cyclosporin A and prednisolone for juvenile cellulitis concurrent with hindlimb paresis in 3 English cocker spaniel puppies. *Can Vet J* 2010; **51**: 1265.

SHAR PEI MUCINOSIS

Definition

Mucin is a clear, viscous fluid made up of glucosaminoglycans, primarily hyaluronic acid.[1] Shar Pei mucinosis is caused by excessive production and deposition of hyaluronic acid in the skin.[2]

Aetiology and pathogenesis

Chinese Shar Pei dogs have been bred to have thick, wrinkled folds of skin, which is a form of generalised cutaneous mucinosis. Inflammation and/or genetics trigger excessive hyaluronic acid production and accumulation in the skin to the point of mucinous vesicles forming.

Clinical features

Vesicular mucinosis is characterised by clear, soft or turgid, thin-walled vesicles full of mucin (**Fig. 10.3**). Mucin may also be expressed from the skin by digital pressure. Dogs with more dramatic folds may be predisposed to vesicular mucinosis. Excessive folding of the skin may cause entropion, corneal ulcers and/or decreased vision. The folding and mucin may predispose to secondary bacterial and *Malassezia* infections. Folding also affects the ear canals, causing narrowing and predisposing to infection. Oropharyngeal folding may cause breathing difficulties.

Differential diagnoses

- Hypothyroidism.
- Inflammation may enhance mucin production.
- Mast cell tumours and cutaneous mastocytosis have been associated with more severe localised cutaneous mucinosis.[3,4]

Diagnosis

Cutaneous and vesicular mucinosis are visually distinctive in this breed, and cytology of a vesicle would reveal an acellular, viscous substance. If necessary, skin biopsy is diagnostic.

Treatment

Mucinosis may indicate underlying inflammation or hypothyroidism. Underlying inflammatory skin diseases (allergic dermatitis, demodicosis and bacterial or yeast infections) should be investigated and treated. Dogs with oropharyngeal, eye or ear problems due to extensive folding of the skin and mucosa should be treated. Excessive mucinosis may improve with age. If needed, prednisone (0.5–1 mg/kg per day for 7 days and then tapered over 1 month) rapidly resolves vesicular cutaneous mucinosis as well as decreasing the thickness of all skinfolds on the body. However, owners may not be happy with their pet's 'deflated'

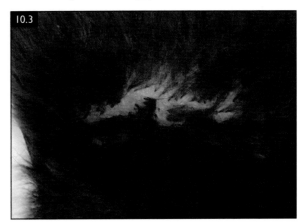

Fig. 10.3 Mucinosis in a Shar Pei dog with excessive folding and bubble-like proliferation of the skin.

appearance during prednisone therapy. When the prednisone is discontinued, the pet's wrinkles usually reform but the mucinous vesicles may not return. Entropion or other fold-related issues often need surgical intervention.

Key points
- All Shar Peis have cutaneous mucinosis to some degree.
- Excessive mucin production may indicate an underlying inflammatory disease.

References
1 Zanna G, Fondevila D, Bardagí M, Docampo MJ, Bassols A, Ferrer L. Cutaneous mucinosis in shar-pei dogs is due to hyaluronic acid deposition and is associated with high levels of hyaluronic acid in serum. *Vet Dermatol* 2008; **19**: 314–318.
2 Zanna G, Docampo MJ, Fondevila D, Bardagí M, Bassols A, Ferrer L. Hereditary cutaneous mucinosis in shar pei dogs is associated with increased hyaluronan synthase-2 mRNA transcription by cultured dermal fibroblasts: Hereditary cutaneous mucinosis in shar pei dogs. *Vet Dermatol* **20**: 2009; 377–382.
3 Madewell BR, Akita GY, Vogel P. Cutaneous mastocytosis and mucinosis with gross deformity in a shar pei dog. *Vet Dermatol* 1992; **3**: 171–175.
4 Lopez A, Spracklin D, McConkey S, Hanna P. Cutaneous mucinosis and mastocytosis in a shar-pei. *Can Vet J* 1999; **40**: 881.

EPIDERMOLYSIS BULLOSA – HEREDITARY

Definition
Hereditary epidermolysis bullosa is a genetic disease of dermoepidermal adhesion that causes skin fragility and blistering in young animals.

Aetiology and pathogenesis
Epidermolysis bullosa is caused by several different genetic mutations affecting dermoepidermal adhesion.[1] There are many subtypes of this disease that reflect the location of the mutation and severity of clinical signs.

Clinical features
This disease is reported in Beaucerons, German Short-haired Pointers, Chesapeake Bay Retrievers, a Toy Poodle, domestic short-haired cats and Siamese cats.[2] It is characterised by blisters and ulcerations of the skin and mucous membranes after minor trauma, often with nail deformity or loss.[1] As a result of this break in the skin barrier and recurrent infections, many animals die or are euthanised at a very young age.

Differential diagnoses
- Trauma.
- In cats, calicivirus and other viral infections can cause oral ulcerations.
- In animals age >2 years old, autoimmune blistering diseases should be considered (see page 167).
- Cutaneous asthenia if no oral ulcerations are present.

Diagnosis
Early onset of non-inflammatory ulcerative lesions induced by trauma is a strong indication of this disease. Biopsy with immunohistochemical staining can confirm the diagnosis, but the stains needed are not widely available.

Treatment
Animals should be treated for secondary bacterial infections and efforts made to avoid trauma.

Key points
- A genetic disease with supportive therapy only.
- The prognosis is poor in severely affected animals.

References
1 Medeiros GX, Riet-Correa F. Epidermolysis bullosa in animals: a review. *Vet Dermatol* 2015; **26**: 3–e2.
2 Miller WH, Griffin CE, Campbell KL, Muller GH. In: *Muller and Kirk's Small Animal Dermatology*. Amsterdam: Elsevier Health Sciences, 2013: 573–617.

EHLERS–DANLOS SYNDROME

Definition

Ehlers–Danlos syndrome comprises an inherited group of congenital connective tissue dysplasias characterised by loose, hyperextensible, abnormally fragile skin that is easily torn by minor trauma.

Aetiology and pathogenesis

Several forms of this syndrome, with different clinical, genetic and biochemical changes, have been recognised in dogs, cats, humans, cattle and sheep.[1] All have a common basis in that they are accompanied by connective tissue weakness due to abnormalities in biosynthesis or post-translational modifications of collagen.[1] The main form of Ehlers–Danlos syndrome in the dog is a dominantly inherited collagen-packing defect characterised by focal or diffuse areas of severely disorganised fibres with many abnormally large fibrils.[1] The tensile strength of affected skin is 4% of that of non-affected skin.[1] Two forms of the syndrome have been reported in the cat: a dominant form similar to the collagen-packing defect of dogs, and a recessive form characterised by a deficiency of N-procollagen peptidase enzyme, which results in collagen that is in the form of twisted ribbons rather than cylindrical fibrils and fibres.[2,3]

Clinical features

Ehlers–Danlos syndrome has been documented in many breeds of dogs and cats.[4] Fragility, hyperextensibility, and sagging or loose skin since birth are the most characteristic clinical findings. Animals may be presented with multiple scars or tears in the skin (**Fig. 10.4**). Joint laxity may be an additional finding that can result in osteoarthritis (**Fig. 10.5**).

Differential diagnoses

The syndrome is clinically distinctive in dogs. Cats may develop fragile skin due to naturally occurring or iatrogenic hyperglucocorticoidism, diabetes mellitus, with excessive use of megoestrol acetate and feline acquired skin fragility syndrome,[5] which should not be confused with Ehlers–Danlos syndrome.

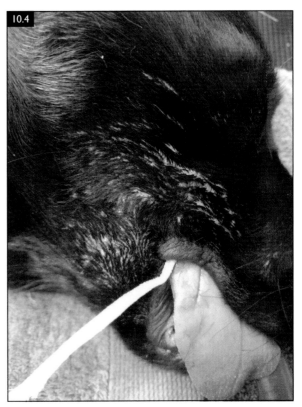

Fig. 10.4 Typical tissue paper scars resulting from multiple episodes of skin tearing in a dog with Ehlers–Danlos syndrome and skin fragility.

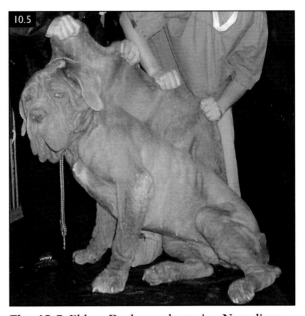

Fig. 10.5 Ehlers–Danlos syndrome in a Neapolitan Mastiff; this dog did not have skin fragility but had marked joint laxity that eventually led to osteoarthritis.

Diagnosis

The diagnosis is based on the history, clinical findings, biopsy for light or electron microscopy, cell culture and biochemical study of collagen.

Treatment

Any tears of the skin that are present should be sutured or glued and the animal's lifestyle adjusted to minimise trauma to the skin. Affected animals should not be used for breeding.

Key point

• Rare congenital disease characterised by fragility and hyperextensibility of the skin.

References

1 Hegreberg GA, Counts DF. Ehlers–Danlos syndrome. In: Andrews ED, Ward BC, Altman NH (eds), *Spontaneous Animal Models of Human Disease*, Vol. II. New York: Academic Press, 1979: pp. 36–39.

2 Patterson DF, Minor RR. Hereditary fragility and hyperextensibility of the skin of cats. A defect in collagen fibrillogenesis. *Lab Invest* 1977; **37**: 170–179.

3 Counts DF, Byers PH, Holbrook KA *et al.* Dermatosparaxis in a Himalayan cat: I. Biochemical studies of dermal collagen. *J Invest Dermatol* 1980; **74**: 96–99.

4 Scott DW, Miller WH, Griffin CE. Ehlers–Danlos syndrome. In: *Muller and Kirk's Small Animal Dermatology*, 6th edn. Philadelphia, PA: WB Saunders, 2001: pp. 979–984.

5 Fernandez CJ, Scott DW, Erb HN *et al.* Staining abnormalities of dermal collagen in cats with cutaneous asthenia or acquired skin fragility as demonstrated with Masson's trichrome stain. *Vet Dermatol* 1998; **9**: 49–54.

CONGENITAL ALOPECIAS

ECTODERMAL DYSPLASIA

Ectodermal dysplasia is caused by heterozygous mutations in the ectodysplasin signalling pathway.[1] Heterozygous mutant dogs have the hairless phenotype and homozygous mutations are lethal during embryogenesis. Abnormalities in dogs with these gene mutations include dental abnormalities (missing teeth, thin, pointed teeth, abnormal angles to the teeth), lack of eccrine glands in footpads, nail abnormalities and a characteristic symmetrical alopecia to varying degrees. Breeds in which ectodermal dysplasia has been selected for include Mexican and Peruvian Hairless dogs and Chinese Crested dogs (*FOXI3* mutation). Mutations can arise spontaneously in other breeds, and there are many different clinical appearances based on the specifically mutated gene. Some dogs with the *EDA1* gene mutation may have striking or mild hair loss on the forehead and dorsal pelvis, chronic ocular discharge and corneal ulceration, chronic upper respiratory disease and predisposition to pneumonia.[2] The hairless and partially haired skin of the affected dogs is predisposed to comedones, milia, follicular hyperkeratosis, bacterial infections and hyperpigmentation due to exposure to ultraviolet light. Treatment for comedones and follicular hyperkeratosis is needed only if the dog has chronic discomfort or infections, and includes oral and topical retinoids, shampoos and other keratin-regulating treatments. Administration of Fc:EDA1 IV proteins in the early postnatal period has improved outcomes in dogs with the *EDA1* gene mutation.[3]

BLACK HAIR FOLLICULAR DYSPLASIA

Dogs with this condition have an abnormality in the growth of the black hairs, perhaps related to pigment transfer abnormalities. These dogs are born normal, but loss of black hairs is noticed by age 2–4 weeks and is progressive. Excessive scaling may occur in areas where hair is lost. Skin scrapes to rule out *Demodex* spp., cytology to rule out staphylococcal folliculitis and culture to rule out dermatophytosis should be performed. On a trichogram, the black hairs show clumped melanin. The appearance clinically is distinctive, but a biopsy may be helpful to achieve the diagnosis (see also page 112).

COLOUR DILUTION ALOPECIA

Colour dilution alopecia is caused by an autosomal recessive *MLPH* gene mutation.[4] The clinical manifestations are caused by abnormal transfer of melanin and follicular dysplasia, resulting in weak hairs and breakage, symmetrically thin hair and predisposition to recurrent bacterial folliculitis, similar to black hair follicular dysplasia. This disease is commonly seen in blue Dobermans, silver Labradors, dilute coloured Dachshunds and Weimaraners, but can be seen in any dilute coat breed. It is very rare in dilute-coated cats. This disease is often first noticed when the dogs are puppies or young adults and tends to worsen with age. In large Munsterlanders, puppies are born grey and white with lighter-coloured eyes rather than black and white, some puppies are deaf and the grey areas become alopecic.[5]

The diagnosis is based on the history, clinical signs and ruling out other causes of symmetrical alopecia. A dull hair coat, easily broken and thinning hair and alopecia in an otherwise normal puppy or young adult dog with a dilute hair coat are fairly diagnostic. Hair plucks will show clumped aggregates of melanin (macromelanosomes). Ruling out endocrinopathies such as hyperadrenocorticism in older dogs and hypothyroidism in dogs aged >2 years with appropriate signs is essential. Skin scrapes and cytology will help rule out other conditions and infections. A biopsy may be helpful to confirm the diagnosis. There is no specific treatment of this condition, only general skin care and management of recurrent infections, if present (see also page 113).

PATTERN ALOPECIA OF SPANIELS

A specific pattern of alopecia is seen in Portuguese Water dogs and Irish Water Spaniels.[6] These diseases appear to be a hair cycling abnormality because hair will regrow spontaneously, but pigment may be clumped and follicles misshapen similar to follicular dysplasia. In affected Portuguese Water dogs, hair loss occurs over the flanks and back. In Irish Water Spaniels, lack of hair on the throat and tail is 'normal' and desirable, but other areas commonly affected are the rump, caudal thighs, dorsal neck and trunk. This is a cosmetic disease and most treatments are unrewarding, although melatonin can be tried (see also page 98).

PATTERN BALDNESS
(Follicular miniaturisation)

Pattern baldness is a condition most commonly seen in small breed, short-coated dogs (Dachshund, Chihuahua, Boston Terrier). It is often first noticed at less than 1 year of age, with no sex predilection. The skin is easily seen through symmetrically fine hairs on the caudal dorsal aspects of ears and distal pinnae, caudal thighs, ventrum and chest. Detecting miniaturised hair follicles on observation or biopsy, along with ruling out other causes of non-inflammatory alopecia are diagnostic. This is a cosmetic disease and no treatment is necessary. Melatonin may be helpful in some cases, with results noticed at 1.5 months and maximal improvement in 3–4 months[7] (see also page 111).

Key point
- In most cases, regrowth of hair is not possible.

References

1 Drogemuller C, Karlsson EK, Hytönen MK *et al.* A mutation in hairless dogs implicates FOXI3 in ectodermal development. *Science* 2008; **321**: 1462–1462.

2 Casal ML, Jezyk PF, Greek JM, Goldschmidt MH, Patterson DF. X-linked ectodermal dysplasia in the dog. *J Hered* 1997; **88**: 513–517.

3 Casal ML, Lewis JR, Maudlin EA *et al.* Significant correction of disease after postnatal administration of recombinant ectodysplasin A in canine X-linked ectodermal dysplasia. *Am J Hum Genet* 2007; **81**: 1050–1056.

4 Drogemuller C, Philipp U, Haase B, Gunzel-Apel A-R, Leeb T. A noncoding melanophilin gene (MLPH) SNP at the splice donor of exon 1 represents a candidate causal mutation for coat color dilution in dogs. *J Hered* 2007; **98**: 468–473.

5 Schmutz SM, Moker JS, Clark EG, Shewfelt R. Black hair follicular dysplasia, an autosomal recessive condition in dogs. *Can Vet J* 1998; **39**: 644.

6 Mecklenburg L, Linek M, Tobin DJ. *Hair Loss Disorders in Domestic Animals.* Oxford: Wiley, 2009.

7 Paradis M. Canine recurrent flank alopecia: treatment with melatonin. In *Proceedings of the 11th Annual AAVD & ACVD Meeting*, Santa Fe, CA, 1995.

CANINE FAMILIAL DERMATOMYOSITIS
(Ischaemic dermatopathy/vasculitis)

Definition

Canine familial dermatomyositis is a hereditary inflammatory disease of skin and muscle that is characterised by symmetrical scarring alopecia about the face and limbs, and atrophy of the muscles of mastication.[1]

Aetiology and pathogenesis

The aetiopathogenesis of canine familial dermatomyositis is unknown. It is postulated that immunological damage occurs to blood vessels, resulting in ischaemic damage to the skin and muscles.[2] The condition is familial in Collies and Shetland Sheepdogs, and breeding studies in Collies support an autosomal dominant mode of inheritance with variable expressivity.[3,4]

Clinical features

The disease occurs more commonly in Collies and Shetland Sheepdogs, but it has also been reported to occur in the Welsh Corgi, Chow Chow, German Shepherd dog and Kuvasz, and may sporadically occur in other breeds.[5] Lesions generally develop before animals are age 6 months, but they can occasionally develop in adults. The face (especially the bridge of the nose, around the eyes and ear tips), carpal and tarsal pressure spots, digital prominences and tip of the tail are typically affected. Scarring alopecia (**Figs. 10.6, 10.7**),

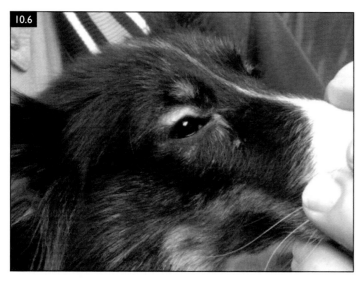

Fig. 10.6 Periocular alopecia in a Shetland Sheepdog puppy with dermatomyosit is.

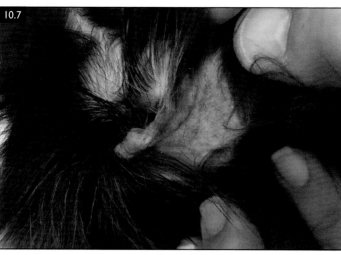

Fig. 10.7 Alopecia at the base of the pinna in a Shetland Sheepdog puppy with dermatomyositis.

erythema, scaling and mild crusting are the most common findings. Occasionally, vesicles, papules, pustules and ulcers may be found.[3] The development and progression of lesions are quite variable, because they often wax and wane and may undergo spontaneous regression. Muscle involvement occurs after the development of skin lesions and correlates with the severity of the skin lesions.[3] It is often minimal and limited to temporal and masseter atrophy. Severely affected dogs have difficulty in eating, drinking and swallowing, and may evidence growth retardation, megaoesophagus, lameness, widespread muscle atrophy and infertility.[3] Skeletal muscle involvement may result in an abnormal gait or poor exercise intolerance. Pruritus and pain are generally not features of the disease.

Differential diagnoses
- Cutaneous or systemic lupus erythematosus.
- Vasculitis.
- Dermatophytosis.
- Epidermolysis bullosa.
- Leishmaniasis.
- Demodicosis.
- Facial pyoderma.
- Pemphigus foliaceus.

Diagnosis
The diagnosis is based on the history, physical exam, compatible histological changes in skin biopsies and electromyographic abnormalities consisting of positive sharp waves, fibrillation potentials and bizarre high-frequency discharges of affected muscles.[4]

Treatment
As the lesions of canine familial dermatomyositis can wax and wane on their own, it is difficult to determine the effectiveness of any particular treatment. No treatment may be needed for cases with minimal lesions as they may spontaneously resolve. Pentoxifylline (15–25 mg/kg po q8–12 h) is effective for many cases[6] (note: generic forms of this drug have been less effective than the name brand Trental®[6]). Oral vitamin E (200–800 IU/day) or marine lipid

supplements may provide some improvement in the skin but not the muscle lesions.[3] Prednisolone (1 mg/kg po q24 h) can be used for the treatment of lesions when they flare, but is not recommended for long-term therapy. Prolonged use of prednisolone is discouraged because it may aggravate the muscle atrophy. Other treatments that may be effective include doxycycline/minocycline 5 mg/kg po q12 h with niacinamide, ciclosporin (modified; 5 mg/kg po q24–48 h), and topical tacrolimus 0.1% q12 h for localised lesions.[1] (See Immunosuppressive Drug Therapy Table, page 289, for more details and doses.)

Treatment will not usually result in complete resolution of lesions, because it minimises only the development of new lesions and lessens the severity of those present. The owners should be warned that scarred skin will not regrow hair. This is a heritable disease, and affected dogs and their offspring should not be used for breeding.

Key point
- Genetic disease that can be managed but not cured.

References
1. Hargis AM, Haupt KH. Review of familial canine dermatomyositis. *Vet Ann* 1990; **30**: 227–282.
2. Gross TH, Ihrke PJ, Walder EJ, Affolter VK. Cell-poor vasculitis. In: *Skin Diseases of the Dog and Cat: Clinical and Histopathologic Diagnosis*, 2nd edn. Oxford: Blackwell Publishing, 2005: pp 247–250.
3. Hargis AM, Mundell AC. Familial canine dermatomyositis. *Compend Cont Educ Pract Vet* 1992; **14**: 855–864.
4. Haupt KH, Prieur DJ, Moore MP et al. Familial canine dermatomyositis: 5 clinical, electrodiagnostic, and genetic studies. *Am J Vet Res* 1985; **46**: 1861–1869.
5. Gross TH, Ihrke PJ, Walder EJ, Affolter VK. Ischemic dermatopathy/canine dermatomyositis. In: *Skin Diseases of the Dog and Cat: Clinical and Histopathologic Diagnosis*, 2nd edn. Oxford: Blackwell Publishing, 2005: pp 49–52.
6. Rees CA. Inherited vesiculobullous disorders. In: Campbell KL (ed.), *Small Animal Dermatology Secrets*. Philadelphia, PA: Hanley & Belfus, 2004: pp 112–119.

CANINE CONGENITAL ENDOCRINOPATHIES
(Pituitary dwarfism)

Definition

Pituitary dwarfism is a hereditary hypopituitarism resulting in a failure of growth with variable coat and thyroidal, adrenocortical and gonadal abnormalities.

Aetiology and pathogenesis

A pituitary gland cyst (Rathke's cleft cyst), resulting in varying degrees of anterior pituitary insufficiency, is responsible for most cases. However, the condition has been described in dogs with either hypoplastic or normal anterior pituitary glands.[1,2] The condition is inherited as a simple autosomal recessive mutation of the *LHX3* gene.[3] Pituitary dwarfism is caused by growth hormone deficiency alone, or in combination with other hormone deficiencies (thyroid-stimulating hormone [TSH], adrenocorticotrophic hormone [ACTH] and/or prolactin).

Clinical features

Pituitary dwarfism is seen primarily in German Shepherd dogs and Karelian Bear dogs (**Fig. 10.8**).[4] Affected dogs often appear normal during the first 2–3 months of life, but then fail to grow and retain their puppy coat. Partial loss of the puppy coat then occurs, resulting in a bilateral symmetrical alopecia over the neck, caudolateral aspects of the thighs and, occasionally, the trunk. Secondary bacterial and/or yeast infections are common. Growth of primary hair is generally limited to the face and distal extremities. The skin becomes hyperpigmented, hypotonic and scaly, and comedones may develop. Gonadal status may be altered with testicular atrophy occurring in males and anoestrus in females. Affected animals may also show evidence of personality changes such as aggressiveness and fear biting.[1] Clinical signs of hypothyroidism and adrenocortical insufficiency will be seen if there is a lack of TSH or ACTH. With thyroid and/or steroid supplementation (if needed), the condition

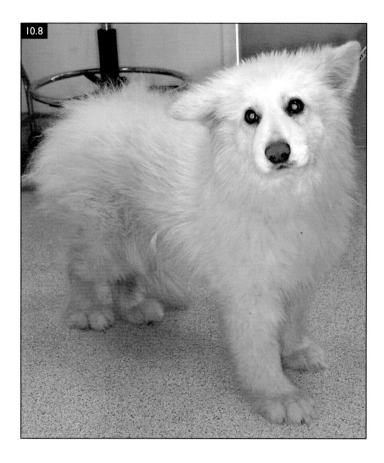

10.8

Fig. 10.8 Pituitary dwarfism with a puppy-like coat in a 4-year-old German Shepherd dog.

is generally compatible with life, but most animals only live to age 3–8 years.[5]

Differential diagnoses

- Congenital hypothyroidism.
- Malnutrition.
- Skeletal dysplasias.
- Gonadal dysgenesis.
- Severe metabolic diseases.
- Congenital alopecias.
- *Demodex* spp.
- Dermatophytosis.

Diagnosis

The history and clinical findings are usually diagnostic of an endocrinopathy and highly suggestive of pituitary dwarfism. There is a genetic test for mutation of the *LHX3* gene available from several commercial labs. Affected dogs will fail to have an increase in plasma growth hormone levels (normal levels 1–2 ng/ml) after the injection of xylazine (0.1–0.3 mg/kg iv) or clonidine (0.01–0.03 mg/kg iv). Low insulin growth factor 1 (IGF-1) levels are also seen in affected dogs. A thyroid panel shows a low TSH level and low thyroxine (T_4) in those also affected with hypothyroidism, and ACTH stimulations tests will be subnormal in dogs with hypoadrenocorticism. Computed tomography or magnetic resonance imaging may show a cyst in the pituitary fossa.

Treatment

Appropriate therapy for adrenocortical insufficiency and/or hypothyroidism, as well as secondary bacterial or yeast infections, should be instituted if necessary. There are many different ways to attempt to replace deficient growth hormone because canine or porcine (identical to canine) growth hormone is not available commercially. However, if available, the dose is 0.1–0.3 IU/kg sc three times weekly for 4–6 weeks.[6] Improvement in the skin and hair will generally be noted within 6–8 weeks after any treatment is given. An increase in stature is generally not achieved unless therapy started very early, because the growth plates close rapidly. Bovine somatotrophin (10 IU sc q48 h for 30 days) can be tried with repeated treatment every 3 months to 3 years.[7] Repeated injections of bovine somatotrophin have the potential to result in hypersensitivity reactions or diabetes mellitus.[6] Progestin therapy, which stimulates the mammary glands to produce growth hormone, has been used to induce hair regrowth and increase body weight and size. Either medroxyprogesterone acetate (2.5–5 mg/kg sc) or proligestone (10 mg/kg sc) can be administered every 3–6 weeks.[8] Progestin therapy may induce diabetes mellitus, acromegaly and, in intact bitches, cystic endometrial hyperplasia and pyometra.

Key point

- A well-recognised disease, but very uncommon.

References

1   Scott DW, Miller WH, Griffin CE. Endocrine and metabolic diseases. In: *Small Animal Dermatology*, 5th edn. Philadelphia, PA: WB Saunders, 1995: pp. 628–719.
2   Lund-Larson TR, Grondalen J. Aetiolitic dwarfism in the German Shepherd Dog. Low somatomedin activity associated with apparently normal pituitary function (two cases) and with panadenopituitary dysfunction (one case). *Acta Vet Scand* 1976; **17**: 293–306.
3   Voorbij AMWY, van Steenbeek VG, Loohuis M *et al.* A contracted DNA repeat in LHX3 intron 5 is associated with aberrant splicing and pituitary dwarfism in German shepherd dogs. *PLoS ONE* 2011; **6**: e27940.
4   DeBowes LJ. Pituitary dwarfism in a German shepherd dog puppy. *Compend Cont Educ Vet* 1987; **9**: 931–937.
5   Feldman EC, Nelson RW. Growth hormone. In: *Canine and Feline Endocrinology and Reproduction*. Philadelphia, PA; WB Saunders, 1987: pp. 29–54.
6   Kooistra HS. Growth hormone disorders in dogs. *World Small Animal Veterinary Association Proceedings*, 2006.
7   Bell AG. Growth hormone responsive dermatosis in three dogs. *N Z Vet J* 1993; **41**: 195–199.
8   Kooistra HS, Voorhout G, Carlotti DN *et al.* Progestin induced growth hormone (GH) production in treatment of dogs with congenital GH deficiency. *Domest Anim Endocrinol* 1998; **15**: 93–102.

ACRAL MUTILATION SYNDROME

Definition
Acral mutilation syndrome is a genetic disease seen in young dogs, which causes self-mutilation of the feet.

Aetiology and pathogenesis
Acral mutilation syndrome is an autosomal recessive genetic mutation causing abnormalities in the sensory neurons of dogs. In tested English Cocker Spaniels in the UK (as of June 2016), 12% were heterozygous carriers and 3% were homozygous affected dogs.[1]

Clinical features
This disease has been reported in French Spaniels, English Pointers, German Short-haired Pointers, English Springer Spaniels and English Cocker Spaniels (**Fig. 10.9**). Other breeds may have similar symptoms but do not share the same genetic mutation.[2–4] The age of onset ranges from 2 months to 12 months, and symptoms consist of licking, biting and self-mutilation of the feet to the point of digit loss. This is usually more severe in the hindlimbs. As this is a genetic disease, several littermates may be affected. Proprioception and motor abilities remain normal. Dogs do not limp on severely affected limbs even with open sores and broken phalanges.[2–4]

Differential diagnoses
- There would be few other dermatoses that cause such dramatic clinical signs in such a young dog, especially when several members of a litter are affected. Acquired neuropathic disease is not usually seen in very young animals or littermates.

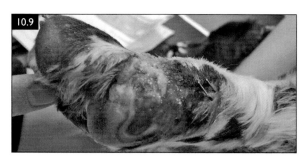

Fig. 10.9 Acral mutilation in a young English Springer Spaniel; the dog had a positive gene test for the condition (photo courtesy of Emma MacFarlane).

- Fishing line, rubber bands, toxins, septicaemia or trauma may cause ischaemic necrosis and slough of the digits similar to this disease. Toxins and septicaemia would also cause necrosis of other distal appendages; constrictions or trauma would usually be restricted to one foot. All of these differentials would cause significant pain, whereas acral mutilation syndrome appears to be painless.

Diagnosis
The diagnosis is based on the history, physical exam and results of genetic testing. Dogs do not show a pain response to noxious stimulus applied to the digits. At necropsy, spinal sensory neurons have characteristic histopathological changes suggestive of decreased neuronal development and evidence of degeneration.[2]

Treatment
Breeding of genetic carriers is not recommended, and carriers can be easily tested for. Treatments are supportive only and include prevention of mutilation by barriers (e.g. muzzles, wraps or Elizabethan collars). Infected lesions should be treated with topical or systemic antimicrobials as appropriate. Gabapentin, pregabalin and amantadine are not consistently effective. Most dogs are euthanised due to the poor prognosis of this disease.

Key point
- Genetic disease with a poor prognosis.

References
1   Figures on AMS in the English Cocker Spaniel in England. (2016). Available at: http://www.antagene.com/en/no/figures-ams-english-cocker-spaniel-england (accessed: 15 April 2018).
2   Paradis M, Jaham CD, Page N, Sauve F, Helie P. Acral mutilation and analgesia in 13 French spaniels. *Vet Dermatol* 2005; **16**: 87–93.
3   Bardagí M, Montoliu P, Ferrer L, Fondevila D, Pumarola M. Acral mutilation syndrome in a miniature pinscher. *J Comp Pathol* 2011; **144**: 235–238.
4   Cummings JF, De Lahunta A, Braund KG, Mitchell Jr WJ. Hereditary sensory neuropathy. Nociceptive loss and acral mutilation in pointer dogs: canine hereditary sensory neuropathy. *Am J Pathol* 1983; **112**: 136.

GENERAL APPROACH TO NODULAR DERMATOSES

Nodular dermatoses may be a precursor to ulcerative dermatoses (see Chapter 7 for additional information about ulcerative dermatoses).

Some nodular dermatoses (such as sebaceous adenomas, page 250, canine viral papillomas, page 252 and cysts, page 251) may be diagnosed with a fine-needle aspirate or physical exam alone. Other nodular dermatoses represent more serious disease and require a biopsy for diagnosis. One of the most

important things to remember when performing a biopsy of a nodule is to include subcutaneous tissue in the sample. Tissue should be obtained for culture and special histopathological stains should be performed on biopsy specimens if a nodule is inflammatory (and not neoplastic) in nature. In addition, immunosuppressive therapy should be avoided until biopsy and/or culture has ruled out infectious disease (see Cryptococcosis, page 259 and Kerion, page 245).

STERILE GRANULOMA/PYOGRANULOMA

Definition

Sterile granuloma/pyogranuloma syndrome is an uncommon immune-mediated disease characterised by skin nodules or plaques with characteristic histopathological features.

Aetiology and pathogenesis

The pathogenesis of sterile granuloma/pyogranuloma syndrome is unknown. However, as no causative agents can be demonstrated and the lesions respond to immunomodulating drugs, an immune-mediated process is suspected.[1-3] In Spain and Italy, where leishmaniasis is endemic, *Leishmania* spp. DNA has been documented by polymerase chain reaction (PCR) and DNA sequencing in 20 of 35 biopsies from dogs that were initially diagnosed as having sterile granuloma/pyogranuloma syndrome.[4] It is therefore important to eliminate *Leishmania* spp. and other infectious agents before concluding that these lesions are sterile.

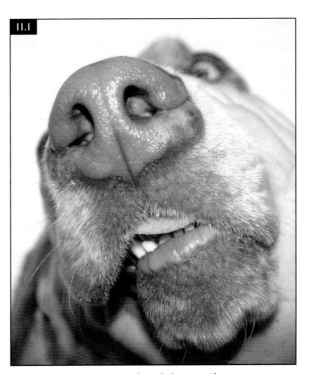

Fig. 11.1 Symmetrical nodular sterile granulomas/pyogranulomas around the nasal planum in a Weimaraner.

Clinical features (Figs. 11.1–11.3)

Lesions consist of firm, non-pruritic (except in cats), non-painful, hairy to alopecic papules,

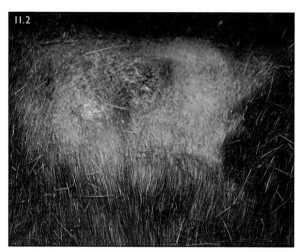

Fig. 11.2 Nodular sterile granuloma/pyogranuloma with early erosions on the dorsal trunk of a Great Dane.

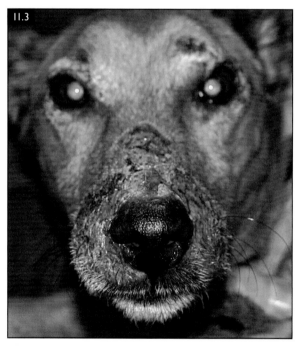

Fig. 11.3 Sterile granuloma/pyogranuloma causing diffuse inflammation and ulceration of the muzzle of a crossbred dog.

nodules and plaques that occur commonly on the head, particularly the bridge of the nose and the muzzle. Less frequently, lesions can appear on the pinna, neck, trunk and extremities.[1-3] The syndrome can occur in any breed, but there is a predisposition for the Great Dane, Boxer, Golden Retriever, Collie and Weimaraner.[1-3] There is no breed predisposition in cats.[5]

Differential diagnoses

- Neoplasia.
- Reactive histiocytosis or histiocytomas.
- Bacterial infection: *Nocardia* spp., *Actinomyces* spp., fast and slow-growing mycobacterial organisms.
- Fungal infection: *Blastomyces* spp., *Coccidioides immitis*, *Histoplasma* spp., cryptococci, *Sporothrix* spp., *Basidiobolus* and *Conidiobolus* spp., and dermatophyte kerions.
- Other infections: *Pythium* and *Lagenidium* spp., *Leishmania* spp.

Diagnosis

The diagnosis is based on dermatohistopathology, with special stains to rule out infectious agents and microbial cultures (tissue) to rule out anaerobic and aerobic bacteria, mycobacteria and fungi. Serology and PCR may also be appropriate to help rule out infections with some organisms.

Treatment

- See Immunosuppressive Drug Therapy Table, page 289, for dosages.
- Doxycycline or minocycline 5 mg/kg po q12 h with niacinamide until resolution and tapering the frequency for maintenance.[6]
- Ciclosporin 5–7 mg/kg po q24 h, tapering to every other day and then twice weekly after resolution.[7]
- Prednisone or methylprednisolone (0.5–2 mg/kg po q12 h) may be administered and lesions generally resolve in 2–6 weeks. The dose can then be changed to alternate-day and, over 8–10 weeks, be tapered to maintenance.
- Azathioprine (2 mg/kg po q24 h or q48 h) may be used along with glucocorticoids in refractory cases.[3]
- The disease has been reported to spontaneously resolve without treatment.

Key point

- This condition is generally controlled rather than cured. However, sterile granuloma/pyogranuloma syndrome is typically quite responsive to therapy.

References

1 Houston DM, Clark EG, Matwichuk CL *et al*. A case of cutaneous sterile pyogranuloma/ granuloma syndrome in a golden retriever. *Can Vet J* 1993; **34**: 121–122.

2 Gross TH, Ihrke PJ, Walder EJ, Affolter VK. Sterile granuloma and pyogranuloma syndrome. In: *Skin Diseases of the Dog and Cat: Clinical and Histopathologic Diagnosis*, 2nd edn. Oxford: Blackwell Publishing, 2005: pp. 320–323.

3 Panich R, Scott DW, Miller WH. Canine cutaneous sterile pyogranuloma/ granuloma syndrome: a retrospective analysis of 29 cases (1976–1988). *J Am Anim Hosp Assoc* 1991; **27**: 519–528.

4 Cornegliani L, Fondevla D, Vercelli A *et al*. PCR detection of *Leishmania* and *Mycobacterium* organisms in canine cutaneous sterile pyogranuloma/granuloma syndrome (SPGS). *Vet Dermatol* 2005; **16**: 235–238.

5 Scott DW, Buerger RG, Miller WH. Idiopathic sterile granulomatous and pyogranulomatous dermatitis in cats. *Vet Dermatol* 1990; **1**: 129–137.

6 Rothstien E, Scott DW, Riis RC. Tetracycline and niacinamide for the treatment of sterile pyogranuloma/granuloma syndrome in a dog. *J Am Anim Hosp Assoc* 1997; **33**: 540–543.

7 Miller WH, Griffin CE, Campbell KL, Muller GH. In: *Muller and Kirk's Small Animal Dermatology*. Amsterdam: Elsevier Health Sciences, 2013: pp. 695–723.

DERMATOPHYTE KERIONS

Canine nodular dermatophytosis

Aetiology and pathogenesis

A dermatophyte kerion is caused by a granulomatous immune response to dermatophytic fungal infection in (primarily) dogs (see Dermatophytosis, page 115, for more details of subcutaneous nodular dermatophytosis in cats). The primary type of dermatophyte may vary regionally.[1]

Clinical features

Dermatophyte kerions are exudative, erythematous, dome-shaped nodules of (most commonly) the haired skin near the nasal planum, head, neck and/or limbs. Dogs with kerions typically present with one to two lesions, but there can be multiple (**Fig. 11.4**).[1] The lesions are generally not pruritic.

Differential diagnoses

• Sterile granuloma/pyogranuloma.
• Histiocytic disease.
• Neoplasia.
• Demodicosis.
• Staphylococcal folliculitis and furunculosis.
• Other deep fungal infections.

Diagnosis

A history of direct contact or environmental exposure to a potentially infected animal (most commonly cats) along with characteristic clinical signs should give a strong suspicion for this disease. Skin scraping will rule out demodicosis. Cytology reveals pyogranulomatous inflammation, with or without bacterial involvement, and, if obtained from exudate expressed from the lesions, will often show fungal arthrospores.[1] A fungal culture for diagnosis and speciation of dermatophyte should be performed, but a negative culture does not rule this condition out. A biopsy is diagnostic and helps rule out other diseases.

Treatment

The following management is for dogs (see Dermatophytosis, page 119 for more information on treatment of nodular dermatophytosis in cats). Lesions may resolve on their own without treatment,[2] but this is unacceptable for most owners. Lesions can be treated with topical antifungals such as clotrimazole, miconazole or terbinafine creams q12 h. This is often

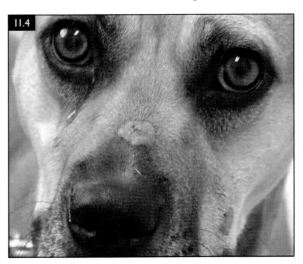

Fig. 11.4 Dermatophyte kerions on the face of a dog.

curative for localised disease. If the disease is extensive, oral antifungals such as itraconazole (5–10 mg/kg per day po with food, although the oral suspension should be given on fasting), or terbinafine (20–30 mg/kg po q12–24 h with food) should be added with the topical therapy until resolution, keeping in mind potential side effects from systemic antifungal therapy. Ketoconazole (10 mg/kg per day po with food) tends to have more gastrointestinal (GI) and hepatic side effects. Lesions typically resolve with therapy in 4–8 weeks.[1]

It is very unlikely that the dermatophyte infection will spread to a human or other animals from the dog's skin lesions[1,3] (probably because the infective spores are in very low numbers[3]). Generally, by the time dermatophyte kerions appear on a dog (1–3 weeks after exposure[2]), quarantining the dog from housemates or household family members is not likely to be useful unless there are specific risk factors for infection (e.g. immunosuppressed, Persian cats or multi-cat households). Bear in mind that lesions on the owner or other animals are more likely to occur after exposure to the original infective source or a fomite 1–3 weeks ago, so all should be monitored and appropriate treatments or prevention performed (see Dermatophytosis, page 115, for more information).

Key point

- Canine dermatophyte kerions can be striking in appearance but contain very few infective fungal spores and respond well to treatment.

References

1 Cornegliani L, Persico P, Colombo S. Canine nodular dermatophytosis (kerion): 23 cases. *Vet Dermatol* 2009; **20**: 185–190.
2 Moriello KA, DeBoer DJ. In: Greene CE (ed.), *Infectious Diseases of the Dog and Cat*. Amsterdam: Elsevier Health Sciences, 2013: pp. 588–602.
3 Mancianti F, Nardoni S, Corazza M, Dachille P, Ponticelli C. Environmental detection of arthrospores in the households of infected cats and dogs. *J Feline Med Surg* 2003; **5**: 323–328.

HISTIOCYTIC NEOPLASIA

Definition

Histiocytes can accumulate in the skin and internal organs. A variety of histiocytic conditions may result and are differentiated based on extent of disease and neoplastic potential.

Aetiology and pathogenesis

Cutaneous histiocytoma is a benign nodular proliferation of Langerhans' cells. Cutaneous histiocytosis and systemic histiocytosis are non-cancerous proliferations of perivascular dermal dendritic cells. Histiocytic sarcomas arise from dendritic cells of the synovial lining of joints. The breed incidence of systemic histiocytosis and histiocytic sarcoma indicates that there is a genetic susceptibility.

Clinical features

Cutaneous histiocytomas are common tumours, usually seen in dogs aged <3 years,[1] although they can be seen in older immunosuppressed dogs. They are typically solitary, small, non-pruritic, non-painful nodules most commonly on the head, ears, neck and limbs). They frequently ulcerate, but in most this precedes rapid resolution.[1] Ulcerated nodules can become infected or a focus for self-trauma. Most solitary lesions resolve within 1–2 months of presentation. Local lymph nodes can be affected, but these cases will still eventually resolve (although rarely this may take many months).[1]

Cutaneous Langerhans' cell histiocytosis is seen most commonly in Shar Peis. This is a condition of multiple rapidly growing, often ulcerated histiocytomas with a worse prognosis than solitary lesions because some of these cases do not have spontaneous regression and have eventual lymph node, lung and internal organ involvement.[2] About 50% of dogs with this condition are euthanised due to extensive ulceration or systemic spread.[2]

Cutaneous histiocytosis is typically associated with one or more firm nodules or plaques, especially around the head, neck, perineum and extremities (**Figs. 11.5–11.7**). They can be hairy or alopecic and erythematous, but are usually non-painful and non-pruritic. More advanced lesions may undergo central necrosis and scarring. There is no apparent age (range 3–9 years), breed or sex predisposition. Spontaneous

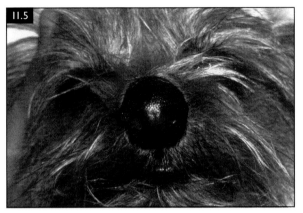

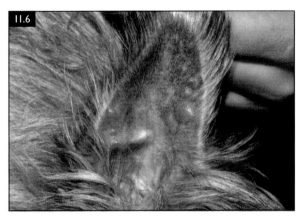

Figs. 11.5, 11.6 Swollen nose (Fig. 11.5) and erythematous nodules on the pinna (Fig. 11.6) of a Yorkshire Terrier with cutaneous histiocytosis.

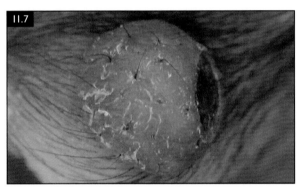

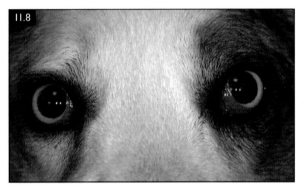

Fig. 11.7 Histiocytoma on the elbow of a dog; it resolved spontaneously over 2 months.

Fig. 11.8 Third eyelid protrusion, conjunctival swelling and conjunctivitis in a Border Collie with systemic histiocytosis.

remission and reoccurrence may occur,[2] but most cases wax and wane without remission. The prognosis is good but needs to be differentiated from systemic histiocytosis, which has similar skin lesions but a worse prognosis.

Systemic histiocytosis is most commonly seen in Bernese Mountain dogs, but also in other breeds including the Golden Retriever, Labrador Retriever, Boxer and Rottweiler. It usually affects adults (4–7 years), but there is no sex predisposition. Skin lesions are similar to those of cutaneous histiocytosis (see above), but there may also be involvement of the conjunctiva (**Fig. 11.8**), sclera, retrobulbar tissues, nasal cavity, lymph nodes and internal organs, including the liver, spleen, lungs and bone marrow. The course of the disease is prolonged, and the prognosis is guarded; most dogs eventually succumb to the disease.[3]

Localised histiocytic sarcomas are focal, rapidly growing and aggressive tumours. They are usually seen in Bernese Mountain dogs, Flat Coat Retrievers,

Golden Retrievers, Labradors and Rottweilers, but other breeds can be affected. There is no age or sex predisposition.[4] The lesions tend to affect the skin, subcutis and deeper tissues on the extremities, often near joints. Despite the local appearance, most of these tumours have already spread and survival times average about 5 months from diagnosis.[5]

Disseminated histiocytic sarcoma is most widely recognised in Bernese Mountain dogs, but has been seen in other breeds including Golden Retrievers, Labrador Retrievers and Rottweilers. There is no age or sex predisposition. This condition is primarily of the internal organs (primary sites are lungs and spleen) and sometimes spread to the skin. Most dogs present with an acute history of lethargy, anorexia, anaemia and weight loss, and other clinical signs depending on the organs affected.[4] In one study of Bernese Mountain dogs, median survival time was 30 days from presentation; <10% live longer than 4 months.[6]

Differential diagnoses

- Bacterial, mycobacterial or fungal granuloma.
- Other cutaneous neoplasia such as nodular epitheliotrophic lymphoma.
- Foreign body granuloma.
- Sterile granuloma/pyogranuloma syndrome.

Diagnostic tests

Aspirates of nodules may reveal atypical histiocytes (**Fig. 11.9**). Lymphocytes are typically present in histiocytomas undergoing regression, but their presence does not indicate regression in the other histiocytic diseases. Neutrophils and bacteria may be present in ulcerated lesions. Biopsy and histopathology with special stains to rule out infectious agents and immunophenotyping to confirm cell type is recommended to confirm the diagnosis. For all cases except a solitary histiocytoma, a thorough physical examination, ocular and retinal examination should be performed, and full blood panel, aspirates of local lymph nodes, ultrasonography of the abdomen and chest radiographs be considered to determine whether there is systemic involvement.

Treatment

- Most **histiocytomas** resolve spontaneously within 3 months.[7] Immunosuppressive drugs that inhibit lymphocyte function may interfere with regression and should be decreased or discontinued if possible. Surgical excision is usually curative for ulcerated and/or persistent nodules.
- For **cutaneous Langerhans' cell histiocytosis**, there are no reported consistently helpful treatments; the lesions may spontaneously resolve over many months, but about 50% of dogs are euthanised due to the disease.[2] Lomustine (CCNU) has been used with some success.[2] There is a report of griseofulvin being helpful in a puppy.[8]
- For **cutaneous histiocytosis**, treatment is typically lifelong. Minocycline or doxycycline at 5–10 mg/kg q12 h with niacinamide is often effective.[9] It may take several weeks for resolution. Ciclosporin (modified) at 5–7 mg/kg po q24 h is another option,[3,9] and it may take several weeks for resolution. Leflunomide has been also reported to be effective.[3] If those options are not available or not tolerated, prednisone or methylprednisolone at 1–2 mg/kg per day is can be used, although animals should be carefully monitored for side effects with daily long-term use.[9] The dose should be tapered to the lowest alternate-day dose possible. Where necessary, steroids can be combined with other immunomodulating and immunosuppressive agents. (See Immunosuppressive Drug Therapy Table, page 289, for dosages.)
- Treatment for **systemic histiocytosis** is similar to that for cutaneous histiocytosis, but the prognosis is more guarded because most dogs seem to eventually succumb to systemic involvement.[3] It is probably best to start aggressive treatment with ciclosporin, leflunomide or CCNU.
- The prognosis for **histiocytic sarcoma**, whether localised or disseminated, is very poor, because metastasis to local lymph nodes or internal organs is very common. Wide surgical resection, sometimes requiring amputation, has been curative in some localised cases without metastases.[4] However, another study showed that 10 of 11 dogs with what appeared to be local disease did have eventual metastases, and of 18 dogs in the study, none lived longer than 16 months after diagnosis. No matter what the treatment, the average time to death was 5 months.[5] CCNU chemotherapy appears to be helpful to achieve partial and short-term remissions in about 30% of local or disseminated cases.[10]

Histiocytic proliferative diseases in cats

Feline progressive dendritic cell histiocytosis is rare and appears to be a slowly progressive indolent form of histiocytic sarcoma. Nodules are first

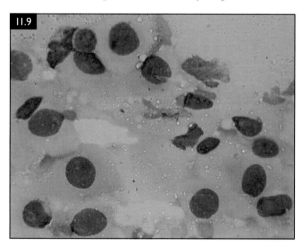

Fig. 11.9 Atypical histiocytes in an aspirate from an histiocytoma.

noticed on the head, neck or lower limbs. Over time, more nodules appear and may ulcerate and coalesce. Eventually internal organs are involved. There do not seem to be effective therapies.[11]

Key points

- Biopsy and histopathological examination are critical for diagnosis.
- The prognosis is good for cutaneous histiocytosis and histiocytoma.
- The prognosis for systemic histiocytosis and histiocytic sarcoma is poor.

References

1 Gross TL, Ihrke PJ, Walder EJ, Affolter VK. Skin diseases of the dog and cat. In: *Clinical and Histopathologic Diagnosis*, 2nd edn. Ames: Blackwell Science, 2005.

2 Moore PF. A review of histiocytic diseases of dogs and cats. *Vet Pathol* 2014; **51**: 167–184.

3 Affolter VK, Moore PF. Canine cutaneous and systemic histiocytosis: reactive histiocytosis of dermal dendritic cellsNANA. *Am J Dermatopathol* 2000; **22**: 40–48.

4 Affolter VK, Moore PF. Localized and disseminated histiocytic sarcoma of dendritic cell origin in dogs. *Vet Pathol* 2002; **39**: 74–83.

5 Craig LE, Julian ME, Ferracone JD. The diagnosis and prognosis of synovial tumors in dogs: 35 cases. *Vet Pathol Online* 2002; **39**: 66–73.

6 Abadie J, Hédan B, Cadieu E, De Brito C *et al.* Epidemiology, pathology, and genetics of histiocytic sarcoma in the Bernese Mountain Dog breed. *J Hered* 2009; **100**: S19–S27.

7 Miller WH, Griffin CE, Campbell KL, Muller GH. Neoplastic and non-neoplastic tumors. In: *Muller and Kirk's Small Animal Dermatology*. Amsterdam: Elsevier Health Sciences, 2013: pp. 774–843.

8 Nagata M, Hirata M, Ishida T, Hirata S, Nanko H. Progressive Langerhans' cell histiocytosis in a puppy. *Vet Dermatol* 2000; **11**: 241–246.

9 Palmeiro BS, Morris DO, Goldschmidt MH, Mauldin EA. Cutaneous reactive histiocytosis in dogs: a retrospective evaluation of 32 cases. *Vet Dermatol* 2007; **18**: 332–340.

10 Rassnick KM, Moore AS, Russell DS *et al.* Phase II, open-label trial of single-agent CCNU in dogs with previously untreated histiocytic sarcoma. *J Vet Intern Med* 2010; **24**: 1528–1531.

11 Affolter VK, Moore PF. Feline progressive histiocytosis. *Vet Pathol Online* 2006; **43**: 646–655.

CANINE EOSINOPHILIC GRANULOMA

Definition

Canine eosinophilic granuloma is a rare syndrome in which nodules or plaques with a characteristic histopathological pattern develop in the skin, oral mucosa or external ear canal.

Aetiology and pathogenesis

Canine eosinophilic granuloma appears to be a hypersensitivity reaction. The precipitating cause is unknown in many instances, but some cases may be hypersensitivity reactions to arthropod bites or insect stings.[1–4]

Clinical features

Siberian Huskies and Cavalier King Charles Spaniels are predisposed, but the condition has been reported in other breeds.[1–8] Dogs tend to be males and aged <3 years. Lesions occur more frequently in the oral cavity, especially on the lateral or ventral surface of the tongue. Oral lesions are friable, bleed easily and often become ulcerated.[3,4,8] Skin lesions consist of solitary or grouped erythematous papules, nodules or plaques on the pinna, muzzle, nasal planum, neck, axilla, flank, prepuce, scrotum or ventral abdomen (**Fig. 11.10**).[1,2,4,6,7]

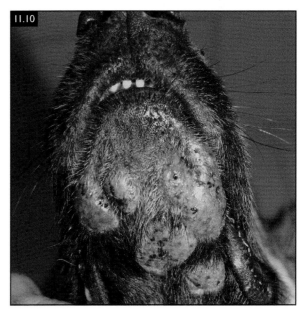

Fig. 11.10 Multiple eosinophilic granulomas in a German Shepherd dog. These were associated with a mosquito bite hypersensitivity.

Differential diagnoses

- Foreign body granulomas.
- Neoplasia.
- Bacterial or fungal granulomas.
- Sterile granuloma and pyogranuloma.
- Histiocytic lesions.

Diagnosis

The diagnosis is based on biopsy, cytology and dermatohistopathology.

Treatment

Small solitary lesions may regress spontaneously.[3,5,7] Methylprednisolone (0.8–1.6 mg/kg po q24 h) or prednisone (1–2 mg/kg po q12 h) may be given. Lesions generally resolve in 2–4 weeks, after which the dose can be changed to alternate-day administration and tapered. Some dogs may need ongoing therapy, but most need treatment only during a flare. Insect repellents can be considered where insect bites are thought to be a trigger.

Key point

- Canine eosinophilic granuloma is diagnosed by biopsy and responds well to corticosteroid therapy.

References

1 Curial da Silva JMA, Kraus KH, Brown TP *et al.* Eosinophilic granuloma of the nasal skin in a dog. *J Am Anim Hosp Assoc* 1998; **20**: 603–606.

2 Gross TH, Ihrke PJ, Walder EJ, Affolter VK. Canine eosinophilic granuloma. In: *Skin Diseases of the Dog and Cat: Clinical and Histopathologic Diagnosis*, 2nd edn. Oxford: Blackwell Publishing, 2005: pp. 358–360.

3 Madewell BR, Stannard AA, Pulley LT *et al.* Oral eosinophilic granuloma in Siberian husky dogs. *J Am Vet Med Assoc* 1980; **177**: 701–703.

4 Norris JM. Cutaneous eosinophilic granuloma in a crossbred dog: a case report and literature review. *Aust Pract* 1994; **24**: 74–78.

5 Potter KA, Tucker RD, Carpenter JL. Oral eosinophilic granuloma of Siberian huskies. *J Am Anim Hosp Assoc* 1980; **16**: 595–600.

6 Scott DW. Cutaneous eosinophilic granulomas with collagen degeneration in the dog. *J Am Anim Hosp Assoc* 1988; **19**: 529–532.

7 Turnwald GH, Hoskins JD, Taylor HW. Cutaneous eosinophilic granuloma in a Labrador retriever. *J Am Vet Med Assoc* 1981; **179**: 799–801.

8 Walsh KM. Oral eosinophilic granuloma in two dogs. *J Am Vet Med Assoc* 1983; **183**: 323–324.

SEBACEOUS GLAND TUMOURS – BENIGN

Including nodular sebaceous hyperplasia, sebaceous adenomas and sebaceous epitheliomas

Definition

Sebaceous tumours are caused by abnormal growth of sebaceous glandular tissue; sebaceous adenomas and sebaceous epitheliomas are likely to start as nodular sebaceous hyperplasia.

Aetiology and pathogenesis

The underlying trigger for this abnormal growth of sebocytes is not known, although certain breeds of dogs (Cocker Spaniels, Poodles) appear to be predisposed and there is evidence that androgens may be involved.[1]

Clinical features

Sebaceous gland tumours are common in dogs and rare in cats.[2] They can be found on almost all areas of the body. Lesions are pinkish/yellowish/whitish, firm, alopecic, warty and multi-nodular or plaque like, hyperkeratotic and greasy (**Fig. 11.11**). They may be pruritic and may ulcerate and bleed easily when the pet scratches them or during grooming. The ulceration and seborrhoea may result in secondary *Malassezia* or staphylococcal infection. Some dogs develop very large numbers of tumours. Affected dogs commonly have concurrent meibomian gland adenomas on their eyelids.

Differential diagnoses

- Large ulcerated lesions may be sebaceous carcinoma.
- Other neoplasia.
- Viral papillomas.

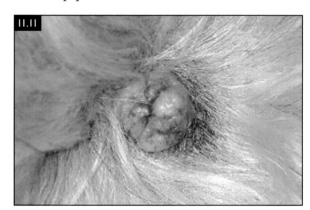

Fig. 11.11 Sebaceous adenoma in an older small breed dog.

Diagnosis

These lesions are usually visually distinctive. Cytology may reveal secondary yeast or bacterial infections and fine-needle aspirates may show sebaceous cells. Histopathology is diagnostic.

Treatment

If lesions are not ulcerated or bothersome, they can be observed without treatment. Surgical excision is curative if all abnormal tissue is removed. Ulcerated or locally aggressive lesions should have margins obtained due to higher likelihood of a carcinoma. Recurrence in the same location is rare with complete removal, but new lesions developing elsewhere is common. CO_2 laser ablation or cautery under sedation and local or general anaesthesia is quick and effective where there are multiple masses and/or sites that would be difficult for surgical excision and closure. Topical application of products containing nitric acid, acetic acid, oxalic acid, lactic acid and zinc nitrate has also been described.

Key point

- Removal or ablation is curative, but there is no known prevention for the common recurrence of lesions elsewhere.

References

1 Sabattini S, Bassi P, Bettini G. Histopathological findings and proliferative activity of canine sebaceous gland tumours with a predominant reserve cell population. *J Comp Pathol* 2015; **152**: 145–152.
2 Gross TL, Ihrke PJ, Walder EJ, Affolter VK. In: *Clinical and Histopathologic Diagnosis*, 2nd edn. Ames: Blackwell Science, 2005.

FOLLICULAR AND APOCRINE CYSTS

Inclusion cysts, infundibular keratinising acanthoma or apocrine cysts

Aetiology and pathogenesis

Cysts are sac-like structures with an epithelial lining caused by abnormal growth of skin structures. As certain breeds seem to be predisposed, it is likely that there is a genetic predisposition in many cases.

Clinical features

Follicular cysts are firm intradermal or subcutaneous nodules ranging from 0.2 cm × 2 cm in diameter (**Fig. 11.12**). There may be a large pore at the top, sometimes with exuding keratin, or no opening. The nodule may have a slight blue or yellow hue due to the cyst contents. The cyst may rupture underneath the skin causing a draining tract and severe inflammation of the surrounding area. The contents of these cysts are thick, caseous and/or granular with a grey, yellow–white or tan colour (typically 'porridge-like').

Infundibular keratinising acanthomas (IKAs) are follicular cysts that may be multiple and problematic in dogs (**Fig. 11.13**). They are 0.5- to 4.0-cm nodules

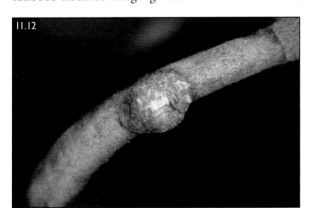

Fig. 11.12 Large follicular inclusion cyst on a dog's tail.

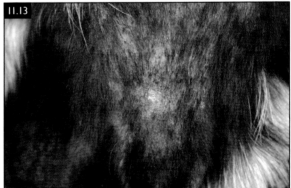

Fig. 11.13 Early infundibular keratinising acanthoma; these lesions often enlarge, rupture and drain a porridge-like material.

with a visible central pore that often has protruding keratin, which forms cutaneous horns. Some IKAs are deep and do not open onto the skin surface. IKAs are located primarily on the dorsal neck and trunk, but can be anywhere. Norwegian Elkhounds, Lhasa Apsos, Pekingese, Yorkshire Terriers, old English Sheepdogs and German Shepherd dogs are predisposed to IKAs.[1]

Apocrine cysts are turgid or soft intradermal nodules that are bluish coloured, thin walled and obviously fluid filled. They are usually on the head and neck, but may occur on the limbs and trunk. Usually the fluid is watery, clear and acellular. Ceruminous adenomas and cysts are found inside and around the ears or on the head of cats and are filled with brown acellular material (see page 279).

Differential diagnoses

- Abscess.
- Deep fungal or bacterial infection.
- Panniculitis.
- Cutaneous neoplasia.
- *Cuterebra* spp. infestation.

Diagnosis

Aspiration cytology usually reveals amorphic keratinaceous and sebaceous debris, sometimes with cholesterol crystals and intact keratinocytes. Neutrophils and bacteria may be present in inflamed and infected lesions. Histopathological examination of excised samples will confirm the clinical diagnosis and exclude epidermal or follicular neoplasia.

Treatment

Observation without treatment is certainly an option for most of these lesions. Lancing and removal of cystic debris alone are not curative, and squeezing these lesions often causes rupture under the skin, resulting in severe inflammation. Surgical excision is curative, although affected animals tend to produce new lesions in due course. Antibiotics may be necessary if lesions become infected. Systemic retinoids such as isotretinoin (1–2 mg/kg po q24 h) or vitamin A (800–100 IU/kg per day) may help in cases with multiple IKAs.[2] These drugs tend to prevent development of new lesions and result in regression of small lesions, but often have little effect on larger lesions.

Key point

- Do not be tempted to squeeze the cysts.

References

1   Gross TL, Ihrke PJ, Walder EJ, Affolter VK. In: *Clinical and Histopathologic Diagnosis*, 2nd edn. Ames: Blackwell Science, 2005.
2   Power HT, Ihrke PJ. Synthetic retinoids in veterinary dermatology. *Vet Clin North Am Small Anim Pract* 1990; **20**: 1525–1539.

VIRAL PAPILLOMATOSIS – CANINE

Definition

Papillomatosis is a typically nodular proliferation of epithelial cells caused by papillomavirus.

Aetiology and pathogenesis

Papillomaviruses are contagious and are introduced through lesions in the skin. Epithelial proliferation is noticed by 4–6 weeks postinfection.[1] Young, social and immunosuppressed dogs are at increased risk of infection. Currently, 14 different canine papillomaviruses have been discovered (CPV1–14).[2]

Clinical features

Viral papillomas are widely variable in appearance. In dogs, typically there is a rapid appearance of papular, nodular, verrucous, fimbriated, donut-like or plaque-like lesions on the skin or mucous membranes. Most lesions are not painful unless on the feet, when infected or if traumatised. Lesions can vary from solitary and pinpoint to large and numerous. There are several different clinical presentations of papillomavirus infections in dogs:

- **Oral papillomas** are the most common type. CPV1 typically causes depigmented shiny plaques on the oral or ocular mucosa, tongue, palate, nares or lips, which progress to nodular fimbriated or cauliflower-like masses (**Fig. 11.14**). Neoplastic transformation has been reported with non-regressing lesions. This virus can infect non-mucocutaneous areas of skin in immunosuppressed individuals.[3] Most spontaneously regress over 1–3 months.

- **Cutaneous inverted papillomas** are 1- to 2-cm raised, smooth, firm lesions with a central pore that often have a donut or cup shape, but can appear as small smooth nodules. They are mostly found on the ventral abdomen but can be seen in multiple locations such as the limbs, head, neck and interdigitally.[4,5] Most spontaneously regress.
- **Papillomavirus pigmented plaques** are most commonly seen in Miniature Schnauzers and Pugs, but can be seen in many breeds (**Fig. 11.15**).[6] These manifest as darkly pigmented plaques with a rough surface and are usually found on the ventrum. Neoplastic transformation has been reported as a rare sequela in several breeds,[7–9] but never in the Pug.[10] They can occasionally be pruritic. These lesions do not undergo spontaneous regression and surgical removal or close monitoring is warranted.
- **Digital/footpad papillomas** – interdigital viral papillomas often appear and regress rapidly, generally within 2 weeks, although 2 months to remission has been reported (**Fig. 11.16**).[11] If they do not regress quickly, a cutaneous horn may form that resembles a toenail. Weight bearing on these lesions can be very painful. Surgical removal or CO_2 laser ablation appears to be curative for footpad lesions.[12] If persistent for many months, digital papillomas may transform to squamous cell carcinoma.[13]
- New research has associated some **footpad corns** in Greyhounds (see page 226) with papillomaviruses.

Differential diagnoses
- Sebaceous adenomas.
- Hair follicle tumours.
- Cutaneous horns.
- Melanocytic neoplasias.
- Squamous cell carcinoma.
- Benign pigmented macule (lentigo).

Diagnosis
The diagnosis may be based on history and clinical appearance of lesions. Excision and histopathological examination are diagnostic and often curative for solitary lesions.

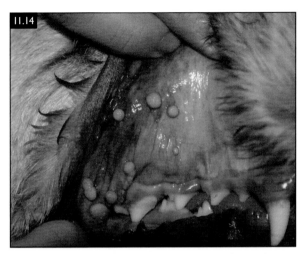

Fig. 11.14 Multiple viral papillomas on the oral mucosa of a dog undergoing chemotherapy.

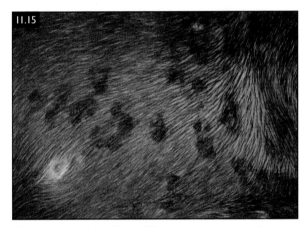

Fig. 11.15 Multiple papillomavirus pigmented plaques in a German Short-haired Pointer.

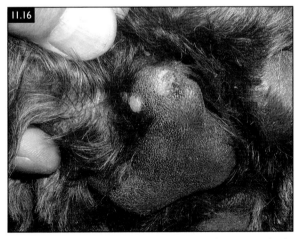

Fig. 11.16 Two viral papillomas on the footpad of a dog.

Treatment

Most papillomavirus infections spontaneously resolve over weeks to months. Neoplastic transformation of non-regressing papillomavirus lesions has been reported with many strains of the virus.[14]

- Observation is the best treatment, because only a small proportion of papillomas do not spontaneously regress eventually. However, pigmented plaques typically do not regress.[10,15] Immunosuppressive therapy must be stopped to permit spontaneous regression, although prednisone therapy does not inhibit spontaneous regression except at high doses (above 2mg/kg per day).[16]
- Interferon should be considered if lesions are still progressive after 3 months, if the pet is on immunosuppressive therapy that cannot be stopped or if the lesions are causing severe pain or disability. There is a report of resolution of severe oral papillomatosis in a dog given 1 MU/kg recombinant feline interferon-ω by subcutaneous injection once daily for 5 consecutive days and the 5-day treatment was repeated 14 days later.[17] Interferon-α-2b has been used orally at an anecdotal dose of 20 000 IU/day po. Lesions often rapidly diminish 2–3 weeks post-treatment. There are no studies of oral interferon for the treatment of papillomas in dogs. Lower doses (as used in studies of other diseases[18]) are anecdotally not as effective for papillomas. There is a report of interferon-α-2A used to treat viral plaques, and it was somewhat helpful at 1000 IU daily po.[9] Side effects are GI, general lethargy or slight fever; these symptoms rapidly disappear on stopping the medication. Clients should be warned that interferon is not an approved therapy and long-term side effects are not known.
- Physical removal with surgery, laser or cryotherapy may be curative with solitary lesions and is the treatment of choice for pigmented papillomavirus plaques. Surgical removal is less helpful for multiple papillomavirus lesions because viral particles are widespread in the surrounding keratinocytes and recurrence is common.
- Imiquimod topically may be helpful for regression of some types of papillomavirus infections.[6] It would be used two to three times a week until complete resolution. The papillomas and surrounding skin may become severely inflamed before resolution. The dog should wear an Elizabethan (e-)collar to prevent licking of the medication, and owners should avoid contact with the medication.
- Topical application of products containing nitric acid, acetic acid, oxalic acid, lactic acid and zinc nitrate has also been described.

Key point

- A common condition that usually resolves spontaneously.

References

1 Favrot C. In: Greene CE (ed.), *Infectious Diseases of the Dog and Cat*. Amsterdam: Elsevier Health Sciences, 2013: pp. 161–174.

2 Lange CE, Tobler, K, Brandes K *et al.* Complete canine papillomavirus life cycle in pigmented lesions. *Vet Microbiol* 2013; **162**: 388–395.

3 Sundberg JP, Smith EK, Herron AJ *et al.* Involvement of canine oral papillomavirus in generalized oral and cutaneous verrucosis in a Chinese Shar Pei dog. *Vet Pathol Online* 1994; **31**:183–187.

4 Shimada A, Shinya K, Awakura T *et al.* Cutaneous papillomatosis associated with papillomavirus infection in a dog. *J Comp Pathol* 1993; **108**: 103–107.

5 Campbell KL, Sundberg JP, Goldschmidt MH, Knupp C, Reichmann ME. Cutaneous inverted papillomas in dogs. *Vet Pathol Online* 1988; **25**: 67–71.

6 Lange CE, Favrot C. Canine papillomaviruses. *Vet Clin North Am Small Anim Pract* 2011; **41**: 1183–1195.

7 Nagata M, Nanko H, Moriyama A, Washizu T, Ishida,T. Pigmented plaques associated with papillomavirus infection in dogs: is this epidermodysplasia verruciformis? *Vet Dermatol* 1995; **6**: 179–186.

8 Walder EJ. Malignant transformation of a pigmented epidermal nevus in a dog. *Vet Pathol* 1997; **34**: 505.

9 Stokking LB, Ehrhart EJ, Lichtensteiger CA, Campbell KL. Pigmented epidermal plaques in three dogs. *J Am Anim Hosp Assoc* 2004; **40**: 411–417.

10 Tobler K, Lange C, Carlotti DN, Ackermann M, Favrot C. Detection of a novel papillomavirus in pigmented plaques of four pugs. *Vet Dermatol* 2008; **19**: 21–25.

11 DeBey BM, Bagladi-Swanson M, Kapil S, Oehme FW. Digital papillomatosis in a confined Beagle. *J Vet Diagn Invest* 2001; **13**: 346–348.

12 Balara JM, McCarthy RJ, Kiupel M *et al*. Clinical, histologic, and immunohistochemical characterization of wart-like lesions on the paw pads of dogs: 24 cases (2000–2007). *J Am Vet Med Assoc* 2009; **234**: 1555–1558.

13 Goldschmidt MH, Kennedy JS, Kennedy DR *et al*. Severe papillomavirus infection progressing to metastatic squamous cell carcinoma in bone marrow-transplanted X-linked SCID dogs. *J Virol* 2006; **80**: 6621–6628.

14 Munday JS, Kiupel M. Papillomavirus-associated cutaneous neoplasia in mammals. *Vet Pathol* 2010; **47**: 254–264.

15 Narama I, Kobayashi Y, Yamagami T, Ozaki K, Ueda Y. Pigmented cutaneous papillomatosis (pigmented epidermal nevus) in three pug dogs; histopathology,

electron microscopy and analysis of viral DNA by the polymerase chain reaction. *J Comp Pathol* 2005; **132**: 132–138.

16 Jahan-Parwar B, Chhetri DK, Bhuta S, Hart S, Berke GS. Development of a canine model for recurrent respiratory papillomatosis. *Ann Otol Rhinol Laryngol* 2003; **112**: 1011–1013.

17 Fantini O, Videmont E, Pin D. Successful treatment of florid papillomatosis in a dog using subcutaneous feline recombinant interferon-omega. *Rev Med Vet* 2015; **166**: 25–29.

18 Cummins JM, Krakowka GS, Thompson CG. Systemic effects of interferons after oral administration in animals and humans. *Am J Vet Res* 2005; **66**: 164–176.

VIRAL PAPILLOMATOSIS – FELINE

Feline fibropapillomas (feline sarcoids), feline viral plaques, feline bowenoid in-situ carcinomas or feline multi-centric squamous cell carcinomas

Definition

Papillomatosis is a crusting, plaque or nodular proliferation of epithelial cells caused by papillomavirus.

Aetiology and pathogenesis

Papillomaviruses are contagious and are introduced through lesions in the skin; epithelial proliferation is noticed by 4–6 weeks after infection.[1] Feline papillomavirus 1 and 2 have been found in viral plaques, bowenoid lesions and cutaneous squamous cell carcinomas in cats,[2] but not in oral squamous cell carcinomas.[3] Bovine papillomavirus-1 has been found in feline fibropapillomas.[4,5]

Clinical features

There are three distinct clinical appearances of papillomaviruses in cats:

Feline fibropapillomas (feline sarcoid) lesions are firm, alopecic, sometimes ulcerated, nodules or small plaques <2 cm, found on the head (lips, nostrils, eyelids, ears), neck, limbs and digits of (most commonly) young cats (<5 years old) that have exposure to the outdoors and often to cattle (**Fig. 11.17**).[5,6] Local recurrence after removal is common.[5]

Feline viral plaques are oval or elongated plaques that are scaly and may be pigmented (**Fig. 11.18**). These lesions are more often seen in older cats or

with poor immune function, and may be associated with *Demodex* mites. These lesions may eventuate to bowenoid in-situ carcinoma or multi-centric squamous cell carcinoma with chronicity, so all three lesions may be present on one cat.[2]

Feline oral papillomatosis is rare and appears as small flat plaques on the tongue.[7]

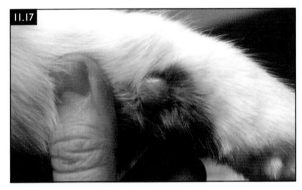

Fig. 11.17 Feline sarcoid.

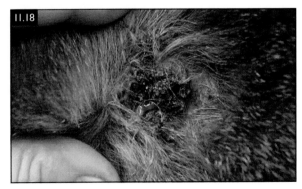

Fig. 11.18 Papillomaviral plaque on a 14-year-old cat.

Differential diagnoses

- Bowen's disease.
- Mycobacterial disease.
- Deep fungal or bacterial disease.
- Squamous cell carcinoma.
- Other neoplasia.

Diagnosis

Biopsy and histopathology are usually necessary for definitive diagnosis of viral papilloma infection in cats.

Treatment

- Spontaneous regression of papillomas typically occurs after the development of a cell-mediated immune response. However, feline viral plaques typically do not regress.
- There are anecdotal reports for the use of interferon at 1.5–2 MU/m^2 sc three times weekly for 4–8 weeks (2 weeks beyond clinical cure) or interferon-α at 30 U/cat po q24 h.[6,8]
- Imiquimod cream (5%) can be applied topically q24–48 h until the lesions regress. An e-collar should be used to prevent ingestion by the cat.[9,10] Owners should avoid contact.
- Surgery, cautery or CO_2 laser ablation can be considered for multiple viral plaques if topical and interferon therapy are not effective or tolerated. Fibropapillomas are frequently recurrent after surgical removal[5] and can be very locally aggressive when disrupted.

Key point

- Viral papillomatosis in cats is widely variable and may cause locally aggressive or neoplastic disease.

References

1 Favrot C. In: Greene CE (ed.), *Infectious Diseases of the Dog and Cat*. Amsterdam: Elsevier Health Sciences, 2013: pp. 161–174.
2 Munday JS, Kiupel M. Papillomavirus-associated cutaneous neoplasia in mammals. *Vet Pathol* 2010; **47**: 254–264.
3 Munday JS, Knight CG, French AF. Evaluation of feline oral squamous cell carcinomas for p16 CDKN2A protein immunoreactivity and the presence of papillomaviral DNA. *Res Vet Sci* 2011; **90**: 280–283.
4 Munday JS, Knight CG. Amplification of feline sarcoid-associated papillomavirus DNA sequences from bovine skin. *Vet Dermatol* 2010; **21**: 341–344.
5 Schulman FY, Krafft AE, Janczewski T. Feline cutaneous fibropapillomas: clinicopathologic findings and association with papillomavirus infection. *Vet Pathol Online* 2001; **38**: 291–296.
6 Miller WH, Griffin CE, Campbell KL, Muller GH. In: *Muller and Kirk's Small Animal Dermatology*. Amsterdam: Elsevier Health Sciences, 2013: pp. 350–351.
7 Sundberg JP, Van Ranst M, Montali R *et al*. Feline papillomas and papillomaviruses. *Vet Pathol Online* 2000; **37**: 1–10.
8 Miller WH, Griffin CE, Campbell KL, Muller GH. In: *Muller and Kirk's Small Animal Dermatology*. Amsterdam: Elsevier Health Sciences, 2013: pp. 153–154.
9 Gill VL, Bergman PJ, Baer KE, Craft D, Leung C. Use of imiquimod 5% cream (Aldara) in cats with multicentric squamous cell carcinoma in situ: 12 cases (2002–2005). *Vet Comp Oncol* 2008; **6**: 55–64.
10 Peters-Kennedy J, Scott DW, Miller Jr WH. Apparent clinical resolution of pinnal actinic keratoses and squamous cell carcinoma in a cat using topical imiquimod 5% cream. *J Feline Med Surg* 2008; **10**: 593–599.

FELINE EOSINOPHILIC GRANULOMA COMPLEX

See Chapter 2 for more details of these lesions with pruritic dermatitis in cats

Aetiology and pathogenesis

The eosinophilic granuloma complex (ECG) comprises three major forms: eosinophilic granuloma, eosinophilic ulcer and eosinophilic plaque.[1,2] These have distinct clinical and histological features, representing different reaction patterns to a variety of underlying causes. Local, uncontrolled recruitment of eosinophils results in the release of potent inflammatory mediators, which initiate ongoing inflammation.[1,3] Underlying causes include adverse food reaction, flea or other insect hypersensitivity, allergic dermatitis, ectoparasites or chronic self-trauma, but some cases remain idiopathic.[2,3]

Clinical features

Some cats suffer single episodes, others exhibit recurrent lesions and a few present with refractory lesions. Combinations of different lesions may be seen in an individual cat.

Linear eosinophilic granuloma

These are distinctly linear lesions that commonly affect the medial forelimbs and caudal thighs. They are more common in cats aged <2 years.[1] The lesions may be alopecic or hairy and may appear whitish or erythematous under the skin. They are often associated with a circulating eosinophilia and allergic or parasitic diseases. Pruritus is variable.

Chin granuloma

This rapid infiltration of eosinophils into the chin and lower lip causes a firm swelling, giving the cat a 'pouting' or 'fat lip' appearance (**Fig. 11.19**). The lesion is usually not ulcerated and does not appear to bother the cat. These often wax and wane and commonly resolve without treatment.

Eosinophilic plaques

Eosinophilic plaques are usually associated with pruritus, although this may not be evident from the history. These are well-circumscribed, ulcerated, erythematous, moist lesions typically found on the ventral abdomen, medial thighs or caudal trunk (**Figs. 11.20–11.23**).[1,2] Adjacent lesions may coalesce, presenting as very large, plaque-like or nodular areas.

Eosinophilic or indolent ulcers

These are well-demarcated unilateral or bilateral ulcers, occurring at the philtrum of the upper lip or adjacent to the upper canine tooth (**Fig. 11.24**).[1,2] The periphery is raised and surrounds a pinkish to yellow ulcerated centre. Large lesions can be very destructive and deforming, but the lesions do not seem to be pruritic or overly painful.

Differential diagnoses

- Trauma.
- Actinic dermatitis.
- Cutaneous neoplasia, especially squamous cell carcinoma.

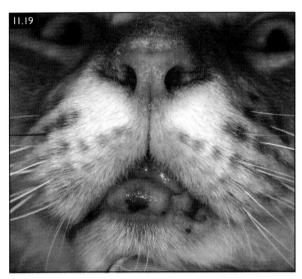

Fig. 11.19 Nodular eosinophilic granuloma on the lower lip of a cat.

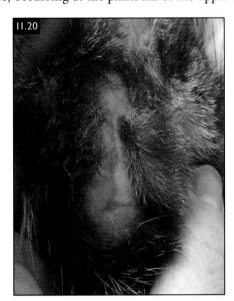

Fig. 11.20 Linear eosinophilic plaque on the caudal aspect of the forelimb in a cat.

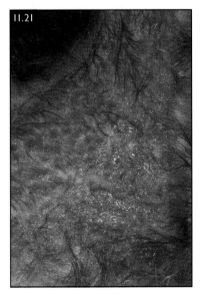

Fig. 11.21 Extensive eosinophilic plaques on the ventral abdomen of a cat.

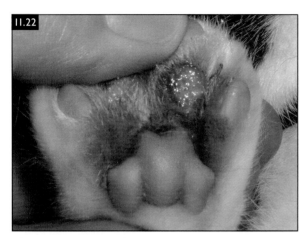

Fig. 11.22 Eosinophilic plaque affecting the interdigital skin.

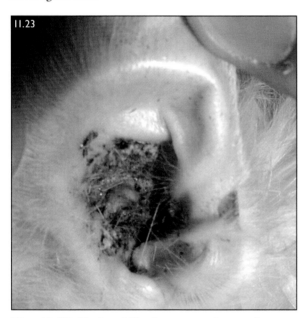

Fig. 11.23 Eosinophilic plaques, erosions and crusts in the vertical ear canal.

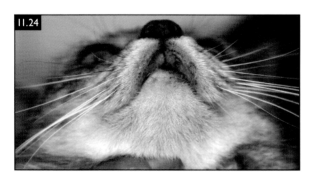

Fig. 11.24 Bilateral indolent ulcers in a cat with an adverse food reaction.

- Dermatophytosis.
- Feline cowpox infection.
- Calicivirus or herpesvirus infection.
- Mycobacterial infection.
- Deep fungal infection.
- Immune-mediated diseases (drug reactions, pemphigus foliaceus, cutaneous lupus).

Diagnosis

The lesions are often very visually distinctive. Cytology shows high numbers of eosinophils, neutrophils and possibly bacterial infection. Biopsy is diagnostic.

Treatment

Ectoparasites must be ruled out with treatment trials. Simple monitoring is appropriate for non-pruritic or non-destructive lesions. ECG may resolve without treatment, but ulcerated or pruritic lesions should be treated. Clindamycin or amoxicillin/clavulanic acid alone have been useful to treat some cases of eosinophilic ulcers of the lips and eosinophilic plaques of the skin that are associated with staphylococcal infection.[4,5] See page 44 for more details of the management of allergic diseases in cats.

Key point

- Common but not well-understood diseases, often related to allergic dermatitis.

References

1 Miller WH, Griffin CE, Campbell KL, Muller GH. In: *Muller and Kirk's Small Animal Dermatology*. Amsterdam: Elsevier Health Sciences, 2013: pp. 695–723.
2 Foster A. Clinical approach to feline eosinophilic granuloma complex. *In Pract* 2003; **25**: 2–10.
3 Bardagi M, Fondati A, Fondevila D *et al*. Ultrastructural study of cutaneous lesions in feline eosinophilic granuloma complex. *Vet Dermatol* 2003; **14**: 297–303.
4 Wilkinson GT, Bate MJ. A possible further clinical manifestation of the feline eosinophilic granuloma complex. *J Am Anim Hosp Assoc* 1984; **20**: 325–331.
5 Wildermuth BE, Griffin CE, Rosenkrantz WS. Response of feline eosinophilic plaques and lip ulcers to amoxicillin trihydrate-clavulanate potassium therapy: a randomized, double-blind placebo-controlled prospective study. *Vet Dermatol* 2012; **23**: 110–e25.

CRYPTOCOCCOSIS

Definition
Cryptococcosis is a deep mycotic disease resulting from infection with several cryptococci fungi.

Aetiology and pathogenesis
Cryptococcus neoformans and *C. gatii* are saprophytic, small, budding yeasts with a global distribution. They are characterised by a mucoid, polysaccharide capsule that can vary in size. The capsule helps to prevent desiccation and also prevents detection by the immune system of the mammalian host.[1] Although these organisms have been isolated from several sources (including soil), they are most frequently associated with pigeon droppings, *Eucalyptus* spp. leaves and decaying vegetation. Based on circumstantial evidence, the most likely route of infection is through inhalation of airborne organisms.[1,2] They may be deposited in the upper respiratory tract, resulting in nasal granulomas, or proceed to the alveoli and induce pulmonary granulomas. Extension of infection from the respiratory tract occurs by local invasion through the cribriform plates to the central nervous system (CNS) or by haematogenous and lymphatic spread,[1,3] Cutaneous infection via traumatic inoculation has also been proposed.[4] Concurrent immunosuppressive diseases (e.g. feline leukaemia virus [FeLV] or feline immunodeficiency virus [FIV] infection in cats and ehrlichiosis in dogs) have been associated with cryptococcal infections. However, underlying diseases are uncommon in companion animals with cryptococcosis. Cryptococci will infect humans, but not normally via an animal host, and are therefore not considered a zoonosis.

Clinical features
Cats
Cryptococcosis is the most frequently diagnosed deep mycotic infection in cats. There is no sex predisposition,[2,3] but young cats (2–3 years) may be predisposed. Signs of upper respiratory disease are most common and include a mucopurulent, serous or haemorrhagic, unilateral or bilateral chronic nasal discharge. Flesh-coloured, polyp-like masses in the nostrils or a firm, hard subcutaneous swelling over the bridge of the nose will be found in 70% of the cases with a nasal discharge. Skin lesions are present in 40% of the cases and are usually papules or nodules that may be either fluctuant or firm and range from 1 mm to 10 mm in diameter (**Fig. 11.25**). Larger lesions often ulcerate, leaving a raw surface with a serous exudate (**Fig. 11.26**).[2,4] Neurological signs occur in 25% of cases and may include depression, ataxia, circling, paresis, paralysis and seizures.[1,3] Ocular involvement (retinitis, optic neuritis, dilated pupils, blindness) occurs in a third of cases and is a marker for CNS involvement. Regional lymphadenopathy, malaise, anorexia or weight loss may occasionally occur.[1]

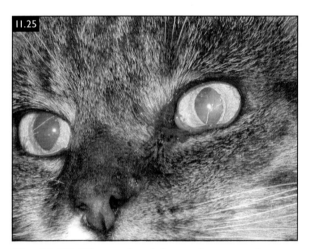

Fig. 11.25 Ulcerated nodules on the nose and periocular skin of a cat with cryptococcosis (courtesy of Peter Forsythe).

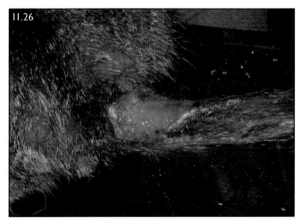

Fig. 11.26 Ulcer on the tail of a cat with cryptococcosis (courtesy of Peter Forsythe).

Dogs

Cryptococcosis is less frequently diagnosed in the dog than in the cat. Most dogs are under 4 years of age at diagnosis. Clinical signs related to ocular and CNS lesions are the most common abnormalities.[3] Skin lesions are rare in dogs, and most commonly consist of papules, nodules, ulcers, abscesses and draining tracts involving the nose, tongue, gums, lips, hard palate or nailbeds.[3]

Differential diagnoses

- Deep pyoderma and bacterial abscessation.
- Other deep mycotic infections.
- Cutaneous neoplasia.
- Histiocytic lesions and sterile nodular granuloma and pyogranuloma (in dogs).

Diagnosis

Cytological examination of nasal or skin exudate or cerebrospinal fluid (CSF) and tissue aspirates generally reveals round to elliptical, 2- to 20-μm diameter organisms with a characteristic capsule of variable thickness, which forms a clear or refractile halo (**Fig. 11.27**). The latex cryptococcal antigen test (LCAT) is a method for detecting capsular polysaccharide antigen in serum,

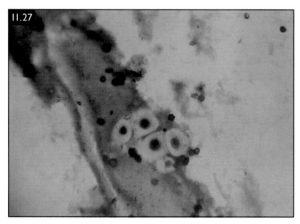

Fig. 11.27 Cytology showing the typical thick-walled capsule of the *Cryptococcus* organisms (courtesy of Peter Forsythe).

urine and CSF. Titres parallel the severity of infection and may be used to monitor response to therapy.[1] Histopathological examination of excision or biopsy samples is diagnostic. Mayer's mucicarmine will differentiate from other similar organisms.[3]

Treatment

An amphotericin B and flucytosine combination is considered optimal therapy for cryptococcal meningoencephalitis.[3] Fluconazole (10 mg/kg q12 h for 2–4 months) is an option for outpatient mono-therapy because it has ocular and CNS penetration. Itraconazole (10 mg/kg po q12 h) has also been reported to be effective. In addition ketoconazole can be used but tends to have more GI and hepatic side effects.[3–6] Therapy should be continued for 1–2 months beyond clinical resolution of lesions or until the antigen titres are negative. See Sykes and Malik[3] for more in-depth details of treatment.

Key point

- The presence of CNS disease negatively affects outcome and neurological damage may be permanent.

References

1   Wolf AM, Troy GC. Deep mycotic diseases. In: Ettinger SJ, Feldman EC (eds), *Textbook of Veterinary Internal Medicine*. Philadelphia, PA: WB Saunders, 1995: pp. 439–462.

2   Ackerman L. Feline cryptococcosis. *Compend Contin Educ Vet* 1988; **10**: 1049–1055.

3   Sykes JE, Malik R. Cryptococcosis. In: Green CE (ed.), *Infectious Diseases of Dogs and Cats*, 4th edn. Philadelphia, PA: WB Saunders, 2012: pp. 621–634.

4   Medleau L, Hall EJ, Goldschmidt MH, Irby N. Cutaneous cryptococcosis in three cats. *J Am Vet Med Assoc* 1995; **187**: 169–170.

5   Legendre AM. Antimycotic drug therapy. In: Bonagura JD (ed.), *Current Veterinary Therapy XII*. Philadelphia, PA: WB Saunders, 1995: pp. 327–331.

6   Medleau L, Jacobs GJ, Marks MA. Itraconazole for the treatment of cryptococcosis in cats. *J Vet Intern Med* 1995; **9**: 39–42.

CHAPTER 12

DISEASES OF ABNORMAL PIGMENTATION

GENERAL APPROACH TO ABNORMAL PIGMENTATION

Depigmentation flow chart (Fig. 12.1)

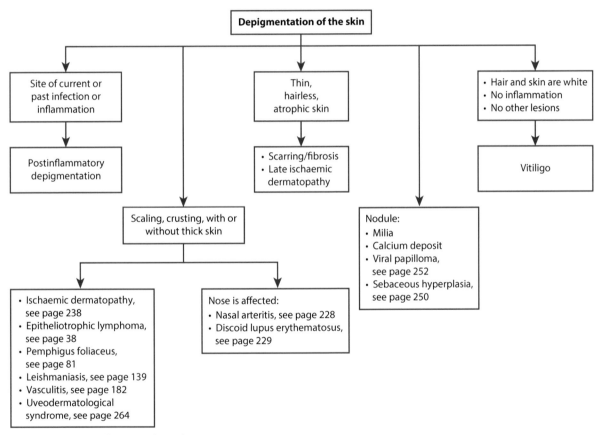

Fig. 12.1 General approach to depigmentation.

Hyperpigmentation flow chart (Fig. 12.2)

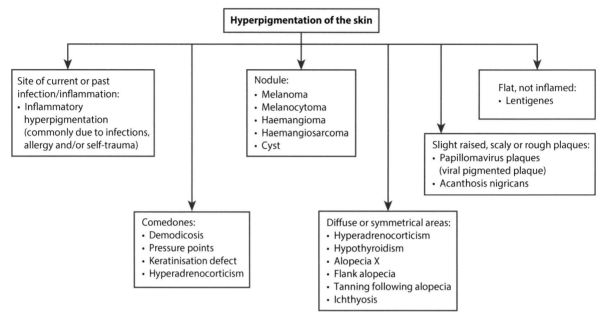

Fig. 12.2 General approach to hyperpigmentation.

VITILIGO

Definition

Vitiligo is an acquired disorder characterised by selective destruction of melanocytes in skin and hair matrix cells; this results in leukoderma (depigmentation of skin) and leukotrichia (depigmentation of hair).

Aetiology and pathogenesis

Vitiligo is thought to result from an aberration of immune surveillance, which allows the development of antimelanocytic antibodies. These antibodies have been demonstrated in dogs and cats with vitiligo, but not in normal animals.[1] Additional theories in humans revolve around the possibility that there is either a neurochemical mediator that destroys melanocytes or inhibits melanin production, or an intermediate metabolite in melanin synthesis that causes melanocyte destruction.[2]

Clinical features

There is a marked breed predisposition for vitiligo in the Belgian Tervuren. Other dogs that appear to

be at increased risk include the German Shepherd dog, Rottweiler, and Doberman Pinscher. It has also been diagnosed in various other breeds and has been reported in Siamese cats.[1,3] Vitiligo generally appears in young adulthood as asymptomatic, well-demarcated depigmented macules on the planum nasale, lips, muzzle, buccal mucosa and footpads (**Figs. 12.3, 12.4**). Leukoderma and, in some cases, leukotrichia occur in affected areas.[4] The progression of the lesions is variable, with lesions in some animals repigmenting whereas others have permanent depigmentation.[4]

Slowly progressive idiopathic depigmentation of the nose is common in dogs. Lay terms for this are 'Dudley nose' and 'snow nose'. There appears to be a predisposition for this in Golden Retrievers, yellow Labrador Retrievers, and Arctic breeds such as the Siberian Husky and Alaskan Malamute.[3] The nasal planum slowly turns brown and then pink. In contrast to vitiligo, the pigment change is usually diffuse and gradual, often depigmenting in the winter and repigmenting in the summer, and affects the nasal planum only. The underlying skin is normal with no evident signs of inflammation and the nose retains its normal 'cobblestone' appearance. Animals do not seem to be affected by the lesions.

Sudden-onset depigmentation of the skin in older animals can be an early sign of epitheliotrophic lymphoma and should be investigated. Depigmentation with smoothing of the nasal planum is an early change in discoid lupus erythematosus. Pigment loss is a postinflammatory change in many immune-mediated dermatoses, particularly lupus erythematosus, and leishmaniasis, thermal and chemical injuries and traumatic scars.

Differential diagnoses
- Canine uveodermatological syndrome.
- Cutaneous lupus erythematosus.
- Dermatomyositis.
- Epitheliotrophic lymphoma.
- Systemic lupus erythematosus.

Diagnosis
The diagnosis is based on history, physical examination and microscopic examination of skin biopsy samples.

Treatment
There is no treatment that has been shown to be of benefit, although the disease is largely only cosmetic. However, depigmented skin may need sun protection.

Key point
- Vitiligo is quite common – client education is important.

References

1 Naughton GK, Mahaffey M, Bystryn JC. Antibodies to surface antigens of pigmented cells in animals with vitiligo. *Proc Soc Exp Biol Med* 1986; **181**: 423–426.
2 Mosher DB, Fitzpatrick TB, Ortonne JP *et al*. Disorders of pigmentation. In: Fitzpatrick TB, Eisen AZ, Wolff K, Freedberg I, Austen KF (eds), *Dermatology in General Medicine*. New York: McGraw-Hill Inc., 1987: pp. 794–876.
3 Gross TL, Ihrke PJ, Walder EJ. Vitiligo. In: *Veterinary Dermatopathology*. St Louis, MO: Mosby Year Book, 1992: pp. 150–153.
4 Guagure E, Alhaidari Z. Disorders of melanin pigmentation in the skin of dogs and cats. In: Kirk RW (ed.), *Current Veterinary Therapy X*. Philadelphia, PA: WB Saunders, 1989: pp. 628–632.

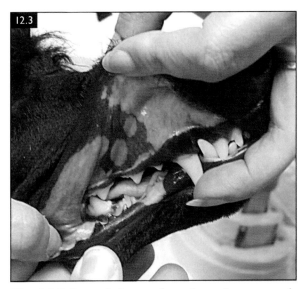

Fig. 12.3 Loss of pigment from the oral mucosa and lips in a standard Poodle with vitiligo (courtesy of Jacques Fontaine).

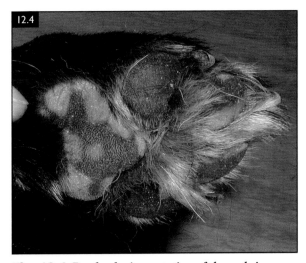

Fig. 12.4 Patchy depigmentation of the pads in a Labrador with vitiligo.

UVEODERMATOLOGICAL SYNDROME
(Vogt–Koyanagi–Harada-like [VKH-like] syndrome)

Definition

Canine uveodermatological syndrome is a rare canine condition that is believed to be an immune-mediated antimelanocyte disease resulting in ocular, dermal and hair abnormalities.[1–4]

Aetiology and pathogenesis

In humans with VKH syndrome there are antibodies and distinct subpopulations of cytotoxic T lymphocytes, with activity against components of melanocytes.[3] Similar mechanisms have been proposed in dogs.[1–3] In humans and Akitas there appears to be a genetic predisposition for this condition.[5]

Clinical features

This condition typically occurs in young to middle-aged dogs. Breeds at risk include Akitas, Samoyeds, Siberian Huskies, Alaskan Malamutes, Chow Chows and their related cross-breeds.[1,3] The syndrome has also been diagnosed in many other breeds. Ocular signs generally precede skin changes and consist of bilateral uveitis progressing to blindness (**Fig. 12.5**). Skin and hair abnormalities include leukoderma and leukotrichia of the eyelids, nasal planum, lips, scrotum, vulva, pads of the feet and scrotal and vulvar areas. Variable degrees of erythema, ulceration and crusting may occur in the depigmented areas (**Fig. 12.6**).[1,3] Depigmentation, erythema, and erosions may occur in the oral cavity.[6] The initial onset ranges from 13 months to 6 years of age.[3] In contrast to humans, neurological signs are uncommon in dogs.

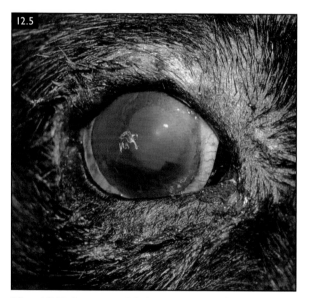

Fig. 12.5 Severe uveitis in a Japanese Akita with VKH-like syndrome; prompt treatment saved this dog's sight.

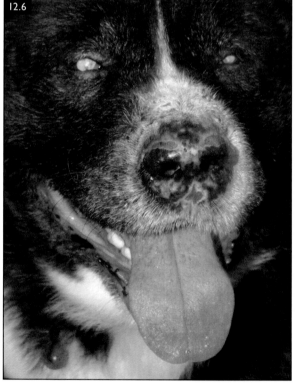

Fig. 12.6 VKH-like syndrome in a Japanese Akita with alopecia, loss of pigment and ulceration of the nasal planum.

Differential diagnoses

- Cutaneous lupus erythematosus.
- Systemic lupus erythematosus.
- Pemphigus foliaceus.
- Pemphigus erythematosus.
- Epitheliotrophic lymphoma.
- Vitiligo.
- Dermatomyositis.
- Leishmaniasis.

Diagnosis

The diagnosis is based on the history, ophthalmic examination, physical examination and histopathological examination of skin biopsy samples. Clinicians should be alert for the combination of ocular and skin disease because immediate therapy is often necessary to preserve eyesight – waiting for histopathological results may affect the outcome.

Treatment

Aggressive topical ocular and oral immunosuppressive therapies are essential to preserve eyesight. Topical or subconjunctival corticosteroids and topical cycloplegics are beneficial in patients with anterior uveitis.[3] Prednisolone, methylprednisolone or prednisone (1–2 mg/kg po q12 h) is usually required to resolve the uveitis and dermatological lesions, and it is recommended to combine steroid therapy with ciclosporin (5–7 mg/kg po q24 h). After resolution of lesions, the steroids should be tapered first to the lowest dose and frequency that maintains remission. Tacrolimus 0.1% can be used to maintain remission in some dogs. The ciclosporin frequency can then be tapered for maintenance. Azathioprine (2 mg/kg po q24–48 h)

or doxycycline/minocycline (5–10 mg/kg po q12 h) with niacinamide, in addition to other therapies, may be needed in cases that do not respond to ciclosporin. Even if the skin is well controlled, periodic evaluation for uveitis is necessary. (See Immunosuppressive Drug Therapy Table, page 289, for dosages and other treatment options.)

Key point

- This condition requires definitive diagnosis and aggressive treatment in order to prevent blindness.

References

1 Gross TH, Ihrke PJ, Walder EJ, Affolter VK. Vogt–Koyanagi–Harada-like syndrome. In: *Skin Diseases of the Dog and Cat: Clinical and Histopathologic Diagnosis*, 2nd edn. Oxford: Blackwell Publishing, 2005: pp. 266–268.

2 Kern TJ, Walton DK, Riis RC *et al*. Uveitis associated with poliosis and vitiligo in six dogs. *J Am Vet Med Assoc* 1985; **187**: 408–414.

3 Morgan RV. Vogt–Koyanagi–Harada syndrome in humans and dogs. *Compend Contin Educ Vet* 1989; **11**: 1211–1218.

4 Murphy C, Belhorn R, Thirkill C. Anti-retinal antibodies associated with Vogt–Koyanagi–Harada-like syndrome in a dog. *J Am Anim Hosp Assoc* 1991; **27**: 399–402.

5 Angles JM, Famula TR, Pedersen NC. Uveodermatologic (VKH-like) syndrome in American Akita dogs is associated with an increased frequency of DQA1* 00201. *Tissue Antigens* 2005; **66**: 656–665.

6 Vercelli A, Taraglio S. Canine Vogt–Koyanagi–Harada-like syndrome in two Siberian Husky dogs. *Vet Dermatol* 1990; **1**: 151–158.

LENTIGENES

Aetiology and pathogenesis

A lentigo (plural lentigines) is a brown–black, circular, hyperpigmented macule or patch. Lentigenes are associated with increased numbers of melanocytes at the dermoepidermal junction, but there is no evidence of focal proliferation or invasive behaviour. Lentigenes are common in orange and tortoiscshell cats.[1] In dogs, these lesions are generally seen in older individuals.

Clinical features

In cats the lesions are first noted on the lips and most affected animals are under a year old. In most cats, these lesions eventually affect all mucous membranes, eyelids, ears and the nasal planum, but are otherwise non-symptomatic (**Fig. 12.7**).

Differential diagnoses

- If solitary and raised, neoplasia such as melanoma is possible.
- Papillomavirus pigmented plaques are seen in dogs and older cats.

Diagnosis

The clinical appearance of flat, non-inflamed lesions on the mucous membranes of young orange cats is highly suggestive and is usually sufficient to make a diagnosis. In older dogs, flat, smooth, non-inflamed greyish or brownish macules or patches are probably ageing changes. Multiple strongly pigmented scaling plaques in dogs may be papillomavirus induced, and these have the potential for neoplastic change. Histopathological examination of biopsy samples will give a definitive diagnosis.

Treatment

Lentigenes in young cats and old dogs are purely cosmetic lesions that do not require therapy.

Key point

- These are benign lesions.

Reference

1   Scott DW. Lentigo simplex in orange cats. *Companion Anim Pract* 1987; **1**: 23–25.

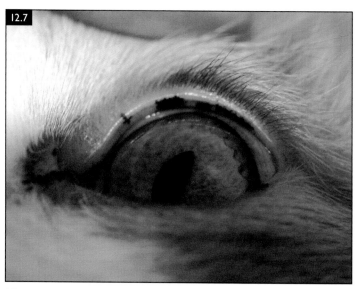

Fig. 12.7   Lentigo simplex on the eyelids of an orange cat.

GENERAL APPROACH TO OTITIS

Cases of recurrent and chronic otitis invariably have primary, predisposing and perpetuating causes in addition to the secondary infection (**Fig. 13.1**).

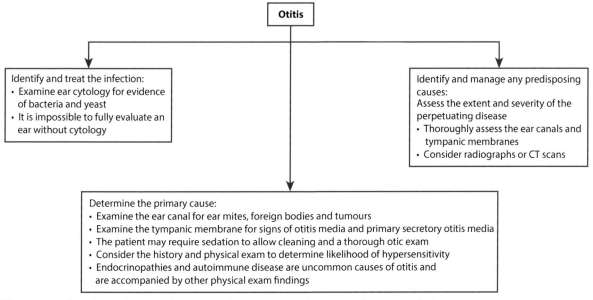

Fig. 13.1 Flow chart showing the approach to otitis. (**CT, computed tomography.**)

OTITIS EXTERNA

Definition

Otitis externa is inflammation of the horizontal and/or vertical ear canal with or without involvement of the pinna. Many primary, perpetuating and predisposing causes exist. Most cases are infected at presentation, but the ears can be inflamed and not infected.

Aetiology and pathogenesis

Infections in otitis externa are invariably **secondary** and most commonly involve commensal (e.g. staphylococci and *Malassezia* spp.) or environmental (e.g. *Pseudomonas* spp.) organisms.

Every case of otitis externa will have a **primary** (underlying) cause. Primary causes of otitis externa include hypersensitivity, ectoparasites, foreign bodies, neoplasia, endocrinopathies, autoimmune disease and keratinisation disorders (**Fig. 13.2**).[1] Hypersensitivity (atopic dermatitis and/or food allergies), ectoparasites (*Otodectes* spp. and, less commonly, *Demodex* or *Otobius* ticks) and foreign bodies are by far the most common primary causes of otitis externa. The only way to manage and prevent recurring otitis externa is to identify and manage the primary cause.

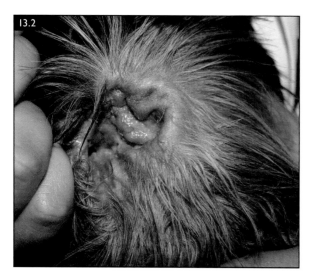

Fig. 13.2 Severe otitis externa in a Cavalier King Charles Spaniel with a primary keratinisation disorder.

Many cases of otitis externa will have a **perpetuating** (secondary) cause that prevents resolution.[1] Perpetuating causes include: maceration or irritation of canal epithelium from medication, altered epithelial migration, ceruminous hyperplasia with excessive cerumen and/or exudate production, oedema, hyperplasia and stenosis of the ear canals, calcification and otitis media. Failure to address all the perpetuating causes of otitis externa commonly results in relapsing chronic otitis. Perpetuating causes can change over the course of chronic otitis and will eventually lead to irreversible changes that require a total ear canal ablation.

Predisposing factors must also be considered when managing otitis externa. Predisposing factors alone do not cause otitis, but combine with primary causes to make the animal more susceptible to it. Predisposing causes include: narrow ear canals, excessive hair, pendulous pinnae, high density of ceruminous glands and excessive cerumen production, hair plucking, and swimming and/or over-cleaning that macerates the ear canal. Predisposing factors may not be easily countered or managed, but should alert clinicians to animals that will be more likely than others to have recurrent otitis.

Biofilms inhibit cleaning, prevent penetration and activity of antimicrobials and provide a protected reservoir of bacteria. They may also enhance the development of antimicrobial resistance, especially in gram-negative bacteria that acquire stepwise resistance mutations to concentration-dependent antibiotics.

All the primary, predisposing and perpetuating causes must be identified and managed as well as the secondary infections for a successful long-term outcome.

Clinical features

The clinical features will vary from individual to individual because of variation in primary cause, predisposing conditions, perpetuating factors, secondary infections and expression of the disease.[2] A few key points include:

- Acute, unilateral otitis externa is common in dogs and typically reflects foreign body penetration. Acute, unilateral otitis externa is unusual in the cat.
- Chronic unilateral otitis externa in the cat is often associated with neoplasia or inflammatory polyp formation, whereas bilateral otitis externa in the cat is most commonly associated with otodectic mange.
- Bilateral otitis externa in the dog, particularly if recurrent, is highly suggestive of hypersensitivity (i.e. atopic dermatitis or cutaneous adverse food reaction). Atopic dermatitis and adverse food reactions can present with unilateral **infected** otitis, but the other ear is almost always also inflamed even if it is not infected. This still represents bilateral otitis – the clinical otitis may also affect each ear sequentially. Atopic dermatitis and food allergies show a characteristic diffuse erythema of the ventral pinnae and ear canals.
- Chronic otitis externa results in a quantitative (more bacteria) and qualitative (initially more gram-positive and eventually more gram-negative bacteria) shift in microbial flora (**Fig. 13.3**).
- Erythroceruminous otitis, with erythema, ceruminous discharge and pruritus is typically associated with a *Malassezia* and/or staphylococcal overgrowth (**Fig. 13.4**).
- Suppurative otitis, with erythema, ulceration, purulent discharge and pain, is typically

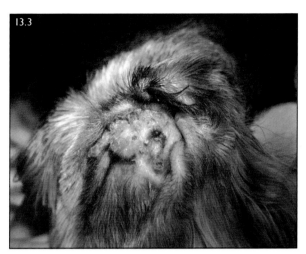

Fig. 13.3 Chronic otitis externa in an atopic Miniature Schnauzer; there is erythema, lichenification, swelling, waxy discharge and stenosis of the ear canal opening. The red papule may be a chronically inflamed polyp or early neoplasia.

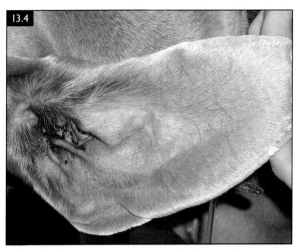

Fig. 13.4 The typical brown discharge that is often associated with *Malassezia pachydermatis* infection. The primary trigger in this case was an adverse food reaction.

associated with a gram-negative (most commonly *Pseudomonas* spp.) infection (**Fig. 13.5**).

- Moist suppurative otitis with a whitish granular discharge can be seen with maceration and/or contact reactions to medication.
- Pustules are rare on the concave aspect of the pinna and are often associated with pemphigus foliaceus or a medication reaction rather than superficial pyoderma.
- Otitis media can cause depression, pain, head tilt, deafness and difficulty in eating, but most cases are difficult to distinguish from otitis externa alone.
- Head tilt, ataxia, nystagmus and Horner's syndrome are associated with severe otitis media and otitis interna, and should be treated as emergencies.
- Very firm, immobile ear canals are often irreversibly fibrosed and/or mineralised.
- Sedation of the animal and cleaning of the ear are often necessary to perform a thorough otoscopic evaluation in severe cases.
- The normal tympanic membrane should be translucent with radiating stria (**Fig. 13.6**).
- The tympanic membrane is more likely to be ruptured in suppurative otitis and where there is stenosis of the horizontal ear canal.

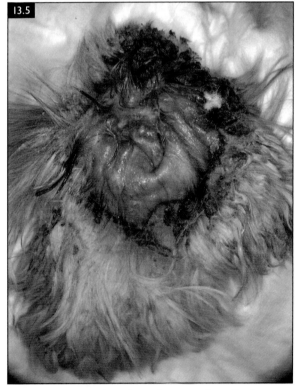

Fig. 13.5 Extensive ulceration, purulent discharge and crusting in suppurative otitis associated with a *Pseudomonas aeruginosa* infection; it is important to remove all the discharge and matted hair during treatment.

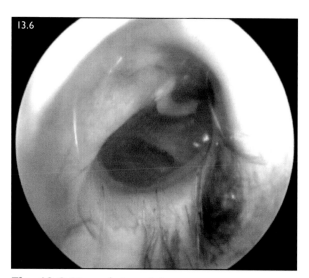

Fig. 13.6 Normal view of the tympanum.

The nature of the discharge can indicate the type of otitis and infection (*Table 13.1*).

The dried material at the opening of vertical ear canal can be misleading and the discharge should always be assessed by otoscopy or taking a sample from the ear canals. These findings are indicative only and cytology should be performed wherever possible.

Diagnosis

A basic evaluation of the ear involves a thorough examination and ear cytology.

Clinical examination

The clinician should examine the patient for evidence of Horner's syndrome or vestibular neuritis. The submandibular lymph nodes should be evaluated for enlargement. Jaw pain should be assessed. The canals should be palpated externally for signs of hyperplasia and mineralisation – healthy ears should be non-pruritic, non-painful, pliable and mobile. The pinnal–pedal reflex should be evaluated. The pinna, vertical canal and horizontal canal should be examined. Some patients may require sedation and cleaning to verify the presence or absence of a foreign body or tumour in the canal.

The tympanic membrane may not be easily visible in diseased ears. This should not preclude treatment, although the possibility of a ruptured membrane should be considered. There are some clues to the position of the tympanic membrane. It sits just inside a short bony tube (the external auditory meatus), which may be palpable with the otoscope tip. There are also some hairs that arise from the ventral ear canal at the insertion of the tympanic membrane.

Cytology (**Figs. 13.7–13.10**)

Cytology is mandatory in all cases of otitis. It can effectively identify the most likely organisms in most cases. This is particularly useful in mixed infections,

Table 13.1 **Nature of discharge from ear**					
Colour	Dark brown	Pale brown to grey	Pale brown to yellow	Yellow to green	Dark green to black
Consistency	Waxy and adherent	Waxy to seborrhoeic	Seborrhoeic to purulent	Purulent	Thick and slimy
Association	Ceruminous otitis	*Malassezia* spp.	Staphylococci	*Pseudomonas* spp.	Biofilm

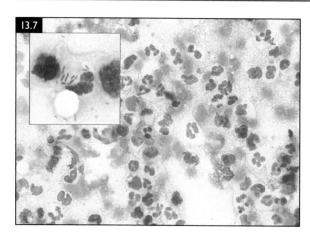

Fig. 13.7 Otic cytology may reveal many leukocytes; in this case with a *Pseudomonas* infection there are numerous degenerate neutrophils – the inset shows intracellular rod bacteria (DiffQuik® stain, ×400/×1000).

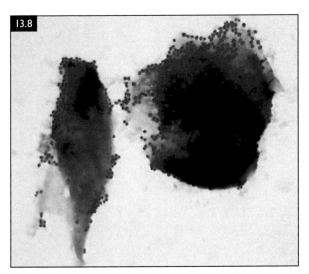

Fig. 13.8 Otic cytology showing a staphylococcal overgrowth (Diff-Quik® stain, ×400).

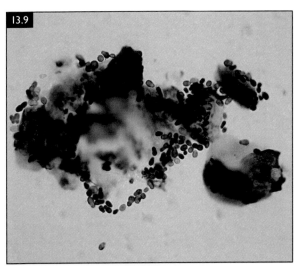

Fig. 13.9 Otic cytology showing a *Malassezia* overgrowth (Diff-Quik® stain, ×400).

where culture may identify several organisms with different susceptibility patterns.

Cytology should be collected from the canal with swabs or curettes and examined microscopically. Mites can be found in material collected in mineral oil under low power (×40). Material air dried or heat fixed and stained with a modified Wright–Giemsa stain can be examined under high magnification (×400 or ×1000 oil immersion) to observe cells and microorganisms. The numbers of yeast, cocci, rods, neutrophils and epithelial cells should be quantified. Biofilms form variably thick veil-like material that may obscure bacteria and cells. Ear cytology is generally more sensitive and specific than culture to determine whether bacteria and/or yeast is present in the ear canal.

Malassezia spp. and staphylococci are straightforward to identify and a good estimate of their probable sensitivity can be made based on knowledge of local resistance patterns and previous treatment. Gram-negative bacteria are harder to differentiate on cytology alone, although *Pseudomonas* spp. are most common.

Using bacterial culture and antimicrobial sensitivity testing

Bacterial culture and sensitivity testing are not necessary in most cases of otitis externa and/or where topical therapy is used. However, it can help identify the

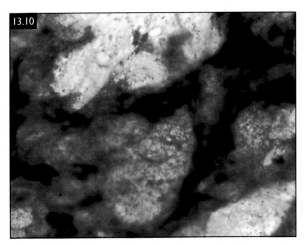

Fig. 13.10 Otic cytology showing a mixed bacterial overgrowth – the thick, dark-staining, veil-like material is a mucoid biofilm (DiffQuik® stain, ×400).

bacteria involved in the infection. This can be useful for less common organisms that are hard to differentiate on cytology, e.g. streptococci, enterococci, *Escherichia coli*, *Klebsiella* and *Proteus* spp., and coryneforms. Knowledge of their probable sensitivity patterns can help guide treatment choices.[3–6] The susceptibility pattern of *Pseudomonas* spp. is harder to predict, although most first-time infections will be susceptible to aminoglycosides, polymyxin B, silver sulfadiazine and fluoroquinolones. However, *Pseudomonas* spp. readily acquire resistance and most isolates from recurrent infections will be multi-drug resistant.

Great care must be taken in interpreting antibiotic susceptibility and resistance results because the susceptibility–resistance breakpoints are based on tissue concentrations after systemic treatment. This does not necessarily mean that the bacteria are resistant to the antimicrobial, because sufficiently high levels may exceed the minimum inhibitory concentration (MIC). Sensitivity data are therefore very poorly predictive of the response to topical drugs because concentrations in the ear canal are much higher than in-vitro tests predict. The response to treatment is best assessed using clinical signs and cytology. Antibiotic sensitivity data can be used to predict the efficacy of systemic drugs, although the concentration in the ear tissues is often low and high doses are needed. No antibiotic withdrawal time is needed before culture, although laboratories should be informed of recent or ongoing therapy.

Treatment

Please refer to the corresponding chapters in this book for detailed information about treatment of the primary causes of otitis externa. In general, treatment of otitis externa is most effective when an ear cleaner, steroid and antimicrobial are combined.

Ear cleaning

Ear cleaning removes debris and microbes from the canal. Some ear cleaners have broad-spectrum antimicrobial activity. Very waxy or exudative ears should be cleaned daily during treatment. Ears that are less exudative can be cleaned less frequently, but at least once a week during treatment. Many types of ear cleaners are available.[6] In many uncomplicated cases of otitis externa, the type of cleaner used may be less important than the actual act of cleaning the ears. It is important to demonstrate effective ear-cleaning techniques to owners.

Ceruminolytic and ceruminosolvent cleaners[7] (i.e. propylene glycol, lanolin, glycerine, squalane, butylated hydroxytoluene, cocamidopropyl betaine and mineral oils) are useful for softening and removing dry waxy debris and/or wax plugs. Surfactant based ear cleaners (i.e. docusate sodium, calcium sulphosuccinate and similar detergents) are better in more seborrhoeic ears and purulent ears. Tromethamine ethylene diaminetetraacetic acid/edetate disodium dihydrate (Tris-EDTA) has very little ceruminolytic or detergent activity, but is soothing in ulcerated purulent ears and is safer if the tympanic membrane is ruptured. Astringents[2] (i.e. isopropyl alcohol, boric acid, benzoic acid, salicylic acid, sulphur, aluminium acetate acetic acid and silicon dioxide) can help prevent maceration of the epithelial lining of the canal. Some astringents also have antimicrobial activity but acids and alcohols may irritate some animals. Antimicrobials[7–9] (i.e. p-chlorometaxylenol [PCMX], chlorhexidine and ketoconazole) are useful for treating and preventing infections. Tris-EDTA has little to no antimicrobial activity by itself, although high concentrations can potentiate the effect of antibiotics and chlorhexidine.

Anti-inflammatory treatment

Steroids decrease inflammation in the ear, which speeds resolution of infection because infectious agents thrive in inflamed tissue. In addition, glucocorticoids (particularly dexamethasone) reverse the ototoxic effect of *Pseudomonas* infections. Steroids are not specifically analgesic, but reduction of the inflammation will reduce pain. However, specific analgesia should be considered in severe cases.

Steroids can be administered as individual topical drops, or as a component of either an ear medication or an ear cleaner. Topical steroids are generally well tolerated, although dermal atrophy of the ear canal epithelium or iatrogenic Cushing's syndrome can occur. These side effects are uncommon and can be minimised by reducing the frequency or potency of the steroid. Hydrocortisone is the least potent steroid. Mometasone and hydrocortisone aceponate are potent anti-inflammatory agents but are also the least likely to cause dermal atrophy. Prednisolone is a moderately potent steroid. Dexamethasone is a highly potent steroid – it is very effective and the injectable preparation can be administered as a topical drop for the ear. Fluocinolone is also a highly potent steroid and when combined with dimethyl sulphoxide (DMSO) it effectively reduces hyperplastic epithelium. However, DMSO may be irritating to an ulcerated ear. Oral steroids are needed if the pet will not tolerate topical steroids, if the ear canal is stenosed or ulcerated, if otitis media is suspected and/or with generalised inflammatory skin disease.

Regular anti-inflammatory treatment is often required to prevent ongoing inflammation once the infection has been cleared (e.g. in atopic dermatitis). Otherwise this leads to a cycle of recurrent infection and chronic inflammation; the progressive pathological changes and end-stage otitis may require surgical intervention. The chronic inflammation makes each bout of infection harder to treat and repeated antimicrobial use may select for resistance.

First-line topical antibiotic treatment (*Table 13.2*)

Many types of antimicrobials are available. In general, topical antibiotics are more effective than oral antibiotics for resolving otitis externa. The high concentration (usually mg/ml) of the antimicrobial can overcome apparent antibiotic resistance – please note that susceptibility tests based on breakpoints established for systemic dosing (in µg/ml concentrations) are poorly predictive of the outcome of topical treatment. It is important to use an adequate volume to penetrate into the ear canals – 1 ml is sufficient

for most ears, but may be too much in very small animals and very large dogs may require more.

The efficacy of concentration-dependent drugs (e.g. fluoroquinolones and aminoglycosides) depends on delivering concentrations of at least $10 \times$ MIC once daily. Time-dependent drugs (penicillins and cephalosporins) require concentrations above MIC for at least 70% of the dosing interval. This is readily achieved with topical therapy, which achieves high local concentrations that probably persist in the absence of systemic metabolism. Most topical medication should be effective with once daily dosing, although some are licensed for twice daily administration. Concentrations of gentamicin were $3-15 \times$ and of miconazole $1.2-2 \times$ the MIC_{90} for canine otic isolates of staphylococci and *Malassezia* spp., respectively, 10 days after a 5-day course of Easotic®. Levels of florfenicol and terbinafine are at least $1000 \times$ the MIC_{90} for staphylococci and *Malassezia* spp. for the duration of treatment with two doses of Osurnia®. Two florfenicol/terbinafine/betamethasone-containing products are licensed for one (Claro®) or two applications 1 week apart (Osurnia®). This can be very useful in stenotic or painful ears where daily administration can be difficult.

Topical antibiotic treatment of multi-drug-resistant bacteria (*Table 13.3*)

If bacteria persist on cytology despite 2–3 weeks of appropriate treatment, then antibiotic resistance should be suspected. Other reasons for treatment failure include: polyps, neoplasia, foreign bodies and other underlying conditions; debris, biofilms and failure to clean the ears; stenosis, otitis media and other perpetuating factors; and poor compliance. *Pseudomonas* are inherently resistant to many antibiotics and they readily develop further resistance if treatment is ineffective.

There is potential for systemic toxicity with silver sulfadiazine and aminoglycosides in extensively ulcerated ears. Systemic aminoglycosides can be nephrotoxic and renal function should be monitored. Systemic fluoroquinolones can cause cartilage damage in dogs <12 months old (18 months in giant breeds), neurotoxicity at high doses and blindness in cats (especially with injectable enrofloxacin).

Table 13.2 **First-line topical antibiotics**	
Gentamicin	Broad-spectrum Ototoxicity rare
Fluoroquinolones	Broad-spectrum and effective against *Pseudomonas* spp. Well tolerated Additive activity with silver sulfadiazine against *Pseudomonas* spp.
Fusidic acid	Gram-positive only Synergistic with framycetin against gram-positive bacteria[10]
Florfenicol	Broad-spectrum but not effective against *Pseudomonas* spp.
Polymyxin B	Broad-spectrum and effective against *Pseudomonas* spp. Inactivated by organic debris and needs a clean ear canal Synergistic with miconazole against gram-negative bacteria Potentially ototoxic
Neomycin	Broad-spectrum but limited efficacy against *Pseudomonas* spp. Can cause contact reactions and potentially ototoxic

Table 13.3 Antibiotics useful in multi-drug-resistant infections[11,12]

ANTIBIOTIC	REGIMEN
Ciprofloxacin	0.2% sol. 0.15–0.3 ml/ear q24 h
Enrofloxacin	15–20 mg/kg po q24 h; 2.5% injectable sol. diluted 1:4 with Tris-EDTA, saline or Epiotic® topically q24 h; 22.7 mg/ml sol. 0.15–0.3 ml/ear q24 h
Marbofloxacin	5–8 mg/kg po q24 h; 1% injectable sol. diluted 1:4 with saline or Tris-EDTA topically q24 h; 2 mg/ml in Tris-EDTA 1 ml topically q24 h; 20 mg/ml sol. 0.15–0.3 ml/ear q24 h
Ofloxacin	0.3% 0.15–0.3 ml/ear q24 h
Pradofloxacin	5–8 mg/kg po q24 h
Carbenicillin	10–20 mg/kg iv q8 h
Clavulanate–ticarcillin*	15–40 mg/kg iv q8 h; 16 mg/ml in Tris-EDTA 1 ml topically q24 h; reconstituted injectable sol. 0.15–0.3 ml/ear q12 h; 160 mg/ml sol. 0.15–0.3 ml/ear q12 h; potentially ototoxic
Ceftazidime*	25–50 mg/kg iv or sc q8 h; 10 mg/ml in Tris-EDTA 1 ml topically q24 h; 100 mg/ml 0.15–0.3 ml/ear q12 h
Silver sulfadiazine	Dilute 0.1–0.5% in saline; additive activity with gentamicin and fluoroquinolones
Amikacin	10–15 mg/kg sc q24 h; 2 mg/ml in Tris-EDTA 1 ml topically q24 h; 50 mg/ml 0.15–0.3 ml/ear q24 h; susceptibility maintained if there is resistance to other aminoglycosides; potentially ototoxic
Gentamicin	5–10 mg/kg sc q24 h; 3.2 mg/ml in Tris-EDTA 1 ml topically q 24; ototoxicity rare
Tobramycin*	Use eyedrops or 8 mg/ml injectable sol. 0.15–0.3 ml/ear q24 h; potentially ototoxic

* Reconstituted solution stable for up to 7 days at 4°C or for 1 month frozen.
iv, intravenous; po, by mouth; sc, subcutaneous; sol., solution.

Systemic antibiotic therapy

Systemic therapy may be less effective in otitis externa because bacteria are present only in the external ear canal and cerumen, there is no inflammatory discharge and penetration to the lumen is poor. Systemic treatment is indicated when the ear canal cannot be treated topically (e.g. stenosis or compliance problems or if topical adverse reactions are suspected) and in otitis media. High doses of drugs with good tissue penetration (e.g. fluoroquinolones) should be considered. (See Superficial pyoderma, page 72 and Otitis media, page 285 for more details.)

Antifungal therapy

Clotrimazole, miconazole, posiconazole, ketoconazole, nystatin and terbinafine are effective against *Malassezia* spp. Antifungals may be administered as individual topical drops, as a component of either an ear medication or an ear cleaner. Antifungal resistance appears to be becoming more common, but choosing an antifungal in a different class tends to be effective if this is suspected. Oral itraconazole (5 mg/kg po q24 h) or ketoconazole (5–10 mg/kg po q24 h) can be administered if systemic therapy is indicated.

Treatment of biofilms and mucus

Biofilms can be physically broken up and removed by thorough flushing and aspiration. Topical Tris-EDTA and *N*-acetylcysteine can disrupt biofilms, facilitating their removal, and enhance penetration of antimicrobials. Systemic administration of *N*-acetylcysteine is well tolerated, and can help dissolve biofilms in the middle ear and other mucous surfaces. Systemic *N*-acetyl cysteine and bromhexine can also liquefy mucus, facilitating drainage in cases of primary secretory otitis media in dogs and feline otitis media due to inflammatory polyps.

Tris-EDTA

Tris-EDTA damages bacterial cell walls and increases antibiotic efficacy, which can overcome partial resistance.[13] It is best given 20–30 minutes before the antibiotic but can be coadministered.

It is well tolerated and non-ototoxic. Tris-EDTA shows additive activity with chlorhexidine, gentamicin and fluoroquinolones at high concentrations.

Ear wicks

Polyvinyl acetate ear wicks can useful in certain cases. These are cut to size and inserted into the ear canal under anaesthesia, soaked with an antibiotic, Tris-EDTA and/or steroid solution and left for 3–10 days, applying the ear solution once daily. The wicks absorb discharge and draw the antibiotic solution into the ear canals. Steroid soaked wicks can resolve stenosis of the ear and prevent stenosis following sharp or laser surgery to remove polyps and other masses within the ear canal. They may prevent drainage from the middle ear in cases of discharging otitis media, however. Ear wicks are well tolerated provided that they are kept moist.

Length of treatment

Acute uncomplicated cases of otitis externa usually resolve within 5–10 days. However, more complex infections with chronic inflammatory changes, multi-drug-resistant bacteria and/or otitis media may require 2–3 weeks of treatment. Severe cases may require 6–8 weeks to fully resolve. Careful clinical examination and cytology are required to determine whether the ear infection has completely resolved.

Long-term treatment

Ear infections will recur unless the underlying (primary) cause is treated. In some cases, i.e. atopy, the primary, perpetuating or predisposing factors for otitis cannot be eliminated or completely controlled. In these cases, continuous ear treatments are often effective. Regular ear cleaning with administration of a topical antifungal and/or steroid once to twice weekly will control inflammation and infection and prevent recurrence of the otitis. It is important to impress on owners the need for regular treatment even if the ears look normal.

Key points

- Ear cytology at every ear examination is essential to determine the status of the infection and to direct treatment. This is true even if the affected ear appears normal on exam.
- Most cases of otitis externa require a combination of cleaning, steroid and antimicrobial to achieve resolution of infection.
- Chronic and recurrent cases need thorough investigation and treatment to identify and manage primary conditions, predisposing factors, perpetuating changes and secondary infections.

References

1 Craig, M. Disease Facts: otitis externa. *Companion Animal* 2013; **18**: 481–483.

2 Zur G, Lifshitz B, Bdolah-Abram T. The association between the signalment, common causes of canine otitis externa and pathogens. *J Small Anim Pract* 2011; **52**: 254–258.

3 Dégi J, Imre K, Catana N *et al*. Frequency of isolation and antibiotic resistance of staphylococcal flora from external otitis of dogs. *Vet Rec* 2013; **173**: 42.

4 Henneveld K, Rosychuk RA, Francisco J *et al*. *Corynebacterium* spp. in dogs and cats with otitis externa and/or media: a retrospective study. *J Am Anim Hosp Assoc* 2012; **48**: 320–326.

5 Mekić S, Matanović K. Antimicrobial susceptibility of *Pseudomonas aeruginosa* isolates from dogs with otitis externa. *Vet Rec* 2011; **169**: 125.

6 Zamankhan Malayeri H, Jamshidi S *et al*. Identification and antimicrobial susceptibility patterns of bacteria causing otitis externa in dogs. *Vet Res Commun* 2010; **34**: 435–444.

7 Nuttall T, Cole LK. Ear cleaning: the UK and US perspective. *Vet Dermatol* 2004; **15**: 127–136.

8 Steen SI, Paterson S. The susceptibility of *Pseudomonas* spp. isolated from dogs with otitis to topical ear cleaners. *J Small Anim Pract* 2012; **53**: 599–603.

9 Swinney A, Fazakerley J, McEwan NA *et al*. Comparative *in vitro* antimicrobial efficacy of commercial ear cleaners. *Vet Dermatol* 2008; **19**: 373–379.

10 Pietschmann S, Meyer M, Voget M, Cieslicki M. The joint *in vitro* action of polymyxin B and miconazole against pathogens associated with canine otitis externa from three European countries. *Vet Dermatol* 2013; **24**: 439–445.

11 Buckley LM, McEwan NA, Nuttall T. Tris-EDTA significantly enhances antibiotic efficacy against multidrug-resistant *Pseudomonas aeruginosa in vitro*. *Vet Dermatol* 2013; **24**: 519–e122.

12 Cole LK, Papich MG, Kwochka KW *et al*. Plasma and ear tissue concentrations of enrofloxacin and its

metabolite ciprofloxacin in dogs with chronic end-stage otitis externa after intravenous administration of enrofloxacin. *Vet Dermatol* 2009; **20**: 51–59.

13 Pye CC, Singh A, Weese JS. Evaluation of the impact of tromethamine edetate disodium dihydrate on antimicrobial susceptibility of *Pseudomonas aeruginosa* in biofilm *in vitro*. *Vet Dermatol* 2014; **25**: 120–123.

Further reading

Harvey RG, Paterson S. *Otitis Externa: An Essential Guide to Diagnosis and Treatment*. Abingdon, Oxon: CRC Press, 2014.

Paterson S, Tobias K. *Atlas of Ear Diseases of the Dog and Cat*. Oxford: Wiley-Blackwell, 2013.

OTIC FOREIGN BODY

Definition

Otic foreign bodies inappropriately occupy the ear canal of dogs and cats. Common types of foreign bodies include grass awns, hair and other organic debris. Malicious or accidental insertion of foreign objects is rare. Iatrogenic foreign material includes cotton wool, cotton bud tips and broken catheters or forceps.

Aetiology and pathogenesis

Grass awns adhere to the coat when a dog or cat is outside. The funnel shape of the grass awn allows it to migrate into the ear canal, but it cannot easily come out on its own (**Figs. 13.11, 13.12**). The foreign body causes variable, acute, and sometimes extreme, pain and pruritus. Most cases are unilateral, but bilateral foreign bodies can be seen.

Foreign bodies are a primary cause of otitis externa.[1] Secondary bacterial or yeast infection may result and perpetuate the otitis. In severe cases the foreign body may penetrate the tympanic membrane and cause otitis media.

Clinical features

Otic foreign bodies generally present with acute-onset head shaking and distress. Otic foreign bodies may also present as a chronic otitis externa that is poorly responsive to treatment. Otoscopic exam will reveal variable amounts of brown, waxy debris and erythema; purulent exudates may be seen with secondary gram-negative infections. The foreign body should be visible on otoscopic exam and if the debris has been adequately removed.

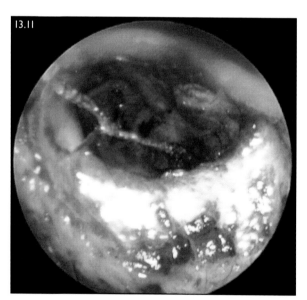

Fig. 13.11 Foreign body in the horizontal ear canal of a dog with acute otitis externa.

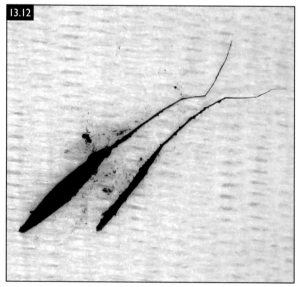

Fig. 13.12 A grass seed removed by video-otoscopy.

Differential diagnoses

The visualisation of the foreign body within the canal is diagnostic, and there are no other differentials. Concurrent otic disease and perpetuating causes of otitis may be present.

Diagnosis

The dog or cat may need to be sedated or anaesthetised to allow complete visualisation of the ear canal. Ear cytology must be examined microscopically to detect the presence of secondary yeast or bacterial infection.

Treatment

The grass awn or other foreign body must be removed using forceps (i.e. alligator forceps through an operating head or video-otoscope) or via flushing. The canal can be flushed using a 5-Fr red rubber or plastic catheter attached to a syringe or irrigation device. Tepid water or saline can be used as a flushing agent. Copious amounts of flushing may be necessary to dislodge the foreign body. Care should be taken to check that the foreign body has been completely removed: a single spike from a grass awn will be enough to perpetuate the problem.

Oral and/or topical steroids may be necessary depending on the amount of erythema, pain and pruritus present in the ear. Bacterial or yeast infections should be treated with topical products (see page 272 for further details about treatment of bacterial or yeast otitis externa).

Key point

- Bacterial or yeast otitis externa may be secondary to an otic foreign body.

Reference

1 Craig M. Disease facts: otitis externa. *Companion Animal* 2013; **18**: 481–483.

FELINE AURAL POLYPS

Definition

Polyps are a common non-malignant tumour found in the ear and/or nasopharynx of cats.

Aetiology and pathogenesis

Polyps originate from the epithelial lining of the tympanic bulla or from the auditory (eustachian) tube.[1] The exact reason for the development of the polyp is unknown, but it may be congenital or a response to inflammation. Polyps cause obstruction of the ear canal, and are a primary cause of otitis externa. Secondary bacterial and/or yeast otitis externa and/or otitis media may occur.

Clinical features

A polyp should be suspected when young cats present with unilateral otitis externa. The polyp may be visible as a flesh-coloured mass in the horizontal canal if the tympanic membrane is ruptured. The polyp may be visible behind the tympanic membrane if this is intact. Polyps tend to fill the entire diameter of the canal, and can grow so much that they extend well into the vertical canal. Polyps are often initially obscured by purulent exudate associated with a secondary bacterial otitis.

Other clinical signs depend on the extent and location of the polyp. These can include an altered voice and snoring with polyps in the nasopharynx. Polyps in the middle ear may cause head tilts, Horner's syndrome, nystagmus and ataxia. Acute otitis media and interna should be treated as an emergency.

Differential diagnosis

- Other aural tumour.

Diagnosis

Most polyps have a pathognomonic appearance with a large, flesh-coloured distal end and a tapering proximal end (**Figs. 13.13, 13.14**). Other types of aural tumours should be suspected if a polyp-like mass develops in older cats. Histopathology confirms the diagnosis.

Diagnostic imaging is useful to determine the extent of the polyps in the nasopharynx, ventromedial compartment of the tympanic bulla, dorsolateral part of the middle ear and/or external ear canal. CT scans are more sensitive and specific than radiographs. In addition, density analysis of the

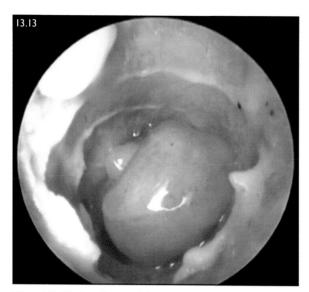

Fig. 13.13 A polyp visible in the horizontal ear canal of a cat.

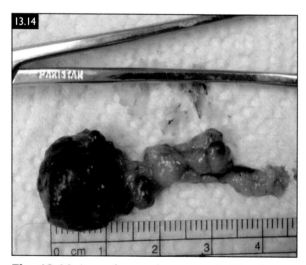

Fig. 13.14 A very large polyp removed with a forceps from a feline ear canal.

soft-tissue patterns can indicate whether it is a solid polyp or mucoid material.

Treatment

Polyps in the nasopharynx, dorso-lateral middle ear and external ear canal can be removed via traction and avulsion with forceps. The cat must be anaesthetised for this. The polyp is grasped firmly with a set of Kelly forceps and slow, continuous traction is applied until the polyp releases from the middle ear. The polyp can usually be removed in one piece,

but sometimes multiple attempts are needed to remove it in its entirety. Small polyps in the horizontal canal can be removed using an alligator forceps through an operating head or video-otoscope.

The ventro-medial compartment of the tympanic bulla is separated from the dorso-medial portion of the middle ear by a bone shelf and, unlike dogs, cannot be accessed through the ear canal. Solid polyps have to be removed via a ventral bulla osteotomy.

Otitis media is often present, so after the polyp has been removed a Tomcat catheter (or similar) should be gently passed into the middle ear. The contents should be aspirated and submitted for culture. Otitis media should be treated with an oral antibiotic (see page 285 for detailed treatment descriptions about otitis media). Topical steroid and antibiotic combinations (e.g. 0.2 mg/ml of dexamethasone and 2 mg/ml of marbofloxacin 0.1–1.0 ml q12–24 h) can be used to manage local infection and inflammation.

Systemic glucocorticoids will decrease pain and inflammation: 2 mg/kg of prednisolone or 0.2 mg/kg of dexamethasone should be given daily until infection resolution (usually 2–4 weeks) and then slowly tapered over 4–8 weeks. N-Acetyl cysteine (600 mg po q12–24 h) or bromhexine (2 mg/kg q12 h) can help liquefy mucus and facilitate drainage from the middle ear. Advanced imaging and a ventral bulla osteotomy should be considered if the polyp recurs.

Horner's syndrome, vestibular syndrome and facial nerve paralysis may occur postoperatively with either technique.[1] These syndromes are temporary, although facial nerve paralysis can uncommonly be permanent.

Key points

- Polyps cannot be managed medically; they must be removed.
- Acute-onset signs of otitis media and/or otitis interna should be treated as emergencies.
- Aggressive glucocorticoid therapy reduces the recurrence rate after removal.

Reference

1   Greci V, Mortellaro, CM. Management of otic and nasopharyngeal, and nasal polyps in cats and dogs. *Vet Clin North Am Small Anim Pract* 2016; **46**: 643–661.

FELINE CYSTOMATOSIS

Definition

Cystomatosis is a non-malignant disorder character-ised by multiple pigmented nodules and/or vesicles in the external ear canal and concave pinna.[1]

Aetiology and pathogenesis

The cause is unknown, but may be degenerative, inflammatory or genetic in origin. The nodules and/or vesicles arise from ceruminous glands in the ear canal and pinna. The vesicles may become so enlarged and numerous that they cause physical obstruction of the ear canal (**Fig. 13.15**).

Cystomatosis is a primary cause of otitis externa. Secondary (perpetuating) yeast or bacterial infec-tions may develop.

Clinical signs

Cystomatosis is characterised by variably sized, pig-mented nodules and/or vesicles in the external ear canal and on the inner aspect of the pinna. The vesicles are filled with brown fluid. Cystomatosis is generally not pruritic or painful unless secondary infections are present.

Differential diagnoses

- Cerumen gland adenoma.
- Cerumen gland adenocarcinoma.

Diagnosis

The appearance of multi-focal pigmented nodules and vesicles in the external ear canal is pathognomonic for pathology of the ceruminous glands. Although a cerumen gland adenocarcinoma is unlikely, it can-not be ruled out based on gross appearance alone. Histopathology of a nodule and underlying cartilage will differentiate an adenocarcinoma, adenoma and cystomatosis. Affected animals should be examined for signs of adenocarcinoma. Signs include metastasis to regional lymph nodes, lungs and viscera.[1] Ear cytology is necessary to identify secondary yeast and/or bacterial otitis externa.

Treatment

Refer to page 272 for details about treatment of yeast and bacterial otitis externa. Three treatment options are available for cystomatosis:

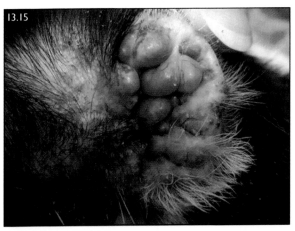

Fig. 13.15 Obstruction of the external ear canal due to cystomatosis (photo courtesy of Lisa V Reiter DVM DACVD).

- Medical treatment to manage and prevent infection in the ears is suitable for early and mild cases. Topical steroids may decrease swelling in the ear. Treatment must be continuous because the primary cause of the otitis externa, the cystomatosis, is not eliminated.
- The second treatment option is ablation of the nodules and vesicles with a CO_2 laser or electrocautery. These are used to ablate all gross evidence of vesicles and nodules in the canal and on the pinna. Topical antibiotics and steroid (see Otitis externa, page 272) should be applied once to twice daily for 2 weeks postoperatively to prevent infection. This treatment modality is very effective with prolonged remission, sometimes for years. These patients should be periodically rechecked to catch any regrowth early. Topical steroids twice weekly may reduce the recurrence rate.
- Total ear canal ablation with lateral bulla osteotomy is the third treatment option. This surgical option should be considered if adenocarcinoma is suspected.

Key point

- The clinician should always evaluate ear cytology to determine whether secondary bacterial and/or yeast otitis is present.

Reference

1 Sula, MJM. Tumors and tumor-like lesions of dog and cat ears. *Vet Clin North Am Small Anim Pract* 2012; **42**: 1161–1178.

EAR MITES
(*Otodectes cynotis* infestation)

Definition
Otodectes cynotis is a surface mite that commonly causes otitis externa in dogs and cats.

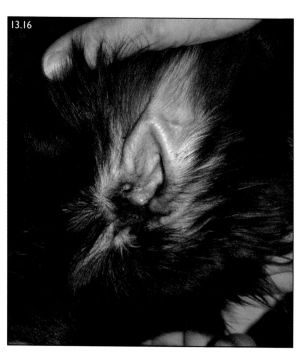

Fig. 13.16 Otitis externa: otic discharge secondary to *Otodectes cynotis* infection.

Aetiology and pathogenesis
Ear mites are contracted via physical contact with an infected mammal. The mites proliferate within the ear canal and cause pruritus, inflammation, waxy debris and secondary yeast or bacterial infections.

Clinical signs
Otodectes cynotis infestation is characterised by large amounts of dry, brown, waxy debris with variable amounts of erythema (**Fig. 13.16**) and pruritus.

Differential diagnoses
* Otitis externa secondary to allergy.
* Otitis externa secondary to other ectoparasites (*Sarcoptes scabiei*, *Demodex* spp. and *Notoedres* spp.).
* Bacterial otitis externa.
* Yeast otitis externa.

Diagnosis
Careful otoscopic examination may allow visualisation of the mites as they move within the canal (**Fig. 13.17**). Mites may also be seen on microscopic examination of swabs of waxy debris collected into mineral oil (**Fig. 13.18**). Swabs of waxy debris must be stained and examined microscopically for yeast and bacteria, because these are a common secondary and perpetuating cause of otitis (see Otitis externa, page 267).

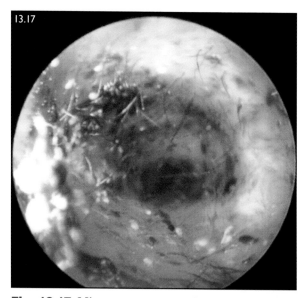

Fig. 13.17 Mites seen on otoscopic examination.

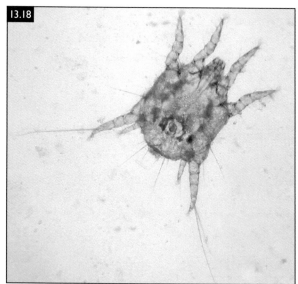

Fig. 13.18 Microscopic examination of mites.

Treatment

Otodectes cynotis is a primary cause of otitis externa.[1] Many types of acaricidal treatments are effective against this mite:

- Sarolaner can be administered orally to dogs at label dose; two doses administered 1 month apart are expected to be >99% effective.[2] Due to mechanism of action, other isoxazolines would also be expected to be effective at label dosing.
- Imidacloprid 0% + moxidectin 2.5% combination products administered topically on two occasions per label directions have at least 82% efficacy.[3]
- Fipronil–(*S*)-methoprene–eprinomectin–praziquantel combination[3] products have >96% efficacy against transmission of ear mites when administered per label dosing.[4]
- Selamectin administered topically on two occasions according to label directions is effective for treating ear mites in both dogs and cats. In some cases, off-label administration of one dose every 2 weeks for three treatments may be necessary.
- Three ivermectin injections administered subcutaneously at 0.2–0.3 mg/kg at 2-week intervals are also effective against ear mites in both cats[5] and dogs.

All cats and dogs exposed to the affected animal should also be treated.

Secondary yeast or bacterial infections may develop and should be treated with topical steroid, antibiotic and/or antifungal and ear cleaning. See page 272 for further details about treatment of yeast and bacterial otitis externa.

Key points

- *Otodectes cynotis* is a primary cause of otitis externa. The clinician must monitor for the development of perpetuating causes of otitis externa.
- *Otodectes cynotis* is transmissible via contact; it is highly contagious and potentially zoonotic.

References

1 Craig M. Disease facts: otitis externa. *Companion Animal* 2013; **18**: 481–483.
2 Six RH, Becskei C, Mazaleski MM *et al*. Efficacy of sarolaner, a novel oral isoxazoline, against two common mite infestations in dogs: *Demodex* spp. and *Otodectes cynotis*. *Vet Parasitol* 2016; **222**: 62–66.
3 Arther RG, Davis WL, Jacobsen JA, Lewis VA, Settje TL. Clinical evaluation of the safety and efficacy of 10% imidacloprid+ 2.5% moxidectin topical solution for the treatment of ear mite (*Otodectes cynotis*) infestations in dogs. *Vet Parasitol* 2015; **210**: 64–68.
4 Beugnet F, Bouhsira É, Halos L, Franc M. Preventive efficacy of a topical combination of fipronil–(*S*)-methoprene–eprinomectin–praziquantel against ear mite (*Otodectes cynotis*) infestation of cats through a natural infestation model. *Parasite* 2014; **21**: 40.
5 Kavitha S, Venkatesan M, Nagarajan B, Thirunavukkarasu PS, Nambi AP. Clinical management of feline otodectosis – a study of 11 patients. *Intas Polivet* 2013; **14**: 331–332.

PSEUDOMONAS OTITIS

Definition

Pseudomonas otitis is infection of the ear by *Pseudomonas aeruginosa* bacteria.

Aetiology and pathogenesis

Pseudomonas spp. are opportunistic environmental bacteria and a perpetuating cause of otitis externa and/or otitis media. Chronically inflamed ears are at risk for developing *Pseudomonas* infections (see Primary causes of otitis externa, page 267). Pseudomonas otitis is more common in dogs than in cats. Infections are invariably secondary to underlying causes of the otitis. Pseudomonas otitis is commonly complicated by biofilm formation. Chronic *Pseudomonas* infections can rupture the tympanic membrane and initiate otitis media. In addition, *Pseudomonas* proteins can be directly ototoxic.

Clinical features

Pseudomonas otitis is most often characterised by acute onset and painful, suppurative, ulcerative and severe inflammation in the external ear canal.

Differential diagnoses

- Other causes of otitis externa (see page 267).
- Suppurative otitis externa with other bacteria.

Diagnosis

The clinical signs of suppurative otitis externa (see **Fig. 13.5**) combined with degenerative neutrophils and rod-shaped bacteria on cytology (see **Fig. 13.10**) are highly suggestive. The diagnosis can be confirmed via culture of the otic exudate. Careful examination of the tympanic membrane with, if necessary, radiographs or CT are necessary to confirm or rule out otitis media.

Treatment[1]

Three components are necessary for resolution of pseudomonas otitis: removal of exudate and biofilm through daily flushing of the ear canal; reduction of inflammation through topical and often oral steroids; and targeting the bacteria with topical antibiotics. (See Otitis externa, page 272 for more details on treatment.)

Ear cleaning

The ear canal should be copiously flushed. The initial clean should be performed under anaesthetic using a catheter through an operating or video-otoscope. It is particularly important to physically remove all the exudate and biofilm, including material from the middle ear if involved. This includes cleaning and removing contaminated hairs and crusts from around the ears.

Ear cleaning should be continued during treatment; once-daily ear cleaning is usually sufficient but sometimes twice-daily cleaning is needed. If the ear is painful or the canal epithelium is macerated, then the frequency should be reduced and non-irritating ear cleaners used. Ceruminolytic ear cleaners are contraindicated with purulent exudates and biofilms. Surfactant (detergent)-based ear cleaners are more effective but may be irritating and potentially ototoxic. Tris-EDTA and acetic acid solutions are safe and non-irritating but have less cleansing and antimicrobial activity. *N*-Acetylcysteine 2% solutions are effective against biofilms. It may be necessary to repeat a full ear flush under anaesthetic two to three times during treatment.

Anti-inflammatory therapy

Oral steroids reduce inflammation of the ear. This will provide some analgesia, but specific pain relief should be administered in severe cases. The reduction of inflammation promotes resolution of infection. In general, prednisone can be prescribed at a dose of 1 mg/kg po q24 h for 1 week, q48 h for an additional 2 weeks and then stopped. The steroid dose and duration may need to change based on patient factors. A variety of topical steroid preparations is available. One option is 2–4 mg/ml of injectable dexamethasone solutions given at 0.2–0.5 ml in the affected ear q12–24 h; as 0.2 mg/ml solutions in Tris-EDTA with or without antibiotics (1.0 ml q24 h); or as 0.5 mg/ml solutions in Epiotic® (ear cleaning with 1–2 ml q24 h). Dexamethasone is the steroid of choice as it can directly counter *Pseudomonas* spp.-associated ototoxicity.

Antibiotic therapy

Bacterial culture and sensitivity testing are helpful to identify *Pseudomonas* spp., and rule out other rod bacteria such as *Escherichia coli*, *Klebsiella* and *Proteus* spp., and coryneforms. Knowledge of the probable susceptibility patterns can help guide treatment choices, but the results of susceptibility test results must be interpreted carefully because the breakpoints are based on systemic treatment and poorly predictive of the response to topical therapy. Most first-time infections will be susceptible to aminoglycosides, polymyxin B, silver sulfadiazine and fluoroquinolones (see *Table 13.2*). However, *Pseudomonas* spp. readily acquire resistance and most isolates from recurrent infections will be multi-drug resistant (see *Table 13.3*).

Myringotomy with flushing of the tympanic bulla flush may be necessary if otitis media is present (see Otitis media, page 285). Topical antibiotics can be instilled directly into the middle ear; fluoroquinolones, gentamicin and ceftazidime appear to be safe, but ticarcillin, amikacin and tobramycin are potentially ototoxic. Systemic antibiotic treatment may be necessary in severe cases, but high doses are required to attain adequate tissue levels in chronically inflamed ears. Drugs with good tissue penetration (e.g. fluoroquinolones) should be considered.

Following up treatment

Pseudomonas otitis may require 6 weeks of treatment to achieve resolution of infection, particularly in chronically inflamed ears and with otitis media. Regular ear cleaning and, if necessary, repeated ear flushing are important. Significant clinical improvement should be observed after 1–3 weeks of appropriate treatment and, if not, the approach to treatment should be re-evaluated.

Repeated cytology to assess the nature of the exudate, and numbers of inflammatory cells and organisms (see Otitis externa, page 270) is very useful. The presence of neutrophils with few to no bacteria indicates ongoing inflammation, over-cleaning and maceration of the ear canals, and/or a contact reaction to medication. A change in the nature of the exudate and organisms indicates that the *Pseudomonas* infection is resolving but the underlying disease is still active. Bacterial culture is useful with pseudomonas otitis because they are not found in healthy ears.

Pseudomonas otitis may recur if the primary reason for otitis is not controlled (see Otitis externa, page 267). It may be possible to remove the source of the *Pseudomonas* spp. by avoiding swimming, cleaning water bowls, and managing lip fold dermatitis and wet 'beards' or body folds.

Key points

- Six weeks of treatment may be required for resolution of pseudomonas otitis externa.
- Steroids promote resolution of infection.
- Pain relief will facilitate topical therapy.

Reference

1 Nuttall T, Cole LK. Evidence-based veterinary dermatology: a systematic review of interventions for treatment of *Pseudomonas* otitis in dogs. *Vet Dermatol* 2007; **18**: 69–77.

PRIMARY SECRETORY OTITIS MEDIA

Definition

Primary secretory otitis media (PSOM) is an accumulation of sterile mucus in the middle ear. PSOM has been reported in Cavalier King Charles Spaniels most often, but this condition is also seen in other brachycephalic breeds such as French Bulldogs and Pugs.

Aetiology and pathogenesis

PSOM is characterised by the accumulation of thick, sterile mucus in the middle-ear cavity. The accumulation may represent an abnormality of the secretory tissue of the middle-ear cavity or a dysfunction of the eustachian tube. Cavalier King Charles Spaniels are over-represented, although PSOM occurs in other brachycephalic breeds. It is probably part of the brachycephalic obstructed airway syndrome (BOAS); the tympanic membrane and middle ears should be assessed in dogs presented with this condition.

Clinical features

The most frequent clinical findings of PSOM include gradual hearing loss and a bulging pars flaccida. PSOM by itself is usually not painful nor pruritic, although head shaking can be seen. The disease is likely to be slowly progressive (possible over months to years). The signs can be subtle and some dogs apparently present with acute deafness, head and neck pain, ataxia, head tilt and/or nystagmus (see **Fig. 13.22**).[1] This should be treated as an emergency because delaying effective therapy may result in permanent neurological deficits.

Differential diagnoses

- Primary bacterial otitis media (rare).
- Bacterial otitis media secondary to otitis externa.
- Cholesteatoma.
- Syringomyelia (when pain and/or neuropathy is present).
- Peripheral vestibular disease (when neuropathy is present).
- Central vestibular disease.

Diagnosis

If pain, pruritus or neuropathy is not present, then the diagnosis is achieved by visualising a bulging pars flaccida (**Fig. 13.19**). Occasionally, the pars flaccida

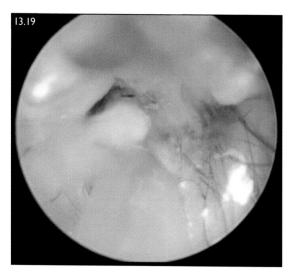

Fig. 13.19 Primary secretory otitis media (PSOM) in a French Bulldog: the bulging pars flaccida is visible at the top right of the image; mucus from the middle ear is appearing from a myringotomy incision in the pars tensa at the left.

will be flat. The pars tensa may be variably bulging or opaque. If PSOM is still suspected despite a flat pars flaccida and normal pars tensa, then the diagnosis can be achieved through advanced imaging (CT).[2] CT or magnetic resonance imaging (MRI) should be strongly considered in patients with neuropathy because syringomyelia may be present.

Treatment

Treatment of PSOM involves a myringotomy (see Otitis media, page 285) and the removal of mucus from the middle ear.[1] The mucus can be suctioned from the middle ear with a 5-Fr red rubber or plastic catheter. Oral steroids (1 mg/kg po q24 h for 1 week, then q48 h for 1 week) and a broad-spectrum antibiotic (see Otitis media, page 286) should be administered for 2 weeks postoperatively to prevent postflushing otitis externa/media. *N*-Acetylcysteine (600 mg q12–24 h) or bromhexine (2 mg/kg q12 h) is well tolerated and can liquefy the mucus, facilitating drainage through the eustachian tube. Affected dogs often require repeated myringotomies and suction to fully remove all the mucus. Tympanostomy tubes can be considered in recurrent cases. These provide egress through the tympanic membrane and prevent the build-up of pressure in the middle ears, but their placement and care require specialist equipment and skills.

Key points

- PSOM should be suspected in Cavalier King Charles Spaniels and other brachycephalic dogs that have reduced or absent hearing.
- Acute-onset deafness, head tilt, nystagmus and/or ataxia is a therapeutic emergency.

References

1 Cole LK. Primary secretory otitis media in Cavalier King Charles spaniels. *Vet Clinics North Am Small Anim Pract* 2012; **42**: 1137–1142.
2 Cole, LK, Samii VF, Wagner SO, Rajala-Schultz PJ. Diagnosis of primary secretory otitis media in the cavalier King Charles spaniel. *Vet Dermatol* 2015; **26**: 459–e107.

OTITIS MEDIA

Definition

Otitis media is inflammation of the middle-ear cavity including the tympanic membrane, tympanic bulla and eustachian tube.

Aetiology and pathogenesis

Otitis media may occur as an extension of otitis externa, through ascension of bacteria from the nasopharynx up the eustachian tube[1] or through haematogenous spread of infection. Primary causes of otitis media include PSOM in dogs (see page 283) and inflammatory polyps in cats (see page 277).

Chronic otitis externa exposes the tympanic membrane (TM) to prolonged contact with exudate. This causes maceration and eventual rupture of the TM. Stenosis of the horizontal ear canal and gram-negative infections are particular risks for rupture of the TM. After rupture, the infection spreads into the bulla of the middle ear. The TM can heal if the otitis externa improves, but the healed TM can trap exudate in the middle ear. This is a common cause of recurrent otitis media in dogs. Chronic inflammation can induce squamous metaplasia of the middle-ear lining leading to a cholesteatoma (the progressive build-up of keratinised and sebaceous material in the middle ear).

Upper respiratory infections or other pathology of the upper respiratory tract lead to inflammation and increased bacterial load in the nasopharynx. The bacteria may ascend up the eustachian tube, leading to an infection of the middle ear. This is a common cause of otitis media in cats.

A retrobulbar abscess or other severe infection involving the head or neck may lead to otitis media through haematogenous spread of bacteria. This is an uncommon cause of otitis media. Middle-ear infections may occasionally spread to the para-aural tissues and/or central nervous system (CNS).

Clinical features

Dogs and cats with otitis media may demonstrate a range of clinical signs. Clinical features include: chronic otitis externa that is refractory to treatment, jaw pain and hesitation to chew, head tilt, Horner's syndrome, facial nerve (cranial nerve VII) neuropathy, signs of otitis interna, opaque and/or bulging TM and/or a ruptured TM. Acute onset vestibular syndrome is a therapeutic emergency.

Differential diagnoses

- Vestibular disease or other neuropathy for dogs or cats with concurrent otitis interna.
- Primary secretory otitis media.
- Inflammatory polyps in cats.

Diagnosis

The diagnosis is based on observing an abnormal TM and/or demonstration of fluid or debris in the tympanic bulla (**Figs. 13.20, 13.21**). The diagnosis of middle-ear disease can also be achieved with imaging such as radiography, CT or MRI, although this must be combined with otoscopy and myringotomy. Imaging is useful when stenosis limits visualisation of the TM and will reveal the extent of the otitis media, and lytic, proliferative and/or expansive changes in the tympanic bulla. Radiography is much less sensitive than CT. MRI is best for evaluation of the soft tissues and nerves around the ears, but will not image bony structures adequately. MRI and CT can use contrast and processing to help identify the type of material in the middle ears.

Treatment

Many cases of otitis media will resolve with medical therapy, but many cases will also require a myringotomy and flushing of the middle ear.

Steroid therapy

In general, oral steroid should be administered for 3–6 weeks, and oral antibiotic should be administered for 6–8 weeks. A typical oral steroid regimen

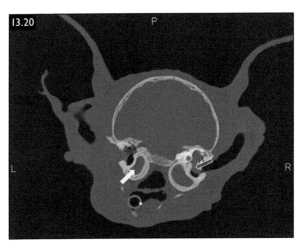

Fig. 13.20 CT scan of a cat with bilateral otitis media: note the soft-tissue filling the ventral–medial (white arrow) and dorsal–lateral (open arrow) compartments of the middle ears; these would be air filled in a healthy cat.

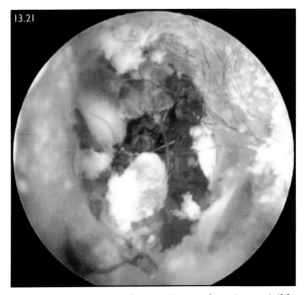

Fig. 13.21 Otitis media in a Boxer: there is no visible tympanic membrane, and there is severe proliferative inflammation of the middle-ear mucosa.

is 1 mg/kg of prednisolone or prednisone po q24 h for 1 week, 1 mg/kg po q48 h for 2 weeks, and then stopped. Steroids should be administered at a lower dose or for a shorter time period if the patient has excessive side effects.

Antibiotic therapy

Oral antibiotics should ideally be selected based on bacterial culture of the middle ear. Staphylococci and *Pseudomonas* spp. are the most common bacteria to cause otitis media. Another consideration when selecting oral antibiotics is the ability of the antibiotic to penetrate the middle ear. Few current data are available with regard to antibiotic efficacy in the middle ear. Antibiotics generally accepted as efficacious for the middle ear include fluoroquinolones, trimethoprim sulfa and cephalexin at label doses, and ceftazidime 30 mg/kg sc q6–12 h.[1] Penetration of antibiotics into chronically inflamed ears is poor and high doses of drugs with a high volume of distribution (e.g. fluoroquinolones) should be considered. Systemic therapy can be challenging if susceptibility is limited to topical and/or parenteral drugs (see below).

Topical therapy

Concurrent topical treatment should be instituted if otitis externa is present, but care should be taken over ototoxicity if the tympanic membrane is ruptured (see Otitis externa, page 267).

Topical antibiotics and glucocorticoids in saline or Tris-EDTA can be directly administered into the middle ear; gentamicin, fluoroquinolones, ceftazidime and dexamethasone do not appear to be ototoxic (see Otitis externa, page 272). It is unclear how long these drugs persist in the middle ear, but, as this is essentially a blind-ended sac, drugs are likely to be active in the middle ear for a few days. Repeated instillation of mg/ml solutions every 5–7 days could therefore be useful in multi-drug-resistant infections that are refractory to oral medication.

Myringotomy and ear flushing

Some cases of otitis media will resolve only if myringotomy and bulla flush are performed. To perform a myringotomy, the patient must be anaesthetised and the ear canal must be free of exudate.

An operating head otoscope or (ideally) a video-otoscope is used to visualise the TM, and an incision or puncture is made in the caudal–ventral pars tensa (avoiding the sensitive structures in the dorsal middle ear). The manubrium of the malleus should be avoided in order to prevent permanent damage to the TM. A spinal needle or a rigid polypropylene catheter with a bevelled tip may be used to perform the myringotomy.

The bulla should be copiously flushed with tepid water or saline. An effective flushing technique involves using a 5-Fr red rubber or plastic catheter in the horizontal canal to direct a continuous stream of tepid water or saline at the myringotomy incision. The free fluid should be aspirated once the middle ear runs clear. Mucus and pus appear white to green–brown, opaque and/or flocculent; clumps of brown waxy material suggest that there is a cholesteatoma. Cholesteatomas require repeated and aggressive cleaning to remove all the keratinised debris.

Systemic antibiotics must be administered 6–8 weeks postmyringotomy, but topical antibiotics can also be directly instilled into the middle ear (see above). Oral steroids should also be administered as previously described. The TM generally heals within 2 weeks.

Refractory otitis media

Chronic otitis media, osteomyelitis of the tympanic bulla and/or cholesteatoma may be refractory to medical treatment. A total ear canal ablation and lateral bulla osteotomy are required in these cases.

Key points

- Otitis media is underdiagnosed.
- Most cases of otitis media require at least 6 weeks of oral antibiotic therapy.
- Acute-onset vestibular syndrome is a therapeutic emergency.
- Prompt identification and management are necessary to avoid chronic irreversible changes.

Reference

1   Gotthelf LN. Diagnosis and treatment of otitis media in dogs and cats. *Vet Clinics North Am Small Anim Pract* 2004; **34**: 469–487.

OTITIS INTERNA

Definition
Otitis interna is inflammation of the inner ear resulting in peripheral vestibular neuropathy.

Pathology and aetiology
Otitis interna is an extension of otitis media.

Clinical features
The affected individual will have signs of otitis media (see Otitis media, page 285). Signs of a peripheral neuropathy will also be present, and include:[1,2] ataxia with loss of balance but preservation of strength, normal proprioception, alert mentation, variable nausea, head tilt towards the affected ear, and spontaneous or positional horizontal nystagmus, with the fast phase away from the affected ear (**Fig. 13.22**).

Signs of central vestibular disease include:[1] vertical nystagmus, proprioception deficits and dull mentation. These signs indicate that the vestibular disease is due to a central lesion such as neoplasia.

Differential diagnoses
- Central vestibular disease.
- Idiopathic peripheral vestibular disease.
- Traumatic injury to the inner ear.
- Otolithiasis.
- Congenital lymphocytic labyrinthitis.

Diagnosis
Diagnosis can generally be achieved through history and physical exam. Advanced imaging may be required in some cases.

Treatment
Otitis interna is an extension of otitis media. Treatment should be instituted as described for otitis

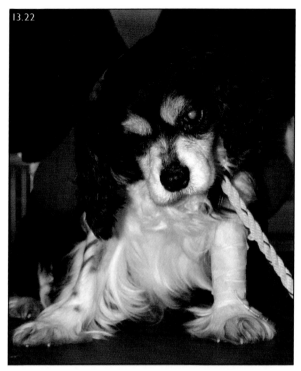

Fig. 13.22 Otitis interna in a Cavalier King Charles spaniel with primary secretory otitis media (PSOM): the dog had acute-onset head tilt, ataxia and nystagmus.

media (see page 285). Prompt treatment is required to avoid permanent neurological deficits.

Key points
- The clinician must differentiate between central and peripheral vestibular neuropathy.
- Acute-onset otitis interna is a therapeutic emergency.

References
1 Cook LB. Neurologic evaluation of the ear. *Vet Clinics North Am Small Anim Pract* 2004; **34**: 425–435.
2 Rossmeisl JH. Vestibular disease in dogs and cats. *Vet Clinics North Am Small Anim Pract* 2010; **40**: 81–100.

IMMUNOSUPPRESSIVE DRUG THERAPY TABLE

DRUG	DOSE	COMMENTS
Pentoxifylline	Dogs: 15–25 mg/kg po q8–12 h	May require 8 weeks for maximum benefit; higher doses can be used
Tetracycline	Dogs >10 kg receive 500 mg po q8 h Dogs <10 kg receive 250 mg po q8 h	This class of antibiotics combined with niacinamide may require 3 months for maximum benefit
Doxycycline	Dogs: 5–10 mg/kg po q12 h	Minocycline may cause more GI upset than other tetracyclines
Minocycline	Dogs: 5–12.5 mg/kg po q12 h	
Niacinamide	Dogs >10 kg receive 500 mg po q8–12 h Dogs <10 kg receive 250 mg po q8–12 h	May cause GI upset and altered behaviour
Prednisone/prednisolone	Dogs: 1–3 mg/kg po	Steroids should be administered q24 h until the disease is controlled. Once the disease is controlled, steroids should be administered q48 h or less.
Prednisolone	Cats: 2–4 mg/kg po	
Methylprednisolone	Dogs: 0.2–1.4 mg/kg po	A slightly higher dose administered q48 h tends to have fewer side effects than a daily dose of steroid – even if the daily dose is lower
Dexamethasone	Dogs: 0.1–0.2 mg/kg po Cats: 1.5–2 mg/average sized cat po	
Triamcinolone	Dogs: 0.3–1 mg/kg po Cats: 0.3–1 mg/kg po	Dexamethasone and triamcinolone have longer durations of activity and should be administered every third day long term
		Dexamethasone is the most diabetogenic
Azathioprine	1.5–2.5 mg/kg po q48 h	Dosing q48 h reduces side effects. Monitor CBC/chemistry q2 weeks for initial 2 months. May require 2 months for maximum benefit
		Do not give to cats
*Ciclosporin	Dogs and cats: 5–10 mg/kg po q24 h	Blood level monitoring is rarely useful when treating skin disease. GI upset is a common side effect. See page 27 for more details about combining this drug with ketoconazole and managing adverse effects.
Hydroxychloroquine	Dogs: 5 mg/kg po q24 h	Monitor CBC/chemistry and perform eye exams. Very few studies on the use of this drug in dogs
Omega 3 fatty acids	Dogs: 180 mg/5 kg (≈10 lb) po q24 h	
Vitamin E	Dogs: 200–800 IU po q24 h	
Chlorambucil	Dogs and cats: 0.1–0.2 mg/kg po q24–48 h	Monitor CBC/chemistry
Mycophenolate mofetil	20–40 mg/kg/day Divide daily dose q8–12 h to reduce GI upsets	Monitor CBC/chemistry
Dapsone	Dogs: 1 mg/kg po q8 h	Monitor CBC/chemistry. Do not give to cats
Tacrolimus 0.1%	Apply topically q12 h	
Betamethasone valerate 0.1%	Apply topically q12 h	Topical steroids are useful for focal skin lesions. Dermal atrophy may occur with prolonged use
Fluocinolone/DMSO (Synotic®, Zoetis)	Apply topically q12 h	

CBC, complete blood count; DMSO, dimethyl sulphoxide; GI, gastrointestinal; po, by mouth.

* In this table and throughout this book ciclosporin refers to veterinary licensed (e.g. Atopica®, Atopica Cat®, Cyclavance®, Modulis® and Sporimune®), human licensed or generic-modified formulations. Clinicians should avoid using non-modified formulations because their bioavailability and efficacy are highly variable.